Multiple Sclerosis:

One Owner's Manual

Andrew Scott

Multiple Sclerosis: One Owner's Manual
ISBN: 978-0-6454680-0-7

To Sarah

Without your help, I would not be here

Contents

Acknowledgments

I started thinking about writing this book in 2018. At that stage, I had been diagnosed for 24 years but common sense now tells me that I had signs of MS well before it was obvious.

Over time, many ideas about how to treat MS have emerged offering the promise of relief. However, the consequences of treatment are still viewed as collateral damage in the war against MS and the long-term effectiveness of the treatments is questionable.

What was missing, to my mind, in the swath of words written on MS, was a basic footprint of knowledge that allowed the patients to access information and question the advice they were receiving. It had to be understandable even though it was about a topic where they lacked background knowledge. It needed to point to scientific literature even if they chose not to read it themselves. That literature needed to reflect what happened in the clinic or the laboratory, not reflect what a mathematician, called an epidemiologist, decided was fact.

Partly to educate myself and partly to fill that void, I decided to write. Having been diagnosed for such a long time and having found my own path through a tortuous track, I decided to include my own experiences. Hopefully, someone will be able to benefit from them. As this book reflects my own journey, some MS symptoms like insomnia and heat intolerance are not included. I am suspicious that what I do negates those problems but here I lack proof. The book is never going to cover every problem. To do that, a much thicker volume is needed.

Writing is harder than I expected. I had to find the basic tools and learn how to include references. I'd like to say someone helped me to do this, but it was a slow process of self-education. The content was easier to manage than the basic setup. However, it soon became apparent that writing is not really a solo enterprise.

After I had disgorged word after word into contorted sentences, I looked for some feedback that what I had written was not unintelligible rubbish to a reader. A lifelong friend, Lachlan Forrest, became my first reviewer. We both laughed when I said to him, "if you can't understand this, no one will!" He quickly confirmed my worst fears that what I had first proposed was completely unintelligible. I thank him for forcing me to pay more attention to the structure of this book.

I showed my revised jottings to a fellow member of the MS community, Eric Johnson. He is based in the United States and has the technical background to have helped me clarify, in my own head at least, how nerve conduction works. It is fascinating to compare our movements to how a crab claw works!

There are others who have helped along the way, including Prof David Small whose comments were very useful.

Above all, you cannot write a book without an editor. Through the services of Olivia Wroth, from SuperScript Writing and Editing, I was introduced to the marvelous, endlessly patient, Ruth Amos from Fix My English. Ruth is the pilot that kept this ship from running on to the rocks. Her PhD in chemistry allowed her to correct the many terminological errors that I made. However, those mistakes were minimal compared to the many grammatical offences that peppered my original offering. On a couple of occasions, she was able to unscramble the ravings of this overwrought writer and find order out of chaos. There would be no book without her.

In 2019, I stopped writing and travelled. I resumed writing in 2020 and 2021 as the Covid-19 pandemic ripped around the world creating enormous heartache and devastating communities. Melbourne attempted to contain this problem by imposing very strict lockdowns. The economic damage that accompanied this was massive. Out of all the businesses I relied on for help with my MS, only one survived the fallout. Luksanaree Phongpheng continues to be the most outstanding remedial masseur I have met.

The team at Pilates on Bourke were all swept away in the economic tsunami that engulfed small businesses. I often think of Tal, Cathryn, Tahlia, Sherrine, Bianca and Elsa. They are all lost to me now but were so important to my recovery. I have a new team now, and they are great, but there is no home base like the old studio provided.

When you are as beaten as I was in 2014, a central core that you can believe in is paramount. For me, that was my children; Emily, James and Alistair. They will be my inspiration forever. I can still remember having a good laugh with Alistair when he said, incredulously, "I never guessed you had MS. I just thought you were crap at sport". Having normal, honest, guilt-free children is a joy.

That's nearly all the people covered. Some, like Paul, David, Lou, Rachana, Dilan and Kwame have shown their true colours by remaining unchanged by the years and treating me as just another person. If you have MS, that is all you really want.

Two other personalities dominated my waking hours through the recovery process; my dogs Doug and the late lamented Pepper. Whether it was demanding a feed, ignoring my commands, going away instead of coming back, looking for a better offer, disappearing into the dark or fretting if I went too far away, these dogs did more for me than any doctor. Only a dog can look at you in exasperation and let you know that life is not just about you. A good dog is a ticket back into society.

None of the chain of events that led to this book would have been possible without the persistence of the girl I knew as Sarah Tarnawsky. Whether it was her visits to the hospital and rehabilitation facility or the work she did in the studio, she never faltered. When everyone else stepped back to see how far I would fall, she stepped forward and changed an unstoppable trajectory. Not many people do that, and rarely are they given the credit they deserve.

Lastly, if you are holding this book, I thank you for being prepared to consider a story that may be different from yours. I do hope you see something that helps you.

Notice of Disclaimer

The contents of this book are not intended to be, and should not be considered, a substitute for medical or other professional advice. The book contains many references to prescription medications and non-prescription supplements. This work does not imply any sort of recommendation, under any circumstances. Neither the author nor any other party involved in this publication warrants that the information contained in this book is in every respect accurate or complete. They disclaim all responsibility for any errors or omissions contained in this work. Every reader is strongly encouraged to confirm the information included in this publication with other sources. The risks of adverse effects resulting from contraindications, inappropriate dosing and unsuitable practices is high. All information provided is intended to create a conversation between those who use this book and their medical providers. As each individual has a unique medical profile, nothing in this book should be construed as personal advice. Readers are encouraged to check the product information included in the package of each drug and to be certain that changes have not been made regarding the recommended dose or the list of known contraindications. Many MS drugs are new and some are infrequently used. It remains of paramount importance that a properly registered medical advisor is involved with their administration.

The author is not a trained medical advisor and does not claim to be any sort of physician. He is an MS patient. This book summarizes his best efforts to provide information that is complete and generally in accord with the standards accepted at the time of publication.

Chapter 1

Why I Have Written This Book

It was December 1994.

I sat opposite the neurologist. Only two weeks before, he had diagnosed me with multiple sclerosis.

"Ideas on MS are like a pendulum," he said, "they swing wildly to the right, then back to the left. The truth is probably somewhere in the middle."

"That sounds profound," I thought, waiting for the next insight.

It never came.

Instead, I was told to go home, resume my normal life, and wait for the next, inevitable attack.

It was not what I expected.

I was ready to tackle this thing. It didn't matter that I knew nothing about it. I'd had time to think, had undergone an MRI (magnetic resonance imaging) scan, and spent three days in hospital being fed steroids through a drip. The next step was up to my neurologist, and I was ready to be a compliant patient.

Then nothing.

"There are no treatments. We don't know what causes this." He spoke with the unquestionable authority of experience. "But there are things we can do."

My wife sat silently in a chair beside me.

Suddenly the whole experience was at an end. We all stood as one, walked to the door, and shook hands.

"You'll know where to find us when you need us," he said, as a farewell.

"How long do you think that will be?" I asked.

"Maybe two years, maybe a bit less. Enjoy life while you can." He paused, then curling up the corners of his mouth, uttered, "Don't worry, we're used to these cases." There was no semblance of reassurance in his voice.

It seemed, until the middle of 1996, that his advice to do nothing was right. Life returned to normal. The double vision had vanished, and my foot no longer hit the floor with a floppy thump when I walked.

Then I became aware of small shudders invading my body. My memory seemed clouded. Simple tasks became just a little "unusual," as though I had never done things quite that way before.

I procrastinated. Was this real? I rang the neurologist.

The receptionist was succinct, "The professor has retired, but the associate professor is now looking after his patients. Would you like to see him?"

It was a yes or no question that seemed to have only one answer.

~

The associate professor was a small man with an officious busyness about him. He reminded me of a small-town railway stationmaster. Everything was under his control. The train did not leave unless he let it; only he could sell you a boarding ticket. His way was the only way. He seemed to enjoy the sense of control.

"You should start using interferon," he declared.

"What's that?" I asked, somewhat befuddled by the lack of discussion leading up to this comment.

He leaned forward and, in his most professorial voice, said, "It's an immune modulator. You inject yourself each day".

I had spent years in financial markets. That sort of answer from a CFO would have sent a share price crashing. I shifted my weight.

Me: "What if I don't?"

Him: "Well, this is the best treatment."

Me: "I don't much care for the idea of injecting myself every day. Is there another way?"

Him: "Well, there is a new product that only requires a weekly injection. I've never prescribed it before, but you could try that. It's the same thing as the daily injection."

He stood up, walked to my side of the desk, and handed me a leaflet and a videocassette.

"There are usually some mild flu-like symptoms, but they will settle down," he said soothingly.

I took the video, which was only a marketing aid, and noticed that both it and the leaflet were for Betaseron (interferon-β-1b), the daily injection.

He looked down at me and indicated the session was at an end. "Anyway, why don't you go home and watch this. Next week we can make a decision."

~

The video did not sit well with me. Everyone in it looked perfect, and its commentary repeated the phrase "mild flu-like symptoms" several times.

I watched it alone. My wife seemed to have no interest at all. The couch felt very big, and the room was empty. I had nothing but my own thoughts to weigh up and make a decision.

In the end, I concluded that he was a professor, and I was a nobody. Why wouldn't I take his advice?

~

The next week I returned to the associate professor's rooms.

He sat like a judge waiting to hear whether I would plead guilty or not guilty. I felt like a prisoner in the dock.

My mind said, "I don't want to do this," but as though I was reading lines from a play I said, "I think I'd like to try the weekly injection. Once-a-week sounds better than once-a-day."

The neurologist's shoulders relaxed, and with a flourish, he wrote the prescription. After admiring his handiwork, he leaned forward and offered it to me.

I stretched out my arm across his desk and took the form.

Me: "Shouldn't we do some baseline tests first?"

Him: "What for?"

Me: "So we have something to compare the outcomes to. Isn't that what you do?"

His demeanor soured. "Your problems are genetic. There's nothing that can be done about that," he snapped.

His color had changed, and his brow was furrowed. The term "small man syndrome" flashed through my mind.

"At least you would have a baseline that we could look back on if we needed to," I said.

He leant back in his chair and sighed. "But we don't know what to look for, so there's no point. I do think it's 100% genetic, but this medication seems to help."

We had reached an impasse.

"Try it," he said, shifting the tenor of the dialogue. "I'll arrange for a nurse from the MS Society to come out and show you how to self-inject."

~

Ten days later, the nurse and I sat in my kitchen. On the table was a big box of the newly released medication. It was a once-a-week injection called Avonex.

Preparing the injection was a complicated process. Avonex (interferon-β-1a) was a new product then, lacking the sophistication of today's formulations. There were two vials—one of sterile water and one of powder. Using one needle, you withdrew the water from one vial and filled the syringe. Then, you injected the water into the powder container and waited until it became a clear fluid. When the mixture settled, you drew it all back into the syringe. Finally, you changed the needle for a fresh one, and the medication was ready for self-injection.

The nurse sent to describe this process was a chirpy man around 40 years of age. Under his guidance, we went through each stage until it was time to change needles for the injection.

"Then you change the needles and inject it into your thigh," he enthused.

I looked at the needles the way a pacifist would eye off an assault weapon.

Me: "You inject it here?"

Him: "Yes. It's really quite simple."

There was a brief exchange, and he reiterated the finer details of how to inject myself.

I sat back from the kitchen table and took a breath. "If it's so simple, let's waste one. How about we fill a syringe with water, and you inject it into your leg while I watch?"

The nurse stared across the table.

"What?" he said uncomfortably.

"You inject a syringe of water into your leg, and I'll watch. You said it was simple. We just waste one vial," I repeated.

Minutes ticked by.

"Touché," he said, "I have to go. You'll be fine."

~

I sat staring at the needle. It was a Thursday night. If I developed mild flu-like symptoms, then I would put up with them at work on a Friday so that the weekends would be free for time with my family.

Clearing my mind, I stood, dropped my trousers, and sat down. My fingers pulled back the skin on my thigh to make it taut, as the nurse had described. I picked up the syringe and plunged the needle into the fleshiest part of my leg.

I had not expected it to be so sharp. To my surprise, the needle buried itself deep in my flesh. I pushed the plunger down and emptied the contents of the vial into my muscle. As I withdrew it, I thought it wasn't so bad. Soon after, I would reconsider my opinion.

~

When you are feeling truly unwell, an ache develops in your muscles.

You know then that bed is the only place you want to be as the pain and weakness starts to envelop you. That ache is interferon at work. An hour after I had injected myself, I was reacting strongly.

My head boomed, and every muscle felt hot, but my body shivered. In bed, I sweated profusely while my teeth chattered. I curled into a ball to stay warm as the blanket over me seemed no more than tissue-thin.

My heart began to pound as though it would explode. It beat with a booming, rapid thud. The pulse of it seemed out of time with the waves of tremors from my spasming muscles. Coincident with this, my teeth chattered on like a wind-up toy gone mad.

This symphony had no conductor. There was no rhythm or pattern to this at all.

My wife gave me paracetamol, and I immediately asked for more. As my mind began to give in to this vicious cacophony, I retreated to the core of my private thoughts. "Is this how it ends?" was my last thought.

I slept until the alarm woke me at 6 am. After 11 hours in bed, I was exhausted and weak. It was only another Friday, so I swallowed some more paracetamol, got up, and went to work. The pain did not leave me until Sunday afternoon. The phrase "mild flu-like symptoms" played over and over in my head.

The next week I did it all again.

~

After six months, my prescriptions had run out. There was no follow-up meeting arranged, no plan for what should happen next. The injections had been universally awful, but I had learned to scoff paracetamol and timetable the injection so that I could sleep through the worst of it.

Unsure about what should now happen, I phoned the associate professor's rooms. His receptionist informed me that he was now the permanent head of the neurology department.

I explained to his secretary that I did not know what I should do now that the prescription had run out. Grasping the situation, she said, "I'll speak to the doctor and ask him what he wants to do."

Two days later, I opened a letter containing a brand-new prescription. There was no accompanying note or "with compliments" slip, only the signed authority.

I stared at it. My mind ran through everything that had transpired.

He had told me that he had never prescribed this product before, so I knew I had to be the first patient he had given it to. I now knew it was hell to take, and it had not improved my quality of life at all. This new prescription implied he didn't have any interest in finding out anything about its effect.

If that was to be his approach, then he was not the man for me. I began to look for a new neurologist.

Who do you ask when you have lost faith in the specialist who is supposed to help you? In medicine, in this country, you have nowhere to go but to a general practitioner (GP)—your local doctor.

Now I sat in front of my doctor and told him the tale of my Avonex experience. He appeared to understand what was needed and gave me the name of a new neurologist.

I did all the footwork, made the appointments, interrupting my working day, hoping to see someone who would take an interest in my health.

Within a minute of meeting this neurologist, I knew I was in the wrong place.

He had no interest in me. I was clearly just another name to add to his revenue roll. He had heard of Avonex but had never prescribed it. This was another "call me when you need me" meeting. I didn't feel like helping to fund his lifestyle, so I asked my GP for another name.

~

I was referred to another associate professor. He was younger than the others, affable, and spoke with a tone that sounded as though he was an authority that I could talk to. The way he flexed my legs, scraped up the sole of my foot, and waved his finger in front of my eyes was no different than the others had done, but he seemed to know more about Avonex.

"I'd like you to keep using Avonex. It is the best thing on the market. Still, there are new treatments in the pipeline, so perhaps I should see you every six months," he said with a confident smile.

A regular appointment schedule sounded like a plan. Finally, I felt I was on the right track. I saw this neurologist twice more at six-month intervals. The first meeting was affable, and he repeated every step he had done before. The second meeting did not go so well.

It was still in the early days of the adoption of the internet. My brand new 486 computer allowed me to use search functions to learn what I could about multiple sclerosis. One search took me to an article published in the magazine *Neurology*. It discussed a review of the incidence of Epstein Barr virus (EBV) infection as a possible indicator of later MS diagnosis, using US army enlistment records. It was a thought-provoking article.

I sat opposite my neurologist and raised what I thought was a harmless question.

"Do you read *Neurology* magazine?" I asked innocently.

"Yes, of course," came the courteous reply.

Now, unknowingly, I hit the detonator. "Did you read last month's article about EBV and MS in the US army?"

I'd had no intention of baiting him, but he reacted as if he had bitten down on a hook.

He responded with a tirade.

"MS is genetic! That other stuff is all rubbish. You shouldn't pay any attention to it. I haven't read the article, but I will. If you want to be treated by me, then don't look at things you know nothing about!" he fumed in indignation.

He was very angry. It was clear to me that though he could access the journal, he rarely did. It seemed he did not enjoy being asked to consider unfamiliar agendas and was determined that I knew it.

I was seething inside but presented a calm exterior. "I need a new prescription for the Avonex." was all I said.

We concluded the ritual of parting, and I walked from his room to see his receptionist.

"Pity I need to come all this way every six months just to get a new script," I muttered.

Sensing the session may not have gone well, she unleashed the collar from my neck. "Your GP can do that; you don't have to come here."

I looked up at her. "Thanks," I said.

I would not see another neurologist for 17 years.

~

So now I was back to my local doctor. How did I find him? And how does he fit into my story?

In the ten-day space between saying I would try Avonex and first using it, I had mulled over the concept of establishing a baseline.

The associate professor had told me that they did not know what to look for, but it also seemed obvious to me that he wasn't interested in looking.

He would always be a follower, not a leader.

His lack of interest was a hurdle I felt I had to clear.

My wife had suffered from allergies, and I knew her allergist quite well. I contacted this specialist with a simple proposition.

"They say MS is an autoimmune disease. You're an allergist. Allergies arise from the immune system. Do you know someone who would test me for anything that's ever been associated with MS?"

She gave me the name of a pathologist who she had heard speak at a conference, so I called and put the proposition to him.

I was happy to pay, and he was curious enough about the idea to agree. So, within a week of being told that there was no point looking, I had found someone who *would* look.

He called about a fortnight later. "Good news," he said cheerfully down the phone, "you have *Chlamydia pneumoniae*. That's sometimes been linked."

"Anything else?" I asked and got a qualified reply. He had not checked for everything, but that was as good as he could do.

"Who knows anything about this?" I asked him. That is how I met my local doctor.

~

My GP was an obsessive man. He was fascinated by infections, in particular, the ones we know little about; the mycoplasmas, chlamydias, rickettsias, bartonella, and the bugs that can bite you long before you know something has gone wrong. Consequently, he was thorough.

He tested me for many things and treated my *Chlamydia pneumoniae*.

Later I developed a stomach ulcer, and he addressed that with a good understanding of its bacterial cause, *Helicobacter pylori*.

However, waiting to see him was painful. Sometimes he would be hours behind. It was common to have a 4.30 pm appointment finally at 7 pm. A consultation could go for over an hour and consisted mostly of long sermons on what he wanted you to know. Sometimes it was interesting, but he often repeated himself, and the magic began to wear off.

He introduced me to an antiviral drug called valaciclovir. My positive response to it led him to try it on other patients, though he never reported any more information than that. He prescribed my interferon-β-1a every six months for about ten years until I tired of taking it.

As useful as he had been, he became a burden. His timetabling became ever more erratic, and he began to see evidence of Lyme disease in every patient. The sermons became longer and longer, and the tests more and more exotic with every negative result. He seemed increasingly like a version of Don Quixote, chivalrously fighting the Lyme disease that had possessed his patients.

One day my GP confided in me that he viewed the pair of us as members of the professional class. His line of logic was he had a duty to charge me the full price so he could subsidize those clients who could not pay. My finance background led me to conclude that he would not be out of pocket under this arrangement. His magnanimous appraisal of my position in life was delivered after a two-hour wait and a one-hour sermon.

I had to bite my tongue. As far as I knew, only he would freely prescribe the valaciclovir that had eased my brain fog and assisted my fatigue.

I began to stretch out the gap between appointments as much as I could.

~

Now it was 2014.

I had three children, two dogs, a stressful job, and a wife who was increasingly remote. My health had been good, so much so that I began to ignore the habits that had kept me well and assumed the worst was behind me. Over the years, I had continued to read and learn about MS whenever I could; sometimes I experimented with various ideas. Some were good. Others caused problems, so I would back off until I recovered.

In late August of that year, I developed a tightness in my side. To compensate, I started to hitch my left hip when I walked. Early on, no one noticed.

Each day I became a bit stiffer; the tight muscles crept around my torso. I developed a terrible stomach-ache, like a bloat. Despite years of doing Pilates, the sudden discomfort was so great that I could not finish a session.

I thought this was just another relapse, and I would shake it off.

Around mid-September, as I sat at my desk at work, a massive thump hit my chest. I continued to sit for a few minutes until someone came up and said something to me. At that point I realized no one had noticed, so I decided to shrug it off. From that moment on, my chest and stomach began to tighten progressively. In the evenings, when I looked in the mirror, I could see how contorted my stomach muscles were becoming. I was finally getting a "six-pack," but not the way I expected.

Each day became more and more difficult. Walking was an issue. The screen on my computer became a haze of white light. Newspapers appeared to hide the print in the same white haze. It seemed impossible to hit the buttons on my keyboard and phone correctly. Every step became a battle with myself. Each movement felt like a shudder. No one noticed.

I continued to drive to and from work each day. There was no refuge at home. At work, the clueless, unpleasant woman who thought she ran my workplace was looking for any excuse to say, "Your time is up," so not being there wasn't a good idea. There was nowhere to rest.

I struggled on like this until Monday the 29th of September. We had been called into a briefing for the float of a major public company. As I had the most experience with this process; I asked the majority of the questions. All the time, I was in real discomfort. In a roomful of 60 people, no one noticed.

Whatever made me decide that I should go to the hospital, I will never know. In an instant, all the faces in the room had gone from the people I was familiar with and had turned into decoration. They looked like so many goldfish just staring through the curve of their bowl of water. "Why am I here?" I thought. "I should be in hospital."

When the meeting concluded, I walked uncomfortably back to my desk and looked down at my assistant. She, at least, had been asking if I was alright.

"I'm going to the hospital and may not be back. I'll let you know."

She nodded.

Trams are 20-ton lurching, noisy, crowded people movers. The people on them are disconnected commuters getting from one place to another as cheaply and quickly as they can. They are no limousine ride.

I had walked out the back of my office and down the hill. The tram would take me to the front door of the nearest hospital. I knew where the tram stop was and wasn't up to a fruitless walk to hail a taxi. As the tram was full, I stood for the whole trip. Several times I nearly lost my balance. Only a firm grip on the strap hanging from the roof prevented me from sprawling over the other passengers. Alighting from the tram was a challenge as it took several downward steps to reach the road.

I walked into the hospital and through its labyrinth of corridors until I reached the emergency department. Eventually, I came to a halt in front of a glass window. The nurse looked up at me.

"I'm four weeks into this MS attack, and I think I need some help," I said as calmly as I could.

She blinked and looked towards a cubicle on the far-left wall. "Come this way," she said. There was no request to complete any paperwork.

~

I had changed into a gown, and a nurse was sticking squares of tape with studs on them all over me. Then, to each metal nipple, she attached a lead. They seemed to be all over me and flowed back to a monitor that was out of my field of vision. She stepped away from me, looked at the screen, turned, and walked through the curtain, out of my cubicle. A moment later, she was back.

"Hold out your hand," she said very firmly and into my open palm poured a pile of pills.

"What are these?" I asked.

"Blood thinners," she said without any humor at all.

"How many do I take?" was my somewhat curious question.

"All of them," was the curt response. Then she was gone.

A moment later, another nurse came in. Then a head popped through the curtain, and a man looked straight at me. I kept popping the pills into my mouth and washing them down with sips of water from a plastic cup.

The head spoke, "You didn't come here looking for a cardiologist, did you?"

"No," I said confidently, "a neurologist, but you'll work it out." Then he disappeared.

My new nurse attended to the monitor, and another head popped through the curtain. "We've got him a bed in cardiology," it said and was gone.

Feeling a little surprised, I turned to the nurse. "What's this stuff about cardiology? I thought you'd get a neurologist."

She pointed at the monitor. "Because of that," she said.

"Well, I can't even see *that*, and I wouldn't know what it meant anyway," was my somewhat dissatisfied reply.

"It's gone crazy," she said with some finality.

"Fair enough," I thought. "At least I'm in the right place."

~

At first, I had thought my visit would be brief. Before the leads were attached, I had sent a text to my Pilates instructor to say I might be late for my lunchtime class.

After all that transpired over the next hour, it was clear to me that I was not going anywhere for a while. I sent a text message to my assistant to say I would be staying in the hospital, and it was unlikely I would soon be back. She confirmed that she would look after things and wished me well.

I sent a follow-up text to my Pilates instructor, Sarah, to confirm that I would definitely miss the class and would be hospitalized for a while. After a few minutes she sent a message back, "Can't come today. I'll come tomorrow."

I was pleased to get such a nice message. What I didn't know was how significant that kindness was to become.

Later I phoned my wife. She came in, but her body language told me she was not pleased to be there. After a time, I said, "You may as well go. There's no point waiting. It could be hours before anything transpires."

She agreed and left.

I waited for a long time for something to happen.

My trolley was wheeled from the ground floor through a series of winding corridors. Then I was taken via a lift to the fifth floor. I was now in cardiology.

The nurses began adjusting my leads, and a man appeared from nowhere. He introduced himself as my cardiologist.

His manner was direct. "Two chambers of your heart have stopped beating properly. We are thinning your blood and giving you some tablets to try to restart them. In the morning, if the tablets haven't worked, we will take you downstairs, stop your heart with paddles and then restart it. If that doesn't kick it back into a normal rhythm, we will give you a pacemaker."

He wasn't asking me. He was telling me. I swore under my breath.

"A pacemaker is an old man thing," I thought. For the first time, all this stuff was irritating me.

~

The following morning, an attendant with a wheelchair was positioned at the foot of my bed. I had already had my preliminary tests, and I was mentally prepared for the paddle procedure. My cardiologist appeared. "Well, your heart has restarted, so we'll just watch things for now," he said.

I was relieved. The paddles did not trouble me as much as the thought of a pacemaker. As far as I was concerned, I had just received a double reprieve.

At about 7 pm, Sarah, as good as her word, came in and stood beside my bed. "How do we get you out of here?" she smiled.

This book is dedicated to her. Over the coming months, no one came close to providing the support and understanding she offered me. When you have been as flattened as I was, you need a champion in your corner. When no one else stood up, she did.

~

After a week, I was introduced to a neurologist. It was many years since I had thought about a specialist, and my views were colored by experience. He seemed more approachable than the doctors I remembered, but I was wary. The cardiologist was now ready to let him treat me, so I began, as I had 20 years earlier, with three days on a steroid drip. Then he tried a small dose of an antidepressant as a muscle relaxant, but I reacted badly after one tablet.

Two days after that treatment, I was still in cardiology. The leads were still hanging from my body. I had been up and had started taking myself to the shower. It seemed that no one paid much attention to me except at mealtimes.

The neurologist stood beside my bed and said, "I think we should start to look at some rehabilitation."

"Why?" I asked.

"Because you can't walk," he answered.

I thought for a moment and realized he was right. When I stood, I had balanced by holding on to a pole. When I thought I had walked, It was only a shuffle. I blamed my slowness on the tangle of wires hanging off me. Most of my day was spent just lying in bed, and it had been like that for over a week.

~

This book is about what I learned from that point on.

None of my neurologists had been articulate enough to clearly explain what was happening to me. During the rehabilitation process, the physical therapists often did more harm than good.

Other health professionals I dealt with had similar communication problems. They could not explain to me why they were trying different medications and treatments. Their skill sets did not overlap sufficiently to allow them to understand clearly what the others were trying to do. Underneath their bravado, they were often just guessing and relying on someone else to take over when they were lost by the complexity of my condition.

MS is often presented as an opaque disease with unpredictable consequences. For a newly diagnosed patient, that is a daunting concept. It offers no pathway to follow and implies a descent into a worsening condition. In truth, a great deal is known.

The processes of fatigue, spasticity, and other associated features are now well understood and taught in universities. They may not always be linked explicitly to MS because many of the condition's features are common to other illnesses. The big wave of better understanding starts in the research of the 1990s, but that means it is still on its way to clinical settings. In the meantime, people with MS have no means of translating what they have been told into something they can understand.

This is not meant to be a simple book. Someone else can provide a high-level overview of what is generally understood about MS. I've never found that those books helped me at all.

This book is not about medications, although obviously, they will be noted. It is not about diet or lifestyle. Try another book for that. It is about the mechanisms at play in your body. Understanding those processes is the only way to empower people who are struggling to come to terms with something they don't yet understand. No one is helped by generalities when they want specifics, so, by necessity, it will be a book you may need to read several times to grasp how everything fits together.

This book is really about communication. If it succeeds, both patients and clinicians will slide it across the table to each other and say, "Read what this bit says." Hopefully, then they can understand each other.

Chapter 2

Things to Remember When it Feels Fruitless

Don't ever think there is a long history behind neurology.

The International Brain Organization was founded in 1961.[1] Its official journal, *Neuroscience*, wasn't established until 1976.

The International Society for Neurochemistry had only 226 members when they had their first conference in Strasbourg in 1967.[2]

The oldest neuroscience society in Europe was established in 1968.[3]

To complete the picture, the world's largest professional body of neurologists, The Society for Neuroscience,[4] only had its first meeting in Washington in 1971.

Neuroscience is a relatively new discipline, and most neuroscientists are not neurologists.

To become a modern neurologist, an undergraduate degree is required, followed by a medical qualification. After that, an internship at a hospital and then a residency often follows. At a minimum, the training will take 12 years. There is a high probability that the people who taught and guided your neurologist were born before some of these neurology societies were even in an embryonic phase.

Today's neurologists are still very much learning on the job. Their opinions and practices have been formed by the guiding hands of doctors who have not been taught any of the knowledge that has flowered since the 1990s. They are making gigantic advances rather than standing on the shoulders of giants. Even then, modern neurology owes much of its foundation to the work of physiologists and anatomists.

A local doctor has followed a different path and is likely to have almost no knowledge of neurology.

~

Charles D. Aring was an early neurologist. In his lifetime, he established the neurology departments of the University of California and the

University of Cincinnati. His involvement at Cincinnati saw him serve as professor and department chairman from 1948 to 1974. He wrote articles on neurology until the end of his life. His obituary in 1998 said, "He inspired those around him, and generations of students revered him. Many entered the field of neurology or psychiatry because of their contact with Dr. Aring."[5]

Nonetheless, in 1965 for the journal *Brain*, he wrote an article, *Observations of multiple sclerosis and Conversion Hysteria*.[6] It's not at all necessary to read the entire article for its thrust to leap off the page.

As an example of how little was known about MS, he quotes from the views of neurologists of the 1940s as follows, "… *symptoms are chiefly if not solely subjective where a superficial though perhaps natural diagnosis of hysteria is apt to be made … Examination discloses no single unequivocal sign of 'organic' nervous disease …*" This view echoed the opinions developed by late 19th century scientists, even though the distiction between lesions as a feature of MS rather than hysteria had already been determined.

While Aring's article is full of compassionate statements about people with MS, he defers to his peers, "*In their studies, they noted the basic hysterical personality structure of certain patients with multiple sclerosis long before they developed signs of the neurological disease.*"

In 2007, over forty years later, Professor Martin L. Pall addressed the article's apparent shortcomings in his excellent book, *Explaining "Unexplained Illnesses"*.[7] Pall summed it up very clearly, "*So here we have MS, a neurological disease now known to be caused by demyelination of neurons and subsequent neuronal dysfunction, ascribed to 'hysteria' …*"

1965 was not that long ago, and opinions can be hard to change.

~

The World Health Organization (WHO) classifies diseases to ensure there are globally recognized standard interpretations of disorders.[8] Its most recently published standard (ICD-11) completely dispenses with any reference to any purported mechanism where a psychiatric disorder presents as an unexplained set of medical symptoms (known as somatoform).

In October 2016, the official journal of the World Psychiatric Association published a review[9] of the major changes that would be implemented in the

WHO's new standard. The term, hypochondriasis, would persist but would now be classified under obsessive/compulsive behaviors. The criterion of "medically unexplained" would be dropped. The review concluded:

> *"It has been argued that patients with medical conditions and with a justifiable reason for somatic complaints may receive an inappropriate psychiatric diagnosis, with the possibility of associated stigma ... A single somatic symptom may lead to a diagnosis of bodily distress disorder or somatic symptom disorder. A good justification for this revision is that a single symptom, for example, pain, may sometimes be as bothersome as multiple somatic symptoms. However, the point has been made that this lowering of the threshold for the diagnosis may lead to an inappropriate labelling of apparently healthy persons as having a psychological disorder."*

In other words, your physician should never describe you as having a somatic symptom disorder. It is an outdated view. You should never be told that your unexplained illness is all in your head. If you, indeed, have an obsessive-compulsive disorder, then it should be treated appropriately. The best way of dealing with an unexplained set of symptoms is to test thoroughly.

You should not accept a casual opinion cast across a clinician's desk that you are imagining your discomfort. The modern practitioner has both tools and referral networks. They should be put to use. Good doctors do inquire.

References

1. *History of the International Brain Research Organisation.* 2018; Available from: https://ibro.org/history/. Accessed March 2021.

2. McIlwain, H. *History of The International Society for Neurochemistry.* Available from: https://www.neurochemistry.org/history. Accessed March 2021.

3. *The History of the European Brain and Behaviour Society.* Available from: https://ebbs-science.org/about.php. Accessed March 2021.

4. *History of the Society for Neuroscience.* Available from: https://www.sfn.org/about/history-of-sfn/1969-2019. Accessed March 2021.

5. Trufant, S.A. and A. Asbury, *Charles D. Aring: 1904–1998.* Annals of Neurology, 1998, **44**(4): p. 710.

6. Aring, C., *Observations on multiple sclerosis and conversion hysteria.* Brain, 1965, **88**(4): p. 663–74.

7. Pall, M.L., *Explaining '"Unexplained Illnesses": Disease Paradigm for Chronic Fatigue Syndrome, Multiple Chemical Sensitivity, Fibromyalgia, Post-traumatic Stress Disorder, Gulf War Syndrome, and Others.* 2007, Harrington Park Press: Binghamton, NY.

8. *World Health Organisation International Classification of Diseases.* Available from: http://www.who.int/classifications/icd/en/. Accessed March 2021.

9. Gureje, O. and G. Reed, *Bodily distress disorder in ICD-11: Problems and prospects.* World Psychiatry, 2016, **15**(3): p. 291–292.

Chapter 3

What Type of MS Do You Think You Have?

When I was diagnosed with MS, I was only offered one classification. So one day, I was surprised when a friend asked me what type of MS I had. To this day, no medical professional has ever bothered to label me as any particular type.

Up until 2001, a diagnosis of MS was either "clinically definite" or "probable MS." There were degrees of confidence around those conclusions related to the testing. The MRI and neurologist's opinions would have confirmed that I was clinically definite, but still, it was just called MS. Different types of presentation were well known before 2001, but they were not significant enough for the clinical practice to raise them with me.

A special report that year[1] tried to standardize a set of factors for determining an MS diagnosis by focusing on the diagnostic criteria.

In particular, they looked at what constitutes an attack, how to separate attacks over time (is it one long attack or more than one?), and the role of the new MRI technology in diagnosis. They replaced the old terms with three new ones: MS, possible MS or not MS. The paper mentioned a variety of presentations:

- monosymptomatic disease suggestive of MS
- disease with a typical remitting-relapsing course
- disease with insidious progression without clear attacks or remissions

The criteria were revised in 2005[2] and again in 2010,[3] and most recently in 2017.[4]

The lead neurologist for the original report was Dr. W. Ian McDonald,[5] a native of New Zealand, who spent most of his working life in England. He was instrumental in establishing that MRI could be used as a non-invasive way of diagnosing MS. The recommendations of the report became known as the McDonald criteria. Later revisions were aimed at clarifying the original definitions and reinforced the role of the MRI as a diagnostic tool.

There is no single test for MS. The first step in diagnosis is to rule out the chance that it might be something else.

The revisions to the McDonald criteria aimed to speed up diagnosis while lowering the risk of a mistake.

~

MS is not easy to diagnose. Laboratory tests are sometimes needed to ensure it is not, in fact, another disease. A diagnosis by a clinician experienced in MS is only one criterion.

Mistakes can be common. A 2016 review[6] by neurologists at four academic MS centers presented data on patients determined to have been misdiagnosed with MS. Of 110 misdiagnosed patients, 36 had been misdiagnosed for ten years or longer. The researchers noted there had been an earlier opportunity to make a correct diagnosis for 79 of the patients. Disease-modifying therapy had been given to 70% of the patients in the study, and 31% had experienced problems with medication. Four people had actually participated in a research study of an MS therapy.[6]

The key feature of MS is the nature of the lesions in the central nervous system. They are usually detected by MRI. Despite the sensitivity of MRI machines, the correlation between the findings of the scans, and the clinical evolution of MS is poor, except in early disease.[7] This discrepancy is usually referred to as the clinical-MRI paradox.[8] A neurologist cannot use an MRI to say with certainty how a disease will progress.

Different diseases can mimic the appearance of a demyelinating plaque such as lupus erythematosus, neuroborreliosis, West Nile virus, Nipah virus, John Cunningham virus, Hendra virus, HHV6, SSPE, HIV, HTLV-1 and HSVs 1 and 2.[9] The list goes on. You can have dominant (Thomsen disease) or recessive genes (Becker disease) that cause mutations in skeletal muscle that make you stiff and weak,[10] but they are not MS.

Lesions in the spine are, perhaps, more telling than lesions in the brain. There does seem to be a better correlation between spinal cord lesions and disability than is seen with lesions in the brain.[7]

For diagnosis, lesions must be observed in more than one location in the brain and/or spinal cord (central nervous system). This is known as dissemination in space. Also, damage from the lesions must have occurred at different points of time. This is known as dissemination in time.

To confirm an MS diagnosis, lesions must demonstrate both time and space dissemination.

MRIs now form part of the diagnostic process. A gadolinium-based contrast agent is often used. The contrast shortens the relaxation rate of tissue. If the blood-brain barrier is leaking (due to inflammation or an illness), an active lesion will show up as a bright area on the scan. This will indicate that the lesion is new or the inflammation is active. Other lesions might be observed, but if they are not bright, then they suggest old damage.

With the latest technology, if the lesions are regarded as symptomatic of MS (i.e., bright), they can be used to indicate dissemination in time. Until the 2017 revision, the neurologist would need to scan at a later date to confirm if there were signs of ongoing damage. Now a single scan is sufficient. This accelerates a diagnosis of MS by around ten months, and studies show that at least 82.5% of patients who would not previously have been diagnosed now get a certain diagnosis.[11]

The attitude among medical professionals towards using the McDonald criteria varies quite a bit. A survey in Scotland of 65 neurologists showed that although 97% of them were familiar with the McDonald criteria, only 53% of them used it in their clinical practice.[12] When presented with a hypothetical first attack, 60% preferred to wait for a second attack rather than rely on an MRI. Only 9% were prepared to say that a diagnosis of MS was likely.

This data could have been skewed by the level of experience of the neurologists. Nonetheless, Scotland has the second-highest incidence of MS in the UK, with 180 sufferers per 100,000 population.[13] Only Orkney, at over 220 per 100,000, is higher in incidence.[14] The surveyed neurologists in Scotland are the local experts, yet they seem reluctant to adhere to a global standard.

The following broad classifications of MS diagnosis remain:

Clinically Isolated Syndrome

If a patient has a first neurological attack, and the lesions don't meet the criteria of dissemination in time, an alternative test can be conducted by testing the spinal fluid for abnormal bands of protein that shouldn't be in the spinal cord. If the bands are present, then dissemination in time is now assumed.

A patient having a neurological event, who does not have the bands or meet the dissemination in time test, is said to have Clinically Isolated Syndrome. This can ultimately develop into MS, but it may not. If you have this syndrome, you may possibly continue to lead a healthy life.

Remitting-Relapsing MS

This is the most common form of the disease. Typically, a relapse occurs that lasts for at least 24 hours, and then there is a remission. Any recovery from an attack may be incomplete. Then there are later attacks followed by recovery. A majority (85–90%) of patients display this pattern.[3]

The typical age of onset of this type of MS is around 30 years. It is reported that women are affected more than men; in some regions by a ratio of three to one. There are indications that there is a trend towards both increasing occurrence and a higher female involvement, again, in some regions.[15]

People with the remitting-relapsing form can develop symptoms collectively called Secondary Progressive MS which lead to a gradual increase in disability over time.[16]

Primary Progressive MS

This form of MS exhibits a slow progressive degeneration of neurological function, usually without any apparent signs of relapses. There is no gender bias apparent, and the onset tends to be around 40 years of age. Approximately 10–15% of patients present as Primary Progressive MS.[17]

The pathology and MRI features of Secondary and Primary Progressive MS are indistinguishable. Some speculate that the lack of a remitting-relapsing pattern is suggestive that attacks may have always been occurring in regions of the central nervous system that are clinically silent in the early stages of the disease. Once damage accumulates, the symptoms of MS become apparent.[18]

~

Neither the original report of the McDonald criteria nor any of the updates go into the specifics of how the neurological problems present themselves. They are purely focused on the recognition of lesions in the central nervous system and rely on the skill of the neurologist to exclude other possible causes of the neurological symptoms. The symptoms themselves are only vaguely alluded to. Measuring disability relies on different criteria.

References

1. McDonald, W., A. Compston, G. Edan, D. Goodkin, H.P. Hartung, F.D. Lublin, H.F. McFarland, D.W. Paty, C.H. Polman, S.C. Reingold, M. Sandberg-Wollheim, W. Sibley, A. Thompson, S. van den Noort, B.Y. Weinshenker and J.S. Wolinsky. *Recommended diagnostic criteria for multiple sclerosis: Guidelines from the International Panel on the Diagnosis of Multiple Sclerosis.* Annals of Neurology, 2001. **50**(1): p. 121–127.

2. Polman, C., S.C. Reingold, G. Edan, M. Filippi, H-P. Hartung, L. Kappos, F.D. Lublin, L.M. Metz, H.F. McFarland, P.W. O'Connor, M. Sandberg-Wollheim, A.J. Thompson, B.G. Weinshenker and J.S. Wolinsky. *Diagnostic criteria for multiple sclerosis: 2005 Revisions to the "McDonald Criteria".* Annals of Neurology, 2005. **58**(6): p. 840-846.

3. Polman, C.H., S.C. Reingold, B. Banwell, M. Clanet, J.A. Cohen, M. Filippi, K. Fujihara, E. Havrdova, M. Hutchinson, L. Kappos, F.D. Lublin, X. Montalban, P. O'Connor, M. Sandberg-Wollheim, A.J. Thompson, E. Waubant, B. Weinshenker and J.S. Wolinsky. *Diagnostic criteria for multiple sclerosis: 2010 Revisions to the McDonald criteria.* Annals of Neurology, 2011. **69**(2): p. 292–302.

4. Thompson, A., B.L. Banwell, F. Barkhof, W.M. Carroll, T. Coetzee, G. Comi, J. Correale, F. Fazekas, M. Filippi, M.S. Freedman, K. Fujihara, S.L. Galetta, H.P. Hartung, L. Kappos, F.D. Lublin, R.A. Marrie, A.E. Miller, D.H. Miller, X. Montalban, E.M. Mowry, P.S. Sorensen, M. Tintoré, A.L. Traboulsee, M. Trojano, B.M.J. Uitdehaag, S. Vukusic, E. Waubant, B.G. Weinshenker, S.C. Reingold and J.A. Cohen. *Diagnosis of multiple sclerosis: 2017 revisions of the McDonald criteria.* The Lancet Neurology, 2018. **17**(2): p. 162–173.

5. Frohman, E.M., O. Stuve and D.H. Miller, *W. Ian Mcdonald, MB, ChB, PhD (1933–2006): The multiple sclerosis physician-scientist of the 20th century.* Archives of Neurology, 2007. **64**(3): p. 452–454.

6. Solomon, A., D.M. Bourdette, A.H. Cross, A. Applebee, P.M. Skidd, D.B. Howard, R.I. Spain, M.H. Cameron, E. Kim, M.K. Mass, V. Yadav, R.H. Whitham, E.E. Longbrake, R.T. Naismith, G.F. Wu, B.J. Parks, D.M. Wingerchuk, B.L. Rabin, M. Toledano, W.O. Tobin,

O.H. Kantarci, J.L. Carter, B.M. Keegan and B.G. Weinshenker, *The contemporary spectrum of multiple sclerosis misdiagnosis: A multicenter study.* Neurology, 2016. **87**(13): p. 1393–1399.

7. Zivadinov, R. and J. Cox, *Neuroimaging in multiple sclerosis.* International Journal of Radiation Oncology, Biology, & Physics, 1999. **45**(5): p. 449–474.

8. Rovaris, M. and M. Filippi, *"Importance sampling": A strategy to overcome the clinical/MRI paradox in MS?* Journal of the Neurological Sciences, 2005. **237**(1–2): p. 1–3.

9. Luque, F.A. and S.L. Jaffe, *Cerebrospinal Fluid Analysis in multiple sclerosis,* in *International Review of Neurobiology.* 2007. **79**: p. 341–356.

10. Portaro, S., O. Musumeci, V. Rizzo, C. Rodolico, M.G. Sweeney, M. Buccafusca, M.G. Hanna and A. Toscano, *Stiffness as a presenting symptom of an odd clinical condition caused by multiple sclerosis and myotonia congenita.* Neuromuscular Disorders, 2013. **23**(1): p. 52–55.

11. Gaetani, L., L. Prosperini, A. Mancini, P. Eusebi, M.C. Cerri, C. Pozzilli, P. Calabresi, P. Sarchielli and M. Di Filippo, *2017 revisions of McDonald criteria shorten the time to diagnosis of multiple sclerosis in clinically isolated syndromes.* Journal of Neurology, 2018. **265**(11): p. 2684–2687.

12. Lumley, R., R. Davenport and A. Williams, *Most neurologists in Scotland do not use the McDonald 2010 criteria to diagnose multiple sclerosis.* Journal of Neurology, Neurosurgery and Psychiatry, 2013. **84**(11): p. e2.

13. Rothwell, P.M. and D. Charlton, *High incidence and prevalence of multiple sclerosis in south east Scotland: evidence of a genetic predisposition.* Journal of Neurology, Neurosurgery and Psychiatry, 1998. **64**(6): p. 730.

14. Fowler, C.J., J.N. Panicker, M. Drake, C. Harris, S.C.W. Harrison, M. Kirby, M. Lucas, N. Macleod, J. Mangnall, A. North, B. Porter, S. Reid, N. Russell, K. Watkiss and M. Wells. *A UK consensus on the management of the bladder in multiple sclerosis.* Journal of Neurology, Neurosurgery and Psychiatry, 2009. **80**(5): p. 470.

15. Hirst, C., G. Ingram, T. Pickersgill, R. Swingler, D.A.S. Compston and N.P. Robertson. *Increasing prevalence and incidence of multiple sclerosis in South East Wales.* Journal of Neurology, Neurosurgery and Psychiatry, 2009. **80**(4): p. 386.

16. Brownlee, W., T.A. Hardy, F. Fazekas and D.H. Miller. *Diagnosis of multiple sclerosis: progress and challenges.* Lancet, 2017. **389**(10076): p. 1336–1346.

17. Lublin, F., S.C. Reingold, J.A. Cohen, G.R. Cutter, P.S. Sørensen, A.J.

Thompson, J.S. Wolinsky, L.J. Balcer, B. Banwell, F. Barkhof, B. Bebo, Jr, P.A. Calabresi, M. Clanet, G. Comi, R.J. Fox, M.S. Freedman, A.D. Goodman, M. Inglese, L. Kappos, B.C. Kieseier, J.A. Lincoln, C. Lubetzki, A.E. Miller, X. Montalban, P.W. O'Connor, J. Petkau, C. Pozzilli, R.A. Rudick, M.P. Sormani, O. Stüve, E. Waubant and C.H. Polman. *Defining the clinical course of multiple sclerosis The 2013 revisions.* Neurology, 2014. **83**(3): p. 278–286.

18.   Palle, P., K.L. Monaghan S.M. Milne and E.C.K. Wan. *Cytokine Signaling in multiple sclerosis and its therapeutic applications.* Medical Sciences, 2017. **5**(4): p. 23.

Chapter 4

Disability and Functional Independence

I remember being told by my neurologist that I could not walk just as vividly as the moment, years earlier, when I had been told I had MS.

In both cases, I didn't know what the doctors really meant. This is part of the dilemma of clear communication between a patient and a neurologist.

I didn't feel that unwell when I was first diagnosed. I thought I would be able to get around when my new neurologist suggested I needed rehabilitation. In both instances, I didn't grasp what disability meant. I didn't understand how it would affect the way I engaged with the world.

~

The treatment of disability falls to physical therapists rather than neurologists. In my case, in 2014, the people working in the rehabilitation facility talked about my 'clonus' but never said what that meant. What they were referring to was the repeated rhythmic contractions around my ankle joint.[1] I had never noticed it, but they were obsessed with it. I was more concerned with the tightness in my torso, but that did not fit their regime.

Some of them talked about my 'Parkinsons', and I guess by that they meant those contractions. It was never explained in a way that I could understand. By implication, being told I also had Parkinson's disease[2] by physical therapists and being given a 'don't argue' response when I queried that claim just added to my confusion. When I checked with my neurologist, he told me that they were wrong, but it was clear that the physical therapist's opinion would never be corrected.

The rehabilitation had one aim: to get me walking normally again. I would come to regard their efforts as a failure. The therapist's focus was on basic muscle movement, but their methods didn't help me. I needed to be shown how to move. I had to activate the muscles in the correct order. They would have claimed credit for any success, but that properly belonged to my Pilates instructor.

The muscles in my back, a few weeks on from the attack, had begun to tighten significantly. The first two days I went to rehab, the physical therapists laid me face down on a bench and applied heat packs to the sorest parts of my back. The heat provided a great deal of relief. However, after those first few sessions, they treated my requests for heat packs as an unnecessary indulgence. The physical therapists made it clear they were too busy, and the request was irksome.

Their only aim was to increase my walking speed. Periodically, I had to walk through and around the building while they timed me and counted the number of steps.

They made me prance on small trampolines, run, in a fashion, up hallways on my toes, and ultimately, they put me on cross-training machines. Part of the process involved walking up and down a staircase. In the early stages, I just kept falling flat on my face. It was my Pilates instructor who taught me how to balance on one leg while moving from step to step. It was never a physical therapist's achievement.

~

One incredibly hot day, after I had already walked my stiff body about one kilometer from the railway station to the hospital, the physical therapists instructed me to use the cross-trainer. The longer I worked, the worse I felt. When I got off, I slumped in a chair, the sweat pouring off me, and asked my case manager if she would take my blood pressure. Although a little put-out, the physical therapist did so.

My reading was 197/110.

So, there we were, sitting in the rehabilitation facility of a hospital. She looked at me and said, "That's not very good. You should see a doctor." Then she summed up her whole approach to the job, "Look, I have to go now as I have another patient in a few minutes."

She knew I had walked from the train station; she knew the day was scorching, and she knew I had to walk back to the station. Despite the obvious fact that my blood pressure was blowing off the charts, she had no time or inclination to direct me to any part of the hospital for assistance.

I walked back to the station in the heat. It was one of the hardest things I've done. At that stage, I was very vulnerable and was incapable of understanding how illogical my decision to do that was.

~

The only measurement that mattered to the physical therapists was how long it took me to walk around the building. Success was measured by how much my speed increased. They were not greatly interested in my repeated complaints about how much my hips and thighs were hurting. The more I did their exercises, the worse I felt. Their protocols were impacting on my Pilates, which was the only program that seemed to help.

In the end, a senior physician of the hospital diagnosed suspected bursitis of the greater trochanter.[3] It is a painful condition caused by repetitive irritation of the tendons and muscles over the bone of the hip. When that diagnosis was relayed to the physical therapists, they concluded that their work was done. I had spent a year as an outpatient of the hospital and was overjoyed that the therapy had ended.

What the physical therapists were trying to do was move me to the lowest Expanded Disability Status Scale score they could achieve. The lower the score, the more likely it was that I could maintain my independence and not be dependent on assistance. For all their good intentions, it isn't possible to tell if time might not have been as significant a contributor to my recovery as their program. I was undoubtedly doing exercises outside the regime they provided.

My physiotherapy treatment was the same as that given to people recovering from other traumas who did not have my neurological profile. Exercise is absolutely fundamental to managing spasticity in MS, but it has to be relevant to the condition.

~

The most common measurement of disability in MS is the Expanded Disability Score Scale or EDSS. Dr. John Kurtzke developed this measurement system in 1955,[4] to objectively measure disability in MS. He divided the scale into a series of steps from 0 to 10. The steps up to 4.5 indicate a high level of ability to walk. The second tier, encompassing steps 5 to 9.5, refers to stages of difficulty walking.

Dr Kurtzke also developed a series of classifications of what is known as functional systems, which are scored from 0 (low-level problem) to 6 (high-level problem). The functional systems cover a range of MS problems, and are classified according to the following categories:

- Motor function (also called pyramidal function)
- Cerebellar
- Brainstem
- Sensory
- Bowel and bladder
- Visual
- Cerebral or mental functions
- and finally, a category for other functions that don't fit into the earlier categories.[5]

In the entire Kurtzke system, fatigue is only mentioned once. However, it is often the most disabling feature of MS. Only the person with the condition can really understand what it means. The description and measurement of fatigue can't be captured by any simple tool or survey.

The total EDSS score is a combination of the scores for gait and functional systems. It may describe your disability, but it won't cure you.

It is a pity that the score rises as the disability increases. Success is often measured in life by achieving higher scores. There is nothing aspirational about a high EDSS score.

There are other measures, such as the Total Functional Independence Measure[6] and the Barthel Index,[7] but, again, these measures are only descriptive.

The list goes on: the ambulation index, the bladder control scale, the bowel control scale, the impact of visual impairment scale, the mental health inventory, the modified fatigue impact scale, the pain effects scale, the paced auditory serial addition test and the sexual satisfaction scale.

In 1964, Bryan Ashworth published a five-step measure of spasticity, from 0 to 4, for the assessment of MS patients. In 1987, two other researchers, Bohannon and Smith, added a step between 1 and 2, called 1+, which is referred to as the modified Ashworth scale.[8] Both versions rely on the observer to determine the score.

There are surveys and inventories for quality of life, tests to see how proficiently you can walk 25 feet and clinical rating scales that are no more than combinations of the different tests. Some tests will produce results that should be called "garbage in/ garbage out". In the end, not even the best of them will make you better. They suit the vast bureaucracy of medicine, but they just reduce the patient to numbers.

Occasionally, something useful is gleaned from all of these measures. A study using an extensive data set known as MSbase[9] concluded that after four years, EDSS scores seemed to become stable. A score at year four was highly predictive of a score at year nine. They also concluded that the risk of progression at year 10 was highly dependent on the score at year five.[10] This highlights that whatever strategy has helped to maintain a low score in the early years after diagnosis becomes critical in the long term.

Where would I fit into that prognosis? I had a major attack at year 20 and now have a low EDSS score again. I couldn't possibly tell.

Kurtzke Expanded Disability Status Scale (EDSS) [4, 11, 12]

These are some of the steps in the Kurtze system.

(FS =Functional Score)

1.0- No disability, minimal signs in one FS (i.e., grade 1).

1.5 - No disability, minimal signs in more than one FS (more than one FS grade 1); or minimal disability in one FS (one FS grade 2, others 0 or 1).

2.5 - Minimal disability in two FSs (two FS grade 2, others 0 or 1); or moderate disability in one FS (one FS grade 3, others 0 or 1); or mild disability in three or four FS (three or four FSs grade 2, others 0 or 1) though fully ambulatory.

3.5 - Fully ambulatory but with moderate disability in one FS (one FS grade 3) and one or two FS grade 2; or two FS grade 3 (others 0 or 1) or five grade 2 (others 0 or 1).

4.0 - Fully ambulatory without aid, self-sufficient, up and about some 12 hours a day despite relatively severe disability consisting of one FS grade 4 (others 0 or 1), or a combination of lesser grades exceeding limits of previous steps; able to walk without aid or rest some 500 meters.

4.5 - Fully ambulatory without support, 'up and about' much of the day, able to work a full day, may otherwise have some limitation of full activity or require minimal assistance; characterized by relatively severe disability usually consisting of one FS grade 4 (others 0 or 1); or combinations of lesser grades exceeding limits of previous steps; able to walk without aid or rest some 300 meters.

5.0- Ambulatory without support or rest for about 200 meters; disability severe enough to impair full daily activities (e.g., to work a full day without special provisions); (usual FS equivalents are one grade 5 alone, others 0 or 1, or combinations of lesser grades usually exceeding specifications for step 4.0).

5.5 - Ambulatory without aid for about 100 meters; disability severe enough to preclude full daily activities; (usual FS equivalents are one grade 5 alone, others 0 or 1, or combination of lesser grades usually exceeding those for step 4.0); or intermittent or unilateral constant assistance (cane, crutch, brace) required to walk about 100 meters with or without resting; (usual FS equivalents are combinations with more than two FS grade 3+).

6.5 - Constant bilateral assistance (canes, crutches, braces) required to walk about 20 meters without resting; (usual FS equivalents are combinations with more than two FS grade 3+).

7.0 - Unable to walk beyond approximately 5 meters even with aid, mainly restricted to a wheelchair; wheels self in standard wheelchair and transfers alone; up and about in wheelchair some 12 hours a day; (usual FS equivalents are combinations with more than one FS grade 4+; very rarely pyramidal grade 5 alone).

7.5 - Unable to take more than a few steps; restricted to wheelchair; may need aid in transfer; wheels self but cannot carry on in standard wheelchair a full day; may require a motorized wheelchair; (usual FS equivalents are combinations with more than one FS grade 4+).

8.0 - Essentially restricted to bed or chair or perambulated in a wheelchair, but may be out of a bed much of the day; retains many self-care functions; generally has effective use of arms; (usual FS equivalents are combinations, grade typically 4+ in several systems).

8.5 - Essentially restricted to bed much of day; has some effective use of arm(s); retains some self-care functions; (usual FS equivalents are combinations, generally 4+ in several systems).

9.0 - Helpless bed patient; can communicate and eat; (usual FS equivalents are combinations, mostly grade 4+).

9.5 - Totally helpless bed patient; unable to communicate effectively or eat/swallow; (usual FS equivalents are combinations, almost all grade 4+).

10.0 - Death due to MS.

Kurtzke Functional Systems Scores

Pyramidal functions

0 - Normal.

1 - Abnormal signs without a disability.

2 - Minimal disability.

3 - Mild to moderate paraparesis or hemiparesis (detectable weakness but most function sustained for short periods, fatigue a problem); severe monoparesis (almost no function).

4 - Marked paraparesis or hemiparesis (function is difficult), moderate quadriparesis (function is decreased but can be sustained for short periods), or monoplegia.

5 - Paraplegia, hemiplegia, or marked quadriparesis.

6 - Quadriplegia.

9 - (Unknown).

Cerebellar functions

0 - Normal.

1 - Abnormal signs without a disability.

2 - Mild ataxia (tremor or clumsy movements easily seen, minor interference with function).

3 - Moderate truncal or limb ataxia (tremor or clumsy movements interfere with function in all spheres).

4 - Severe ataxia in all limbs (most function is challenging).

5 - Unable to perform coordinated movements due to ataxia.

9 - (Unknown).

Brainstem functions

0 - Normal.

1 - Signs only.

2 - Moderate nystagmus or other mild disabilities.

3 - Severe nystagmus, marked extraocular weakness, or moderate disability of other cranial nerves.

4 - Marked dysarthria or other marked disability.

5 - Inability to swallow or speak.

9 - (Unknown).

Sensory functions

0 - Normal.

1 - Vibration or figure-writing decreases only in one or two limbs.

2 - Mild decrease in touch or pain or position sense, and/or moderate reduction in vibration in one or two limbs; or a vibratory fine motor competence (such as figure writing) decrease alone in three or four limbs.

3 - Moderate decrease in touch or pain or position sense, and/or essentially lost vibration in one or two limbs; or a mild decrease in touch or pain and/or moderate decrease in all proprioceptive tests in three or four limbs.

4 - Marked decrease in touch or pain or loss of proprioception, alone or combined, in one or two limbs; or moderate decrease in touch or pain and/or severe proprioceptive decrease in more than two limbs.

5 - Loss (primarily) of sensation in one or two limbs; or moderate decrease in touch or pain and/or loss of proprioception for most of the body below the head.

6 - Sensation essentially lost below the head.

9 - (Unknown).

Bowel and bladder function

Rated based on the worse function, either bowel or bladder

0 - Normal.

1 - Mild urinary hesitance, urgency, or retention.

2 - Moderate hesitance, urgency, retention of bowel or bladder, or rare urinary incontinence (intermittent self-catheterization, manual

compression to evacuate bladder or finger evacuation of stool).

  3 - Frequent urinary incontinence.

  4 - In need of almost constant catheterization (and constant use of measures to evacuate stool).

  5 - Loss of bladder function.

  6 - Loss of bowel and bladder function.

  9 - (Unknown).

Visual function

  0 - Normal.

  1 - Scotoma with visual acuity (corrected) better than 20/30.

  2 - Worse eye with scotoma with maximal visual acuity (corrected) of 20/30-20/59.

  3 - Worse eye with large scotoma, or moderate decrease in fields, but with maximal visual acuity (corrected) of 20/60-20/99.

  4 - Worse eye with a marked decrease of fields and maximal visual acuity (corrected) of 20/100-20/200; grade 3 plus maximal acuity of better eye of 20/60 or less.

  5 - Worse eye with maximal visual acuity (corrected) less than 20/200; grade 4 plus maximal acuity of better eye of 20/60 or less.

  6 - Grade 5 plus maximal visual acuity of better eye of 20/60 or less.

  9 - (Unknown).

Cerebral (or mental) functions

  0 - Normal.

  1 - Mood alteration only (does not affect EDSS score).

  2 - Mild decrease in mentation.

  3 - Moderate decrease in mentation.

  4 - Marked decrease in mentation (chronic brain syndrome - moderate).

  5 - Dementia or chronic brain syndrome - severe or incompetent.

  9 - (Unknown).

References

1. Manella, K.J. *Operant conditioning of tibialis anterior and soleus H-reflex improves spinal reflex modulation and walking function in individuals with motor-incomplete spinal cord injury*, E.C. Field-Fote, Roach, K.E., Thomas C.K. and T.G. Hornby, Editors. 2011, ProQuest Dissertations Publishing.

2. Ebadi, M.S., R. Pfeiffer and Z.K. Wszolek, *Parkinson's Disease (Second Edition)* 2013, Boca Raton, Fla.: CRC Press.

3. Newson, L., *Trochanteric bursitis.* 2012: Available from https://www.gponline.com/trochanteric-bursitis/musculoskeletal-disorders/article/1130005 Accessed January 2021.

4. Kurtzke, J.F., *Rating neurologic impairment in multiple sclerosis: an expanded disability status scale (EDSS).* Neurology, 1983. **33**(11): p. 1444–1452.

5. *US Department of Veterans Affairs multiple sclerosis Centers of Excellence : Kurtzke Expanded Disability Status Scale.* 2018.

6. Rabadi, M. and A. Vincent, *Comparison of the Kurtkze Expanded Disability Status Scale and the Functional Independence Measure: measures of multiple sclerosis-related disability.* Disability and Rehabilitation, 2013. **35**(22): p. 1877–1884.

7. Tanovic, E., D. Vrabac, A. Kadić and A. Rama. *Evaluation of the treatment efficacy of patients with multiple sclerosis using Barthel index and Expanded Disability Status Scale.* Journal of Health Sciences, 2014. **4**(2): p. 110

8. Harb, A. and S. Kishner, *Modified Ashworth Scale*, 2020, StatPearls Publishing: Treasure Island (FL)

9. Butzkueven, H., J. Chapman, E. Cristiano, F. Grand'Maison, M. Hoffmann, G. Izquierdo, D. Jolley, L. Kappos, T. Leist, D. Pöhlau, V. Rivera, M. Trojano, F. Verheul and J.P. Malkowski. *MSBase: an international, online registry and platform for collaborative outcomes research in multiple sclerosis.* multiple sclerosis, 2006. **12**(6): p. 769–774.

10. Hughes, S., T. Spelman, M. Trojano, A. Lugaresi, G. Izquierdo, F. Grand'Maison, P. Duquette, M. Girard, P. Grammond, C. Oreja-

Guevara, R. Hupperts, C. Boz, R. Bergamaschi, G. Giuliani, M.E. Rio, J. Lechner-Scott, V. van Pesch, G. Iuliano, M. Fiol, F. Verheul, M. Barnett, M. Slee, J. Herbert, I. Kister, N. Vella, F. Moore, T. Petkovska-Boskova, V. Shaygannejad, V. Jokubaitis, G. McDonnell, S. Hawkins, F. Kee, O. Gray, H. Butzkueven and MSBase Study Group. *The Kurtzke EDSS rank stability increases 4 years after the onset of multiple sclerosis: results from the MSBase Registry.* Journal of Neurology, Neurosurgery and Psychiatry, 2012. **83**(3): p. 305.

11.   *National Multiple Sclerosis Society Functional Systems Scores and Expanded Disability Staus Scale.* Available from: https://www.nationalmssociety. org/For-Professionals/Researchers/Resources-for-Researchers/Clinical-Study-Measures/Functional-Systems-Scores-(FSS)-and-Expanded-Disab. Accessed November 2020.

12.   Haber A. and N.G. LaRocca, Editors. *Minimal Record of Disability for Multiple Sclerosis.* 1985; National multiple sclerosis Society: New York. Available from https://www.nationalmssociety.org/For-Professionals/ Researchers/Resources-for-MS-Researchers/Research-Tools/Clinical-Study-Measures/Functional-Systems-Scores-(FSS)-and-Expanded-Disab. Accessed January 2021.

Chapter 5

Indications of Multiple Sclerosis

I didn't just wake up one morning in late 1994 and say to myself, "Oh, I must have MS."

On that December morning, I swung my feet out of bed. As I did so, my left foot felt odd, as though I had pinched a nerve. When I tried to walk, my ankle was floppy. Each step meant my foot hit the ground with a slap.

The night before, I had felt quite unwell when I had tried to complete a circuit at a gym. Although I was no fanatic, it was evident to me that my sedentary desk job wasn't optimal for fitness. My assumption that morning was that during the circuit, I had pinched a nerve.

When someone asked me why I was walking differently, I laughed it off as a silly gym injury.

~

Later that day, I attended a lunch presentation and sat at the midway point of a long table. My head was turned to the presenter.

Someone asked a question, so I turned towards the speaker. When I did this, I saw two images of everyone to my right. It was a sudden and unexpected change. I turned my head back to the left and saw only a single clear-cut image.

Whatever the lunch presentation was about suddenly became entirely uninteresting to me. I didn't quite believe what I was seeing, so I entertained myself for the balance of the lunch by swinging my head from side to side to test the limits of what was happening. When the lunch ended, I had already concluded that my floppy foot and the double vision were somehow related.

Although I felt quite well, I left work and went to the hospital. That visit led to a diagnosis early the following week.

While some people report that a diagnosis makes them burst into tears, I didn't react like that. My first thought was, "Well, that explains a lot."

MS doesn't fall from the sky; it creeps up on you. Often over a very long period of time. At first, the changes it brings are subtle, almost imperceptible reference points. Without the benefit of hindsight, the variations are so small you discount them. Sometimes those moments of clumsiness and tiredness pop back into your mind. What you couldn't explain at the time becomes rational with hindsight.

~

When I was 14 or 15, I recall lying down at school on a bench and falling into a deep 20-minute sleep. As I awoke, I saw a teacher walk past with a quizzical look on his face. What I had done must have looked odd, but, by then, I was awake and seemed healthy. This sudden need to sleep was something that often arose over the next few decades. I recall doing it in Malaysia when I was backpacking in my 20s. When I woke, a fellow traveler was looking at me. He said there was something odd about what I had done. I assured him I was fine, and that it must have been the heat.

My build suggested I should have been a reasonable sportsman. Instead, I was clumsy, slow, and often unaware of where my body was in space. Not surprisingly, I was the first one offered up if an opposing team was short a player.

In my 20s and early 30s, my physical awkwardness increased. Although I knew I was not stupid, I only scraped through my exams because I struggled to process information quickly enough.

Often I became woozy if I changed position too suddenly. Sometimes I just ran out of steam and needed to sleep.

There were things I couldn't recall, people I couldn't name. I lived with an awkwardness that made me feel like a fool. Often, I had a sense of not being connected to anything or anyone around me. A veil was between me and everything else.

Despite all those things, I thought I was normal. If something wasn't quite right, I was sure it was my fault. Despite all my social connections, all my activities, and all the camaraderie, I stood alone, never sure what separated me from everyone else. Sometimes I wore a veneer of confidence, sometimes a cloak of silence. A question I asked myself over and over with increasing frequency was, "Why am I so tired?"

As my 20s gave way to my 30s, this issue of tiredness became a constant. I went to doctors, paid to be tested in clinics, tried diets, and all sorts of exercise. Each time I asked about my tiredness, the answer came back as a question, "What's your job?" Then a definitive, "That'll be it." In my gut, I knew that was nonsense.

My friends rolled their eyes when I would retire to the couch for a quick sleep. The standing joke was that I couldn't handle a drink. Through their half-drunk reverie, they were always surprised by how well I bounced back. They paid little attention except to comment on what poor form my sleeping was.

In the year before my initial diagnosis, I'd started to wonder if I was some sort of weird mental case. Crowds began to trouble me. I didn't object to them being around me or behind me, but I hated walking towards them. The people seemed almost to shudder or jump from spot to spot as they approached me. It threw my sense of balance awry.

I thought I might have some deep-seated psychological problem that I just couldn't admit to myself. In truth, the problem was that my eye muscles moved at different speeds, and my mind struggled to reconcile all the erratic, moving images. Thankfully, that problem resolved itself and never came back.

When I was younger, slow people used to frustrate me. I'd duck around them and shoot down the path. As my undiagnosed condition worsened, I found myself being overtaken by everyone, and I couldn't keep up with them. I'd try to stride out and catch them but kept falling further behind. A friend who had a chance meeting with me in the street said, "What's the matter with you? You're walking like an old man."

All this time I thought I was healthy, and that all my problems were my fault. I just needed to try harder.

So, MS doesn't just appear. It silently wraps itself around you, feeding on your self-worth, your energy, and your wit. It seduces you into not questioning what is happening, and, for some, a diagnosis comes as a complete surprise. It has, nonetheless, been your companion for some time.

Common Early Signs of MS

Fatigue.

Visual disturbance (loss of vision, double vision, eye pain, color blindness).

Altered sensation, including numbness and tingling, burning, pins, and needles, hugging, or squeezing.

Muscle spasms (often very painful).

Muscle stiffness.

Muscle weakness.

Clumsiness, shaking, and tremors, coordination issues, vertigo.

Pain.

Facial pain.

Cognitive disturbance (usually short-term memory, attention span, spatial awareness, problem-solving).

Depression and anxiety (including mood swings).

Sexual problems.

Bladder retention and control.

Bowel motility problems (both constipation and incontinence).

Speech and swallowing problems.

All these symptoms can arise from causes that have nothing to do with multiple sclerosis. What defines MS is the damage done to the myelin sheaths that surround the portions of neurons called axons. The scarring, called a sclerosis, is indicative of a deterioration called demyelination.

NHS, U.K. *Symptoms of multiple sclerosis.* 2019. Available from: https://www.nhs.uk/conditions/multiple-sclerosis/symptoms/. Accessed November 2020.

Chapter 6

Myelin in the Central Nervous System

What goes wrong in MS?

MS is a disease where the fatty material covering part of a neuron, called an axon, in the central nervous system (the brain and spinal cord) becomes damaged. That covering, which looks more like a string of sausages than a continuous film, helps transmit signals through our nervous system.

When the covering is damaged, the nerve signals are interrupted.

~

All the messages that pass along the surface of the axons of our neurons are pushed by small electrical impulses. The speed of the impulse depends on the surface area of each axon. The larger the surface area, the faster the signal travels. Many axons have a fatty layer that increases the surface area and this speeds up the signaling capability.

The fatty covering, made up of a precise arrangement of proteins and fats, is called myelin. The myelin covering the axon is not a continuous film. It is made up of discrete packages separated by gaps. These gaps between the fatty segments are called nodes of Ranvier[1] after the scientist who discovered them in 1878.

The strength of the signal is conserved at the node by the activity of sodium ion channels. These channels help build electrical charges. The charged signal then leaps from node to node.

Myelin acts as insulation to prevent potassium ion channels from receiving the charged signal. If the protective myelin flanking a node, called a paranode, is damaged, the signal may find a way to flow under rather than over the myelin. Worse still, if the next sequence, called the juxtaparanode, is damaged then potassium ion channels are exposed and the insulating property of myelin is lost. The consequence of this is that the signal is diverted to the potassium ion channels rather than to the next node and does not continue to travel along the axon.[2]

Neurons don't make myelin. In the central nervous system, another cell called an oligodendrocyte makes it. The oligodendrocytes wrap myelin around an extension of each neuron, called an axon.

There are millions upon millions of neurons in the brain. Nearly all of them have at least one axon growing away from the cell body. Some axons are small, but some can extend for over a meter. The axon carries the impulse of the neuron. If one cell fails, it can affect a whole chain.

~

When you are born, the process of coating axons with myelin (myelination) is still near its beginning. Its genesis is in the fourteenth week of fetal development. The process takes time, and there is minimal myelin formation in the brain at birth.[3] Growing myelin depends on dietary fats,[3] and is a process that takes until adolescence to complete.

Types of fats (cholesterol, phospholipids, and glycolipids), collectively called lipids, make up about 70% of a sheath of myelin, and the remaining 30% is protein. This ratio of lipids to protein is the inverse of the ratio found in the membranes in other cells of the body.[4] Cholesterol is essential in myelin formation as it allows the myelin basic protein to be stacked in layers to become a membrane.[5]

Oligodendrocytes are only found in the central nervous system. In the peripheral nervous system (the rest of the nervous system), a different cell, called a Schwann cell, performs a similar role.

Schwann cells can be replaced, but for oligodendrocytes replacement is a far slower process. As an example, if you damage your leg, the nerves can, possibly, recover, but if you damage your spinal cord, the consequence is more likely to be permanent.

Myelin basic protein (MBP) is the major structural protein and accounts for 30% of the protein in myelin.[6] It belongs to a group called intrinsically disordered proteins (IDP). The proteins in this group lack a rigid structure, and this suppleness helps them bind more easily to targets. MBP is, in effect, a molecular glue.

MBP is observed only in the oligodendrocytes that have migrated into axonal pathways, and it is produced just before they bind to the axon.[5]

Within myelin, most attention has been focused on a protein called 18.5-kDa MBP.[7] This form of MBP consists of 168 amino acid residues.[5] It is not a simple substance.

> The cardinal feature of multiple sclerosis is damage to the myelin in the central nervous system. Electrical pulses running to and from the brain along the nerves cannot get past the damaged area.

Unmyelinated Nerves

In both the central and peripheral nervous systems, many axons are unmyelinated. The speed of a nerve signal depends on two factors: the diameter of the nerve fiber and the involvement of myelin. Signal conduction occurs along the surface of the fiber, not deep inside it. The addition of myelin to an axon speeds up the signal.

However, not every function in the body requires a fast signal. Digestion, for example, does not. Myelinated fibers are concentrated where speed is essential – in our sensory nerves and the motor functions that drive our muscles.[3]

Demyelination

When myelin degrades, the process is called demyelination. Everyone is continuously demyelinating and remyelinating as new myelin is laid down. In MS, this normal process is disrupted. The myelin degrades faster than it is replaced, creating permanent damage. Some demyelination is transitory but permanent damage leaves a scar, called a sclerosis.

As the signals to and from the brain are affected, any part of your motor or sensory pathways may become impaired. Stiffness, weakness or impaired sensation can arise. You may experience this in your limbs, your torso or your eyes. It may affect your bowel, your bladder, your speech or your expressions and how you move. It can contribute to enduring, crippling fatigue. Collectively, these outcomes may reduce your sense of self-worth.

There was an interesting observation made in 1994. When scientists analyzed the components of myelin and separated them into the smallest elements, they found that people with MS had a higher proportion of a less dense form of myelin, similar to that found in children under the age of six.[8] The authors of the study concluded that this myelin may be prone to degradation by one or more factors. If the myelin were to deteriorate, it could provide the initial conditions to trigger a profound response. What is uncertain is whether the stripping away of mature myelin is a consequence, or a cause of disease. What resembles a less mature form of myelin may represent an early stage of remyelination.

~

Later in this book, there is a note about citrullination, sometimes known as deimination (Note 15). It is the process by which the amino acid arginine is converted into citrulline. Arginine is a large, positively charged amino acid. This positive charge makes it electrostatic, and that contributes to the structure of its associated protein. Citrulline, by comparison, is uncharged. The conversion from one amino acid to the other can cause a protein structure to unfold, increasing the risk of degradation.[9]

The same scientists noted that when 50% of the myelin basic proteins were deiminated, the patient was chronically ill with MS. In a healthy brain, usually only 20% is deiminated. In a very rare, fatal demyelinating disease called Marburg Syndrome, the proportion of deiminated MBPs reaches 90%.[9] This suggests a correlation between demyelination and deimination.

~

Myelin oligodendrocyte glycoprotein is a component of the outer layer of the myelin sheath. It is well known by the acronym MOG. In animal models of MS, it is the most prominent target of demyelinating antibodies. Anti-MOG antibodies are found in MS patients, but they are not unique to the disease. They may play a secondary role but are not the cause of MS.[6]

References

1. Barbara, J-G. *Louis Antoine Ranvier (1835-1922)*. Journal of Neurology, 2006. **253**(3): p. 399–400.

2. Arancibia-Carcamo, I.L. and D. Attwell. *The node of Ranvier in CNS pathology*. Acta Neuropathologica, 2014. **128**: p. 161–175.

3. Saladin, K.S., *Anatomy & Physiology : The Unity of Form and Function (Third Edition)*, 2004. McGraw-Hill Higher Education: Boston.

4. *2 - Neuron-Glial Cell Cooperation*, in *Cellular and Molecular Neurobiology (Second Edition)*, C. Hammond, Editor. 2001. Academic Press: London. p. 24-35.

5. Harauz, G. and J.M. Boggs. *Myelin management by the 18.5-kDa and 21.5-kDa classic myelin basic protein isoforms*. Journal of Neurochemistry, 2013. **125**(3): p. 334–361.

6. Nikbin, B., M,M. Bonab, F. Khosravi and F. Talebian. *Role of B cells in pathogenesis of multiple sclerosis*, in *International Review of Neurobiology*. 2007. **79**: p. 13–42.

7. Kattnig, D.R., T. Bund, J.M. Boggs, G. Harauzc and D. Hinderberger. *Lateral self-assembly of 18.5-kDa myelin basic protein (MBP) charge component-C1 on membranes*. Biochimica et Biophysica Acta, 2012. **1818**(11): p. 2636–47.

8. Moscarello, M.A., D.D. Wood, C. Ackerley and C. Boulias. *Myelin in multiple sclerosis is developmentally immature*. The Journal of Clinical Investigation, 1994. **94**(1): p. 146–154.

9. Musse, A.A. and G. Harauz, *Molecular "negativity" may underlie multiple sclerosis: role of the myelin basic protein family in the pathogenesis of MS*. International Review of Neurobiology, 2007. **79**: p. 149–72.

Chapter 7

Stiff and Sore

The messages delivered by nerve impulses either excite or inhibit. The effect depends on what chemical, or neurotransmitter, is delivered.

The purpose of neurotransmitters is to permit neurons to communicate with each other. Neurotransmitters are made in the cell body of each neuron. They travel along an extension of the neuron, called an axon, until they reach the furthest point. Here, they wait in many small membranous sacks, called vesicles, to be released from the axon by an electrical nerve impulse. When a neurotransmitter is pushed out of the axon, its target will be a receptor on an adjacent neuron, gland or muscle cell. When the neurotransmitter binds, it triggers a change in the electrical activity of the target neuron. What leaves the neuron and doesn't bind to a target, either dissipates or is reabsorbed by the neuron.

When receptors open, they allow specific molecules that are outside a cell to enter. It is the new molecules that have the effect of changing the electric charge inside the target cell. That, in turn, starts a cascade of actions.

~

There are many neurotransmitters, but we will only look at two.

Acetylcholine

The neurotransmitter acetylcholine is the primary agent that activates the skeletal muscles—the muscles connected to bones.

Receptors that open when activated by acetylcholine create a channel in the cell membrane that allows only sodium ions to enter the cell. When sodium does this, it makes the inside of the cell become less negatively charged than when it was resting. The change triggers a wave of actions that result in muscle contraction.

GABA

In contrast to this, another neurotransmitter in the central nervous system, called gamma (γ) aminobutyric acid (GABA), reverses the effect of acetylcholine. It opens a different receptor that can allow only chloride ions (and sometimes potassium) to enter the cell. Chloride has the opposite effect to sodium and makes the charge inside the cell more negative. The impact of this is that the activating signal desists. Chloride is like an "off switch" that ends the activation. Potassium has a similar but more muted effect.

For skeletal muscle, pathways from all parts of our body allow the control systems of the brain to coordinate these opposing signals to give us a smooth, coordinated movement. When myelin is degraded in the central nervous system, these pathways become dead ends before the messages are delivered.

~

When skeletal muscles move, some of their actions are just reflexes. The primary intention of a reflex is to make a muscle contract even before any sensory message passes to the brain. That reflex is driven, in part, by acetylcholine.

When a reflex makes a muscle tighten, the coordinating parts of our brain respond by sending an impulse to release GABA. We don't need to tighten endlessly, and we do need to maintain our balance. The brain intends to switch the reflex off.

GABA passes along neurons of the spinal cord to inhibit the tightening of a muscle. When this message is corrupted by damaged myelin, the muscles do not receive this signal and the muscle stays tight. Alternatively, if damage were to stop the muscle from informing the brain about a contraction, then the brain would be unaware. Communication between the brain and the muscle can be affected in either direction.

If we plan to move in a certain way, we need some muscles to tighten while others relax to create a smooth, balanced action. When a muscle does not receive a GABA-driven message to relax, it remains tight because the only message the muscle is receiving is one that is signaling it to contract.

Consequently, when we are trying to tighten another muscle that needs to contract, we cannot instruct the opposing muscles to relax. We become stiff, and this often becomes painful.

That is what damage to the myelin coating does to the way we move.

It is a significant problem and needs to be treated as a specific issue.

The neurons that drive movement in our body are called motor neurons. When their cell body is inside the brain or spinal cord, they are called upper motor neurons. These ultimately connect to neurons that are outside this privileged area. This second group is known as the lower motor neurons. These make up the nerves that take the messages to our muscles.

Lower motor neurons have connections to muscles that allow them to activate by reflex without asking the brain for permission. To make the reflex response appropriate, the muscles will then send messages to the brain through sensory connections. Our brain responds by telling the muscle to stop contracting.

If a sensory neuron is damaged, the brain does not receive a signal about the muscle contraction. When the upper motor neuron is damaged, the signal to relax does not arrive, so the muscle stays tight. That is what happens with MS.

If the damaged motor neuron were outside the central nervous system, it wouldn't tighten the muscle. That would lead to a floppy muscle and some wasting from disuse. MS is an upper motor neuron disease. Lower motor neuron problems present as flaccid muscle responses.

~

No one ever gave me the dignity of making sure I understood this principle. I have had to read multitudes of research papers and watch countless videos and lectures in order to understand this. But it is so fundamental. Knowing about GABA and reflex tightening helps me to make sense of my own body and treat the tightness correctly.

The reality of life with MS is that you are told very little, often nothing at all, and are left in an information limbo.

~

Some researchers say muscle stiffness and cramp occurs in up to 90% of MS patients.[1] I'm not sure how they get their numbers, but spasticity does affect me.

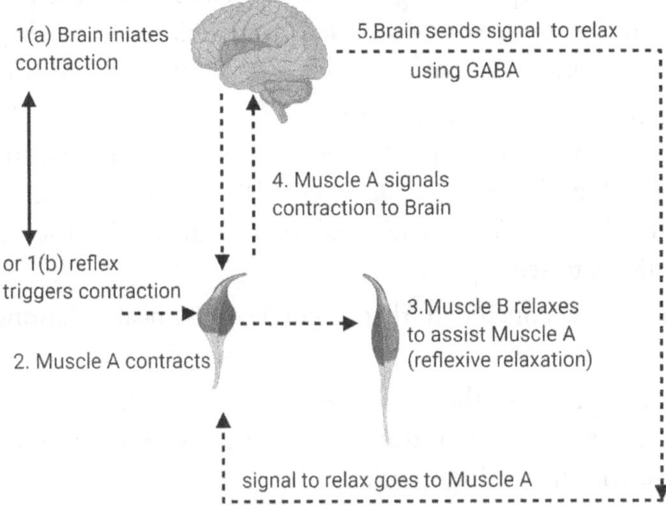

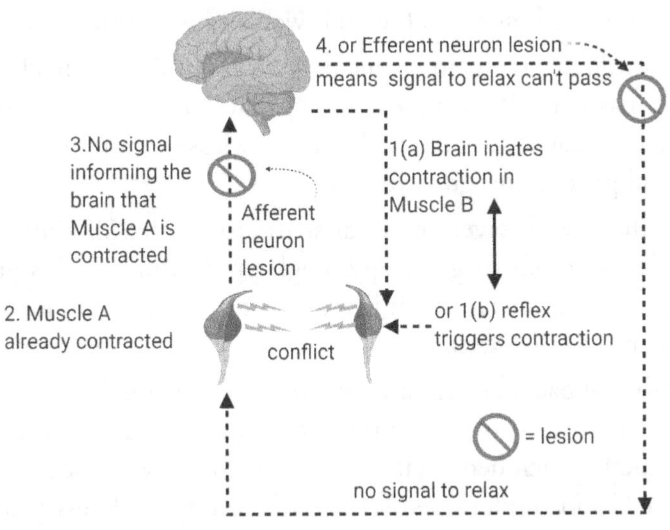

Figure 7.1 When the brain is unaware that a muscle is contracted or is unable to send a message to that muscle to relax, the result is that two or more muscles cannot signal each other to reflexively relax to create smooth, controlled movement. We become stiff. Efferent neurons can also send activating signals (not shown here).

Created with BioRender.

A study in 2004[2] looked at data on spasticity and how it was treated. The results are kept in a registry called NARCOMS (the North American Research Committee on MS). There were 20,380 patients whose data they could draw on. Those patients update their information twice a year.

Despite this big number of interested patients, the study invited only 330 of them, who already had an implanted anti-spasticity drug called intrathecal baclofen, plus another 660 randomly selected patients to respond. All up, 665 patients took part in the study. The survey required the patients to self-report.

The study concluded that there was a linear relationship between spasticity scores and the length of time since diagnosis.

More than half the replies that indicated there were no spasticity problems at all were remitting-relapsing cases. Worsening MS went hand in hand with increasing spasticity.

The respondents to the survey showed that people with higher levels of spasticity were more likely to be male, disabled, and unemployed. Generally, they had been diagnosed with MS for longer than the average and experienced more relapses and worsening symptoms.

According to the study, females were about 80% as likely to experience severe spasticity. Remitting-relapsing patients were 70% as likely to be affected by spasticity compared to those whose condition was worsening or who had primary progressive MS.

Of those with severe or total spasticity related disabilities, 47% were on a disease-modifying therapy. High proportions of this group were on specific medications for their loss of motor function (because they were the dominant group asked).

Both oral baclofen and implanted devices that deliver that drug directly to the spine were more than twice as frequently used as other treatments. The study concluded that this medication was "often sub-optimally managed" and "underdosed for fear of ensuing weakness and fatigue."

Rather than using baclofen, my preference is to use dantrolene sodium. This drug didn't even make it into the study tables. I feel as though it is mentioned in some reports for completeness, but very few doctors use it.

Another study, published in 2005[3] used an 88 item Multiple Sclerosis Spasticity Scale (MSSS-88) to measure the condition of the participants. This confusing study was wholly based on self-reported data. The study sent several surveys by post, and the results were returned the same way. The report described the process of self-reporting as a "reliable and valid, patient-based, interval-level measure of the impact of spasticity in MS."

In the first survey, the respondents didn't reply as the researchers had expected. The answers didn't fit neatly into the boxes provided. The researchers concluded that the MS patients couldn't reliably distinguish between words like "little" or "moderately" and "quite a bit".

In their second survey, 32% of MS patients who used wheelchairs described their spasticity as "moderate". Maybe self-assessment is unreliable.

Even the authors of the study concluded their survey had limitations.

How can anyone know what proportion of the MS population has problems with spasticity? I know that I have some. If you have spasticity issues, you need focused strategies to deal with it. Even if spasticity doesn't trouble you now, you should plan for it to arise. It is easier to prepare for it than wait until it happens.

References

1.   Portaro, S., O. Musumeci, V. Rizzo, C. Rodolico, M.G. Sweeney, M. Buccafusca, M.G. Hanna and A. Toscano. *Stiffness as a presenting symptom of an odd clinical condition caused by multiple sclerosis and myotonia congenita.* Neuromuscular Disorders, 2013. **23**(1): p. 52–55.

2.   Rizzo, M.A., O.C. Hadjimichael, J. Preiningerova and T.L. Vollmer. *Prevalence and treatment of spasticity reported by multiple sclerosis patients.* multiple sclerosis, 2004. **10**(5): p. 589–595.

3.   Hobart, J.C., A. Riazi, A.J. Thompson and I. Styles. *Getting the measure of spasticity in multiple sclerosis: The Multiple Sclerosis Spasticity Scale (MSSS-88).* Brain, 2006. **129**(1): p. 224–234.

Chapter 8

Dealing with Medical People

In 1997, a wonderful Australian film called "The Castle"[1] was released. It is a very gentle but humorous story built on the premise that a man's home is his castle.

In this film, a very simple family, called the Kerrigans, headed by the ever-optimistic Darryl, a tow truck driver, suddenly find that a building inspector has condemned their family home and the land is to be acquired for an extension of the adjacent airport. Darryl decides to fight this injustice and recruits the best legal mind he knows.

Unfortunately, Darryl is coming from a very uninformed background. He only knows a bumbling lawyer who is stretched to his limit by petty criminals, property conveyancing, and his unfathomable photocopier.

Despite all his limitations, the lawyer, Dennis Denuto, finds himself standing before the bench of one of Australia's highest courts, trying to argue that the acquisition of the Kerrigan family home breaches the principles of the Australian constitution.

He has a very vague idea about a landmark native title case known as the Mabo decision.[2] Apart from that inkling of information, he finds himself clueless and being judged on the quality of his argument by the best of the judiciary.

As the pressure mounts, he utters these words that have become part of the lexicon of Australia's comedic folklore:

"In summing up, it's the constitution. It's Mabo. It's justice. It's law. It's the vibe, and … aah, no, that's it. It's the vibe. I rest my case."

Dennis is way out of his depth. He is caught out by the knowledge that the bench he is addressing understand that he doesn't know what he's talking about.

People with MS haven't built a lifetime of in-depth medical knowledge about the illness to be able to judge the advice they receive from medical professionals. Most doctors call MS an autoimmune disease, some don't but defer to the term if pressured.

~

When I was in the hospital, I shared my room with a man who had received lower back surgery. At each change of nursing staff, there was a handover procedure. The old shift would run through, in detail, the recent history of the patients. Often, I could hear a detailed description of the medication and the history of my roommate.

However, when my medical history was described, there was far less detail. They may as well have said, "He's an MS patient, he's one of those." The response was always the same, "Oh yeah, hmmm."

~

When I had left the hospital and, later, had moved on from the spasticity clinic, I reached the point where I needed more of the medication the clinic had given me. This was called Dantrium (dantrolene sodium).

I gave the old container to a doctor who had never heard of it. He freely admitted he knew nothing about MS.

Although I asked for a medication he was clueless about, he had no problem prescribing it for me. The label told him who had given it to me previously. He rang a designated phone number, obtained the government authority, and wrote out the prescription. As he handed it to me, he said, "You should be on some vitamin D."

"Why?" I asked.

"They say people with MS have low vitamin D." He said with great certainty.

"Thanks, but I'll be right," I replied.

He did not know me, had never heard of the medication he had just authorized, and told me he knew nothing about MS. It did not stop him confidently advising me I needed vitamin D.

One of the problems I suffered after my 2014 attack was elevated blood pressure. My cardiologist tried several different medications to bring it down, but none were sustainably effective. My blood pressure would sometimes be almost normal, and then out of nowhere it would skyrocket. At the time, I gave little thought to the impact an outstanding legal fight over my insurance was having. Since that has been resolved, my blood pressure has been much better.

When I saw my cardiologist, I warned him I was on dantrolene sodium. He didn't know of it.

He was an associate professor, highly regarded and well known by the medical community. The dantrolene manufacturer's advice contained precise warnings not to use calcium channel blockers with dantrolene sodium, but I still had to tell him that. As well, a common ACE inhibitor had an unambiguous warning from the governing advisory authority that it was not to be used with dantrolene. He was never going to check.

I do like him and have no issue with him.

At one meeting, in his rooms, he said to me, "I know nothing about MS."

A fortnight later, I saw my neurologist and mentioned the blood pressure problem.

He said, "I know nothing about cardiology."

On both occasions, I thought to myself, "Well, you should."

~

This is what I know about the general immune system response:

The immune system is made up of a complex set of interactions. At our most basic level, we are protected by the barriers of our skin, the acidity of our digestive system, the mucous that clears our body's pathways, and the chemistry of our secretions.

The function of the immune system is to deal with pathogens or injury. It may be dealing with viral or bacterial invaders. It may have to respond to physical shock.

Some significant parts of the immune system are the thymus, the spleen, the lymph nodes, and bone marrow. These elements are connected by different means and are usually called the organs of the lymphatic system.

There are types of bacteria that have a symbiotic role, such as gut bacteria, and contribute to our good health.

The immune system can recognize the difference between what is "self" and "non-self." It will ignore elements of what we are, rather than attack them. If it detects a "non-self" pathogen, it will initiate an attack. If it does not recognize a "self" element and attacks it, the reaction is called an autoimmune response.

At its highest level, the immune system is classified by the speed of the response. The quickest responder is the innate immune system. It is our most basic first level of defense. This system contains defenses such as macrophages that can engulf and consume invaders, mast cells that release molecules that regulate the function of tissues and organs, complement proteins which can destroy invaders, and we have chemical mediators. These elements are part of a chain that will lead a dendritic cell to communicate with T cells, triggering the slower adaptive immune system.

The second level of defense, the adaptive immune system, is activated when a T cell signals a B cell, which can then secrete antibodies. The antibodies bind to a pathogen so it can be identified by white blood cells and eliminated. The T cell can also activate other T cells. Both T and B cells rapidly expand in number once they are activated.

There are many types of T cells. Some of the activated T cells can differentiate into T killer cells or T helper cells (that help other immune cells).

The adaptive immune system can be divided into further divisions:
1) The humoral response, which is driven by B cells
2) The cell-mediated response, which is driven by T cells.

These two responses have to work together and often recruit the innate immune system. Everything should work together to eliminate infection and create a memory to respond more quickly to a second infection.

Nearly all major MS drugs target T or B cell activity. The interest is in the adaptive immune system. The innate system mainly gets academic attention.

My neurologist once said to me, "You should be on something."

I had tried interferon-β-1a for ten years. Briefly, at his behest, I tried dimethyl fumarate, but it didn't agree with me.

He mentioned a few different drug names, and each time I came up with a reason not to take it.

Progressive multifocal leukoencephalopathy (known as PML) is one of the reasons I gave for not taking the drugs he offered. PML is a demyelinating disease that is derived from a widespread infection called John Cunningham virus (JCV). Many people have a JCV infection and never realize it.

No one knows how JCV reaches the brain. It is assumed that T cells control JCV and limit its activity. When the virus replicates inside oligodendrocytes, they cannot produce myelin. Replicating JCV becomes aggressive. It is then called PML.

PML affects individuals who lack JCV-specific T cells in the brain. The basis of many MS drugs is to deplete the activity of those types of immune cells. MS itself is not a risk factor for PML, but the use of some MS drugs has been noted as a risk.[3]

If PML is recognized and treated, you might survive with significant neurologic deficits. Untreated, it is fatal.[4]

When you are offered an MS drug, you are not being offered a lolly. It will be a potent medication. You should always ask about PML and ask to be tested for JCV before you start taking anything that targets T and B cells.

~

A lot of medical advice is offered on the basis that you are like the uninformed Darryl Kerrigan. You simply do not know the risks and, consequently, you trust the advice of someone who is supposed to be qualified.

No matter how skilled they are, how warm the manner of presentation, or how professional they seem, they may not have all the answers. MS remains a disease of unknown origin and the topic of considerable speculation.

Sometimes if you dig in and ask why a particular treatment is preferable, you can hear a whisper in the answer, "It's the vibe."

References

1.   Cilauro, S., J. Kennedy, J. Kennedy, T. Gleisner, R. Sitch, M. Marusic, ... E. Choi, (Writers), R. Sitch, (Director) and M. Hirsh, D. Choate, C. Kennedy, B. McRieson and K. Stuckey, (Producers). 1997. *The Castle*.

2.   *Mabo v Queensland (No 2) ("Mabo case") [1992] HCA 23 1992 175 CLR 1*, in *High Court of Australia*. 1992. High Court of Australia.

3.   Alstadhaug, K.B., K.M. Myhr and C.H. Rinaldo, *Progressive multifocal leukoencephalopathy*. Tidsskr Nor Laegeforen, 2017. **137**(23–24).

4.   Clifford, D.B., *Progressive multifocal leukoencephalopathy therapy*. Journal of Neurovirology, 2015. **21**(6): p. 632–636.

Chapter 9

Environment or Inheritance

The endless question that MS throws up is, "How did I get this?"

Was it genetic? Did I inherit it? Will I give it to my children? Am I infectious? Did I do something wrong? Did I eat the wrong thing? Have I exposed myself to something? Who gave it to me? Have I maltreated myself? Or am I just stressed?

These are all questions that follow the first question, "Why me?"

The standard answer is, "We don't know."

Science has three avenues to explore:

Did you:

1)   inherit it.

2)   acquire it.

3)   or was it a mix of the two?

I was born in 1957, so I am a middle to late entry into the baby boom. In that post-war world, everything pre-war was old. Transport, foodstuffs, social values, communication, materials, agriculture, shopping, and medication were all changing. Populations were uprooted and settling in new places. No one from pre-war 1939 would have foreseen how altered the world would become.

An Illustration - My Family History

My father was born in 1913. He was the only child of five to reach adulthood. All his siblings died of common childhood diseases. In 1940, as the war became more obviously a significant event, he joined the army. Almost immediately, he was given leave because he contracted mumps. After 86 days of training, he was shipped out to Malaya. On the 15th of February 1942, he was ordered, along with thousands of others, to surrender to the Japanese at the fall of Singapore.

Three days later, at 28 years of age, he was exposed to his first taste of life as a POW. His Japanese conquerors began executions on Changi beach. He was imprisoned, with many others, at Changi, then was forced to help construct the infamous Burma-Thailand death railway. As an officer, he would, many times, have a Samurai sword presented to his neck and be told, "Your men no work, you get choppy choppy." He was beaten, starved, and saw brutality and death dished out daily.

After 1,545 days overseas, he was discharged as medically fit. He had been fattened up, so he then weighed six and a half stone, about half my weight now. His discharge record notes ulcer scars on both legs. There is no mention of malnutrition or disease. Nor is there any hint of the heaviness and disillusionment he must have felt with life. Like other soldiers, he took all that silently to his grave.

At 45, he had his first heart attack. Seven years later, he lay dying at my feet.

~

My mother raised my brother and me by herself. She carried a heavy bitterness about how life had turned out, and, as a child, I was well aware of it. Her father had been in the trenches of France in World War One. He was 47 years old when she was born. His view of the world was forged in an earlier century and tempered by the savagery of the fields of France. He had been gassed and hospitalized. As a child, my mother became ill with rheumatic fever. The memory of that never left her. It was almost always the first part of her life that she would recall.

In the early war years, she became a nurse, mainly as a way to leave a family that belonged to a different age. Her work years were very stressful. She was matron-in-charge of a tuberculosis chalet in her 20s. The exposure to those patients ultimately led to her own TB infection. She spent three years in hospital as each lung was independently deflated, and a cure was provided. Every scan of her chest always showed the dark shadows of that infection.

She was a great believer in the power of antibiotics and took what would now be regarded as too many, too often.

The best of times for my parents must have been short. Before I was a year old, my father had his first heart attack, and until his death, a bitter shroud of fate enveloped our family.

For me, life was always stressful. My parent's history, though not spoken about often, hung like a pall over everything. My father's early death was very isolating; my mother's grief and anger was my daily trial. I suppose there was love, but it was not warm.

There was always respect and a black humor. When she was 89, my mother had a stroke. The following day, I leaned over her hospital bed and said, "Is there anything you want?"

She looked up at me and, with a slurred voice, said, "A scotch and soda and a cigarette."

"I don't think that's going to happen," I replied.

She resigned herself to the situation. "Hmm, a brandy and dry then," was her last reply.

~

I was the product of two people who endured many illnesses, infections and stress. Both of them had stared their own possible death in the face day after day. For long periods they had dealt with never-ending horrible deaths all around them. Both of them absorbed that and just moved on.

Life leaves scars. We can't see all of them, but they change the people who wear them. If our parents are changed, do we carry the consequences?

~

We inherit characteristics from our parents. Their DNA fuses to become the blueprint for our own. Sections of our DNA are transcribed to messenger RNA in the nucleus of the cell and are then transported to our ribosomes to make proteins.

Imagine you were born as one of two identical twins that were separated at birth. Would the two of you remain identical as your lives diverged? Before birth, the genetic code, like a string of letters, was identical in both of you.

Although the letters remain the same, do the spaces between the letters change? Do the commas, full stops, the paragraphs and sentence structure of the same string of letters alter as the experience of life writes a different story for your genetic twin compared to you? Do the punctuation marks of events make you into different people?

Every cell in your body contains the same genetic blueprint. The code is your DNA. As it can be quite long, it is packaged like a ribbon wound around a protein spool called a histone. This winding conserves its length, compacting it into tightly bound packages. When enough packages are bound together, they are called chromosomes.

If all your cells have the same code, how do they know if they should become a liver cell or a heart cell? Compounds made of carbon and hydrogen provide the instructions.

A key compound for instruction is called a methyl group. It binds to a gene and, by doing so, blocks it and stops it from being expressed. The methyl group binds differently in each type of cell. The interplay between proteins and genes is influenced by the methyl group.

The histone protein plays an essential role in this. If the DNA is tightly wound around it, there is no room for the methyl group to bind. The histone can change to have a lower electrostatic charge so that the DNA ribbon can loosen to provide an access point for a methyl group.

The methyl group behaves like a switch, and sometimes like a lock, and the histone behaves like a dial that can be turned.

In computing terms, the DNA is your hardware. It is not the language of your life. That role belongs to your Epigenome, the compounds that instruct your DNA and determine how tightly bound it is to your histones. That is your software.

~

As your hardware, the DNA never changes. But the epigenetic tags that instruct it do change. Not only do they change throughout your life, but they can be inherited.

Sometimes, the changes can be temporary, to accommodate developments like puberty or pregnancy. They reflect what we do. If our diet is poor, the methyl groups bind to the wrong place. Smoking is a disaster. Stress alters the epigenetic tagging.

Most of the epigenetic tags from a parent are stripped from an embryo in the first few days of life. However, researchers can now see that some parental tags stay stuck on the embryo.[1] What happened to my parents can, possibly, affect me. Just as what happened to their parents may have impacted on them. It becomes inescapable that what happened to my grandparents could also affect me.[2]

These aberrant tags are not exclusively passed from mother to offspring. Researchers have found evidence of neurogenetic disorders linking the paternal grandmother to a current disease. The father can carry a maternal imprint to a new generation.[3]

Many "modern" diseases look more and more likely that they were passed on to us from earlier generations. The twentieth century saw more migration and dislocation, more war, more changes in diet, more medical innovation and more changes in lifestyle than any time before it. What happened in the three or so generations that lived through that time was profound.

Is MS a modern disease? The first description of its hallmark features is generally thought to come from a researcher named Charcot in 1868.[4] There are only scattered references before that but no-one doubts that it may have existed for thousands of years.

The First Record of an MS Patient?

The earliest record of a person who had symptoms that modern physicians would regard as consistent with MS concerns St. Lidwina the virgin, of Schiedam (1380–1421).[5]

At the age of 15, she fell on ice whilst skating and may have broken a rib. Following this accident, she remained largely bedridden for the remainder of her life. Intermittently, she seemed to recover and then would relapse. She had a sharp pain in her face attributed to a tooth problem (trigeminal neuralgia?), partial loss of sight, trouble walking, and sensory issues, including heat intolerance. Supposedly, she did not sleep for the last seven years of her life (insomnia?).

Her bones, which were found in 1947 and examined in 1957, revealed changes consistent with paralysis of the legs and right arm.

Her capacity to appear to have recovered to only repeatedly relapse has attracted modern physician's interest as a possible early example of MS.

Although she was one of nine children of a humble laborer, the story of her strange illness became well known throughout Holland.

Her steadfast refusal to entertain marriage and her continued suffering (which probably included non-MS symptoms) was regarded as consistent with piety. The unusual nature of her illness attracted the famous physicians of the time who considered her untreatable. Her supporters believe she was called upon to suffer for the sins of others.

Legend suggests she performed miracles from her bedside and saintly characteristics were attributed to her.

In 1890, she was canonized by Pope Leo XIII and is known as the patron saint of ice skating and the chronically ill.

Perhaps MS is a modern disease. Maybe it isn't. In the early 21st century, millions of people have it.

Our DNA is made up of arrangements of nitrogenous bases. These bases are called adenine (A), thymine (T), guanine (G), and cytosine (C). They are bound together by hydrogen bonds. There is a strict pairing pattern.

A methyl group can bind to the cytosine base. This union blocks an enzyme involved in protein synthesis from attaching to the cytosine. The gene related to the local sequence around that cytosine that has been blocked is termed a "silenced gene". It is turned off and can't create a protein.

The methyl group also makes the ribbon of DNA coil more tightly to the histone, making it harder for enzymes to gain access.

An acetyl group is similar to a methyl group, but it has an extra carbon and oxygen atom. When it binds to the DNA this loosens how tightly the DNA adheres to the histone.

Genes are continually being modified by methylation and acetylation. The processes start and stop and then repeat. Diet, environment and toxins can cause both of these modifiers to bind in the wrong place, influencing the wrong genes. These factors become significant in maternal health, but they can be passed on through a paternal line.[3]

A maternal diet that is "methyl sufficient" would contain adequate zinc, B12, folic acid and betaine.[6] All these nutrients affect the level of DNA methylation in the early embryo. The consequences of inadequate levels can be lifelong. The folates, in particular, along with methionine, affect the synthesis of embryonic proteins and the DNA that drives them.[6]

I have no idea whether my mother was adequately provided with those nutrients. Neither can I tell if she had, in her early life, received sufficient quantities from her mother. All I know is that I was provided with less than six weeks breastfeeding and then stuck on whole cow's milk. The consequence was that I was a sickly infant. Until the cow's milk was removed, I had spindly limbs and a distended belly. My mother always referred to me as a hellish baby who screamed.

~

After we are born, we lose some methyl groups. This step encourages certain receptors to develop. Research suggests that early maternal care is fundamental to this process.[7] If this is diminished, it may lead to conditions like anxiety and depression, and this may explain why these have been an increasing phenomenon.[8]

I doubt my mother did breastfeed me for as long as six weeks. She gave me enough excuses to make me wonder why she kept mentioning it. It must have preyed on her mind. I never raised the subject, but she often did. Soon after my birth, her attention must have turned to her sick husband. They had only recently moved to the town for his work, so there was no network she could call on.

Eighteen months after I was born, my mother prematurely gave birth to my brother. All her life, she talked about how intensively she nursed him in his first year. Confronted with a sick husband and a premature baby, I was not her primary concern.

I wonder what happened to my methyl groups back then.

To date, there is no epigenetic model of MS. Gene variations, sometimes called alleles (or allelomorphs) on the genes HLA-DRB1*1501, -DQB1*0301, -DQB1*0302, -DQB1*0602 and -DQB1*0603 may influence an MS prognosis of patients who present more severe clinical outcomes. The cause of variation is unknown.[9]

References

1. Chong, S. and E. Whitelaw, *Epigenetic germline inheritance.* Current Opinion in Genetics & Development, 2004. **14**(6): p. 692–696.

2. Green, W.H. *Epigenetics.* 2102. Available from: https://www.youtube.com/watch?v=kp1bZEUgqVI. Accessed January 2021

3. Buiting, K., S. Gross, C. Lich, G. Gillessen-Kaesbach, O. el-Maarri and B. Horsthemke. *Epimutations in Prader-Willi and Angelman Syndromes: A molecular study of 136 patients with an imprinting defect.* The American Journal of Human Genetics, 2003. **72**(3): p. 571–577.

4. Kornek, B. and H. Lassmann, *Axonal pathology in multiple sclerosis. A historical note.* Brain Pathology, 1999. **9**(4): p. 651.

5. Murray, T.J. and W. I. McDonald, *Multiple Sclerosis: The History of a Disease.* 2005, Demos Medical Publishing.

6. Wolff, G.L., R.L. Kodell, S.R. Moore and C.A. Cooney. *Maternal epigenetics and methyl supplements affect agouti gene expression in Avy/a mice.* FASEB Journal, 1998. **12**(11): p. 949–957.

7. Zhang, T.-Y., I.C. Hellstrom, R.C. Bagot, X. Wen, J. Diorio and M.J. Meaney. *Maternal care and DNA methylation of a glutamic acid decarboxylase 1 promoter in rat hippocampus.* The Journal of Neuroscience, 2010. **30**(39): p. 13130–13137.

8. Bagot, R.C., T-Y. Zhang, X. Wen, T.T.T. Nguyen, H-B. Nguyen, J. Diorio, T.P. Wong and M.J. Meaney. *Variations in postnatal maternal care and the epigenetic regulation of metabotropic glutamate receptor 1 expression and hippocampal function in the rat.* Proceedings of the National Academy of Science, 2012. **109**(Suppl 2): p. 17200–17207.

9. Zivadinov, R., L. Uxa, A. Bratina, A. Bosco, B. Srinivasaraghavan, A. Minagar, M. Ukmar, S. yen Benedetto and M. Zorzon. *HLA-DRB1*1501, -DQB1*0301, -DQB1*0302, -DQB1*0602, and -DQB1*0603 Alleles are Associated With More Severe Disease Outcome on Mri in Patients With Multiple Sclerosis.* International Review of Neurobiology. 2007. **79**: p. 521–535.

Chapter 10

The Building Blocks of Biology

If you want to know why you are tired or why you lack the energy to do things, you need to understand how life derives its energy.

The Constituents of Life

There are not many elements that constitute living organisms. Nearly everything is composed of arrangements of around 16–18 elements.

Roughly, 99% of all living matter is made up of hydrogen, oxygen, carbon, and nitrogen.

All elements are made up of atoms. At the most basic level, atoms have three subatomic particles. Two are in the nucleus of the atom—a cluster of positively charged protons and uncharged neutrons. The third component, in a halo around the nucleus, is one or more negatively charged electrons.

Some atoms share their electrons with other atoms to form bonds. This alignment of atoms creates molecules.

When molecules are drawn diagrammatically, carbon is so promiscuous as part of almost every bond that it is assumed to be at each joint of the molecule. As it is involved in so many structures, it is not often labeled like the other elements are. Carbon is, nonetheless, the basis of the molecules of life. Its structure is tetravalent, which means one carbon can make four bonds. If it binds with another carbon, they can rotate around each other. This characteristic helps make biomolecules flexible. Carbon can also form double and triple bonds making the structures immensely strong.

The glue that holds the bonds together is the electrons. Breaking these electron bonds releases the energy that drives organic life.

Biomolecules

Carbon forms stable bonds with five other elements: hydrogen, oxygen, nitrogen, phosphorus, and sulfur. The nature of a carbon molecule means that chains, rings, or branched molecules can be created from the arrangement of these elements. This results in a vast number of potential molecular structures. Roughly 15,000 molecules in living organisms can be made from the different arrangements of just these six elements. For simplicity's sake, the atom combinations are classified into 30 functional groups. You have met some of these functional groups already—a methyl group is a functional group, and so is an acetyl group. These groups maintain their properties wherever they occur.

Biomolecules are the building blocks for larger molecules called macromolecules. Some macromolecules, called polymers, are repeating arrangements of functional groups. As each group is added to the polymer during formation, a water molecule is removed. Examples of these polymers are DNA, proteins, sugars (polysaccharides), and nucleic acids. Adding back a water molecule, called hydrolysis, is a process that breaks up the structures during, for example, digestion.

Nucleotides

The nucleotide is the basic unit that forms nucleic acids. It has three parts:

1) a nitrogenous base made up of carbon and nitrogen atoms,

2) a five-sided sugar (ribose), which may have lost an oxygen molecule (deoxyribose), and

3) a phosphate group.

The nitrogenous bases form either one or two rings. If there is one ring, the base is called a pyrimidine. If there are two rings, it is called a purine.

The double-ring structures, when bound to a sugar, are known as adenine (A) or guanine (G). The single-ring structures, also bound to a sugar, are known as uracil (U), cytosine (C), or thymine (T). These are the building blocks of nucleic acids.

When the base and the sugar join, the nitrogenous bases become nucleosides. When the phosphate joins the nucleosides, they become nucleotides. That gives rise to a change in the name of the base (e.g., adenine becomes adenosine).

Up to three phosphates can form a tail on these molecules. Each phosphate is more loosely bound than the preceding phosphate. The nature of this binding becomes a critical part of metabolism and energy production.

Adenine plays a major role in energy production. If one phosphate is added to adenine, it becomes adenosine monophosphate (AMP). Two phosphates make it into adenosine diphosphate. A three-phosphate chain creates an unstable group called adenosine triphosphate (ATP). This instability makes the molecule ideal as a donor of phosphate to drive reactions. Breaking this phosphate bond is the most dynamic reaction in the human body. If ATP fails to be always available, we fail.[1, 2]

Thermodynamics[3]

There are well-understood rules about energy. When discussing energy, and why people with MS seem to lack it, two fundamentals underpin every aspect:

1)   Energy is neither created nor destroyed. It is only converted from one form to another.

2)   There is a conservation of energy (it is somewhere)

Given these two rules are always true in biology, we can now ask questions about the energy use in our bodies.

Does each chemical reaction in our body require or release energy?

If there is a reaction, how fast is it? How far does it extend? How great is the energy of the outcome compared to the energy of the reactants that caused it?[2]

Are reactions spontaneous, or do they need energy to drive them?

~

In a landslide, energy is released as the rocks and boulders tumble down the hillside. To put them back at the top of the hill would require a great deal of energy.

But the landslide wasn't instant. For millennia, the rocks did not fall. The energy in them was always there, but something needed to cause them to start sliding. Something had to be a catalyst. The catalyst did not need to be as "energetic" as the landslide. It may have been a minimal reaction, but it started a profound release of energy as everything tumbled down. Catalysts promote change. The energy release they can trigger can be far more than the catalyst can generate itself.

Is all the energy from the reactants useable? How much is free to be converted? How much is unusable? Does the temperature where the reaction is happening influence the reaction? What happened to the energy in the landslide?

Some proteins are the catalysts for the reactions in our bodies.

Proteins can bind together to form complexes called enzymes that react to drive consistent reactions. The very building blocks of life, the ribbons of nucleic acids called RNA, can also act as enzymes.

Enzymes

In life, enzymes are particular. They bind only to specific reactants. The reactants are called substrates. An enzyme preferentially binds to a substrate. The shape of the enzyme and the molecules that make up the substrate create unique partnerships.

Sometimes enzymes can bind loosely to other partners if the shapes are similar enough, but the union will be short-lived. Not all binding is sufficient to trigger a reaction.

To drive a reaction, the substrate must fit into part of the enzyme (protein) called the active site, like a key in the lock of a door. The key is the enzyme, the lock is the binding site, and the door is the substrate. Nothing happens to the door unless the key is a "good enough" fit in the lock.

If the binding site on a substrate is small, then what is the function of the rest of the protein? In biology, the bulk of the substrate is regulating how the binding site is functioning.

It does this by expressing molecules called inhibitors. They are either reversible or irreversible inhibitors. The two types may be competing with each other. If they compete, they will bind to the active site. If they are non-competitive, they bind to some other part of the protein, which can change the shape of the protein and therefore the shape of the binding site. Sometimes this leads to another activation or an inhibitory action (allosteric regulators).

How enzymes work depends on the environment they exist in. The level of acidity (pH) makes a significant difference. Temperature affects enzymes. The environment can change the structure of the protein, and this changes its function. The introduction of cofactors, coenzymes, and prosthetic groups will all change how the protein works.

Enzymes are not loose cannons. They are not vigilantes roaming the wild, untamed landscape. Their specific nature means they are more like a line of factory workers.

Depending on which line of enzymes interacts with a substrate, a pathway to a particular product develops. Sometimes what is made will shut down another pathway that uses the same substrate, sometimes it will stimulate a pathway.

Everything involved in building or breaking down molecules in a cell requires a spark of energy. That comes from breaking the phosphate bonds of that unique molecule adenosine triphosphate (ATP). Without that catalyst, there is no life.

If MS has robbed you of energy, the greatest service you can do for yourself is to understand how fundamental ATP is. Your whole body is driven by chemical reactions that are the endless series of biological landslides that represent life. ATP is the spark of energy that starts each one.

References

1. Knox, B.A., *Biology: an Australian Focus (Fifth Edition)*. P.Y. Ladiges, B.K. Evans and R. Saint, Editors. 2014. McGraw-Hill Education: North Ryde, N.S.W.

2. Ingwall, J.S., *ATP and the Heart*. 2002. Springer: Boston, MA

3. Haynie, D.T., *Biological Thermodynamics*. 2001. Cambridge University Press: Cambridge, UK.

Chapter 11

Making ATP

The Basics of Energy

Every process going on in our body needs energy.

To consume foodstuffs, to extract the goodness from them, to add what we obtained to our body's stores, all this requires energy. Every movement, each aspect of growth, our whole life needs energy to sustain it.

Where does the energy come from? What is the basic unit of energy?

~

Imagine you are a gambler. You enter a gaming hall intent on playing a poker machine, the infamous one-armed bandit.

In your wallet, you have $100 in notes. The machine only takes tokens. Notes are unrecognizable to the machine. The paper money needs to be exchanged for tokens.

You can only spend tokens in the machine. Sometimes the machine will pay you, but in the long run, it is the ability to keep exchanging notes for tokens that keeps you in the game.

This is like the dilemma our bodies face when we consume food. How do we reduce what we eat to an energy currency our bodies will recognize?

~

In the gaming hall, we take our notes to the cashier. If we have notes of different denominations, then each value will return a specific number of tokens. The cashier has a process for determining what each note can be exchanged for. Still, every note, ultimately, becomes a series of tokens.

Fats, proteins and carbohydrates (including sugars) are the currency denominations we offer our body's cashier. Our need for a common base in energy metabolism means we must convert the inputs into ATP, the body's energy token. But this does not happen immediately.

First, we convert some of the inputs into glucose. As a molecule, this is still too big a denomination for our metabolism to harness. It is made up of six carbons attached to twelve hydrogens and six oxygen atoms.

A glucose molecule needs to split and split again to break its six-carbon sugar structure into two three-carbon sugars. This process, called glycolysis, is independent of oxygen.

There are 11 enzymes involved in the stages of glycolysis. Three steps produce irreversible outcomes. Irreversible reactions create molecules that just can't be added back to create the original molecule. The process happens in the cytosol, which is the intracellular fluid of a cell. A few tokens of energy (ATP molecules) are used to start the process of glycolysis, but a small net surplus of the ATP tokens are made (actually, it makes two ATPs).

Each three-carbon sugar, now called pyruvate, then is stripped of one carbon atom and becomes Acetyl-CoA. In this form, it can be used by ingenious factories within the cell, called the mitochondria. Beyond this step is where the bulk of ATP is released by utilizing two complexes: the Krebs cycle and, ultimately, the electron transport chain (usually to net 34 to 36 ATPs per glucose).

Fatty acids can also release Acetyl-CoA, skipping glycolysis. Burning fatty acids in the presence of oxygen, called β-oxidation, yields the most ATP.

ATP is the universal token you can spend in the casino of life.

There is very little ATP stored in the human body. In a 250 g human heart, for example, there would only be about 0.7 g of ATP at any one time. There is an absolute need to keep replenishing the ATP pool. A human heart beats 10,000 times a day. The amount of stored ATP in a heart is about enough for ten beats. The weight of ATP our heart would use is about 6,000 g a day.[1]

We need to be able to synthesize ATP on-demand rapidly. The supply always needs to meet the demand. The level of ATP should stay constant. Its concentration can't ebb and flow. The usage and manufacture of ATP happens in parallel. There is not a sequence of rises and falls.[1]

All the steps of cellular respiration need to work perfectly. If they don't, you have no energy to draw on. You are fatigued. Endlessly exhausted. Many systems in your body will fail.

Making ATP from Glucose- How we get energy from Carbohydrates
One glucose makes about 38 ATP

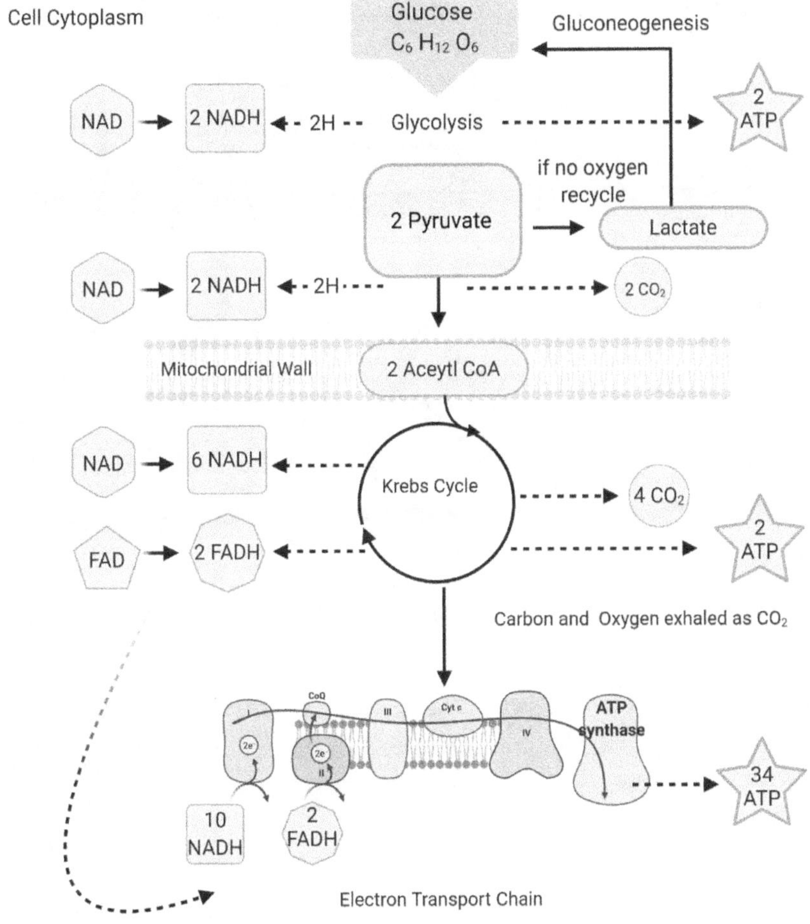

Figure 11.1 Glucose is broken down to form acetyl CoA. In this form it enters the mitochondria where the hydrogen atoms are used make ATP and the carbon and oxygen are exhaled as carbon dioxide.

Created with BioRender.

References

1. Ingwall, J.S., *ATP and the Heart*. 2002. Springer: Boston, MA.

Chapter 12

Fatigue

How do you describe fatigue with MS?

It is not the tiredness you feel at the end of the day. Nor is it the slump as energy is spent, either during or after strenuous exercise.

It is darker, heavier, all-consuming, and endless. Sleep is not a respite from it. You feel clothed in its dense, heavy folds, smothered by it. You carry it but can never put it down. So often you wish you could reach out and give it to someone and say, "Here, feel this so you can understand."

MS fatigue robs your memory. There are names you cannot put to faces, no matter how long you have known them. Sentences you read, but, by the last word, you cannot remember what came before. Places you find yourself standing, and you have no idea why you are there. Sometimes you stop speaking mid-sentence, and, as a listener stares, you realize you don't recall what you said.

There is no fabled light at the end of a tunnel that you are striving to reach. You are facing a wave that pushes against you, but it comes from all directions. It has no end. Your limbs, though lifeless, are a burden that somehow you can move. You are isolated by your vagueness, yet, when someone speaks, you answer their question with a smile.

Others see you as they are, but they are light, almost dancing in front of you. A deadweight has sucked all the joy of being from your deepest recesses. You are a husk.

No matter where you are, your world is a deep pool, and you are far from the edge. Sometimes you reach out, but there is only a tide of steady resistance against your body, and emptiness inside you.

Over and over, you are attacked by drowsiness. Your consciousness starts leaking from you, so you choose to lie down. You don't just have a little nap. Your body collapses in on itself, and you succumb to the sensation, entering a deep, dark place. Sometimes you crave this, welcoming the descent into nothingness.

Maybe a short time later, you awake. For a moment, you feel energized. Then the weight of the wave returns.

Like a faintly glowing globe, you crave energy. But there is none.

In the midst of all this, your legs start to throb, or your eyes lose their focus.

As you move, your hand reaches for a reference point: a wall, a door, a rail. You search for something real to tell you where you are in space. Your foot starts to drag, trying to grip the earth and upend you.

It is not a life you can share. Others are intolerant if you describe it, so you are condemned to a silent, solitary, half-world.

You are trapped between conversations, not belonging to one or to another. Too slow to process, too dull to respond, too tired to care. You learn to be polite and smile.

All this repeats, and repeats, and repeats.

~

I did not know real fatigue until after I had started interferon-β-1a. The tiredness I felt before my diagnosis was fatigue, but it felt more or less conventional. Interferon-β-1a brought with it an added dimension that is sometimes likened to a migraine.[1–5]

Real fatigue became my constant companion. Sometimes it embarrassed me. More often though, it threatened my livelihood. There is no empathy in the workplace for weakness. Your disability threatens everyone you interact with. You become a dangerous link in the chain. There is no sympathy or tolerance for you. It becomes a life of "shape up or ship out."

In my family, it was the same. Although not intentional, there was no tolerance.

Everyone sees the world through their own eyes, and you spoil that view. Silence, good humor, and diligence are your true friends.

An MS diagnosis can be an employment shield. If you can honorably do your job, then removing you opens an employer to the full force of anti-discrimination legislation.

Nonetheless, no matter how energetic you feel at any time, your fatigue sits like a guillotine blade above you.

Although honesty and openness about MS help you deal with all relationships, there is a dark side in most people. You cannot show them the blade is there.

~

The year after I left the hospital was probably the most mentally fatiguing time of my life. It was up to me to make all my own decisions. There was no one to double-check and correct my mistakes.

A long time later, a friend of mine reminded me that during that year I had told him that the gas bill was too difficult to work out. I knew what it was, and I had the money to pay it, but I couldn't understand how to do it.

Paperwork started to pile up next to my laptop. I'd open an envelope and stare at the contents. Usually, I decided that today wasn't the day to try to do something with any bill or letter. Maybe tomorrow would be better. For months, I just opened envelopes and piled the paperwork on top of earlier letters. Nothing stayed in my mind long enough for me to understand what was written on any paperwork.

I could organize myself to travel to and from my Pilates classes. If I needed to pay a bill there, I just flashed a card. When the card statements came in, I added them to the growing pile. I could read a word, but its meaning was almost immediately gone from my mind.

Melbourne has a vast railway network. Sometimes I would catch a train on the Glen Waverley line to the city. On the return trip, I would travel on the Lilydale line and get off at a station that was miles from where I lived. After searching the car park for my car, I would realize I was in the wrong place. Then the issue was remembering how to get back to where I had started.

None of this was dementia. It was all fatigue.

Neurologists' Approach to Fatigue

Neurologists and those treating MS rarely think about how energy is created. Perhaps they are not trained to look at it. It could be that the topic was such a small part of their education that it has slipped between the cracks.

Their focus has two main categories:

1) Lassitude—the overwhelming tiredness that has no cause, and

2) Nerve fiber fatigue, sometimes called Uthoff's sign. This is often associated with heat stress or exertion.

While these two are logical, convenient, and reasonable categories, they don't sit well with me. They help the decision-making process for a neurologist, but, as a patient, I don't find my real-world experience fits easily into these descriptions. They make me feel like I've been told a street shoe is perfect for a marathon.

~

Neurologists can't look at an MRI and predict if lassitude will arise. This exhaustion doesn't correlate with disease or disability. Your deficits that can be measured might be minimal, but fatigue can hang on to you. You exist wearing a coat of heavy wet cement. Your body just doesn't respond to your mind's desire. Some researchers speculate that the activity of cytokines (the cells messengers) dictates this.

In 1889, Wilhelm Uthoff, a German ophthalmologist, described a relationship between exercise and a temporary loss of vision.[6] Now this relationship is associated with neurological deficits brought on by changes in body heat. The observation has been adapted to justify how an MS gait worsens the further the distance traveled.

The accepted explanation of Uthoff's sign is that the loss of myelin affects the transmission of electrical impulses along nerve cells during a process called saltatory conduction. The nerve impulses are supposed to jump rapidly from node to node assisted by the existence of myelin (see Chapter 6 for more detail). Damage to myelin upsets this and results in those nodes seeming to be too far apart. Heat exaggerates the worsening of the signal. The movement of impulses changes and the message is likely to be lost. If the body temperature returns to normal, the function is restored. Heat does not damage the pathway; it just worsens the signal.

Neurologists' treatment of Fatigue

1) Exercise

In a complete about-face from earlier decades, neurologists now approve of and recommend exercise. However, what they mean by exercise has no standard definition.

How does an unfit, greying, haggard neurologist convince a low energy MS patient that exercise is beneficial? Do they say, "Don't do as I do, just do what I say"?

How can a super fit neurologist who thrives on the endorphin rush convince someone who will never get that surge that exercise will help?

Neither type of doctor is likely to say, "Join my class, and we will do this together."

There is no meeting of the minds. No agreement exists on what "exercise" means.

"What's the point?" becomes the common refrain.

2) Medication

Lassitude is sometimes treated with an old Influenza-A drug called amantadine. Anecdotal evidence suggested that it helped fatigue in MS. There was no certainty that it was effective in Influenza-A, so it is no longer prescribed for that. Sometimes it is used for parkinsonism to reduce the side effects of other treatments. [7] The evidence that it helps with fatigue is unconvincing.[8] It may be no better than aspirin. [9]

The relationship between fatigue and sleepiness is still unclear to researchers. Narcolepsy drugs, modafinil and armodafinil, seem to promote wakefulness. According to one report,[10] the optimal dosage is uncertain. This research speculated that an "inverse U" effect might mean higher doses of these drugs are less meaningful than low doses.

For nerve conduction fatigue, the drug 4-aminopyridine can be prescribed. This is a potassium channel blocker. It binds to the exposed nerve where myelin has been stripped away to patch the damage and help the signal to continue. The drug, Ampyra, is an extended-release version of 4-aminopyridine. This is a serious drug. Your creatine clearance rate should be determined before you start taking it. Pre-existing renal impairment needs to be considered. There are numerous side effects, so you should be aware of the prescribing notes. Seizures and anaphylaxis are known outcomes. Dosing needs to be correct. Amprya's stated objective is only to improve walking, where possible. The word "fatigue" does not appear on the highlights for prescription information.[11]

3) Depression

After I had left the hospital, commenced rehab, and started to look around at my new life, my neurologist wanted to see me. I had already come off dimethyl fumarate as it didn't agree with me, so in his mind, I was not on any MS treatment.

I stepped into his office, and we shook hands. He indicated we should sit.

Looking across his desk at me, he wasted no time.

"You seem depressed," he said, looking concerned.

I looked back at him and tilted my head slightly to the side.

"Nup," I said with a grin, "Don't think so. Just a bit tight."

His shoulders sagged, and he noticeably aged before me. The Grand Master had played his most certain opening move in what should be a masterful game of chess. The philistine before him refused to play. His next move was no longer certain.

"You should be on something," he suggested.

"Why?" I replied. "How about we do nothing and see what happens? I'm not stupid. I'll come to you if I realize I need to."

I was aware that depression is a natural reaction to a significant shock to your system, but I wasn't going to be led into following a well-worn path.

"What about pain?" he asked.

I replied with what could be my philosophy. "I would rather have pain and know who I am, than have pain and not care about it. How can I recover if I don't care?"

It was his turn to tilt his head. A gentle smile creased his face. At least, on this point, we agreed.

Depression is common in MS. To a casual observer, it may be difficult to separate the tiredness called lassitude from depression. A lack of desire to participate is very different from being too fatigued to be involved. Anhedonia is a state of mind where the desire to enjoy life is absent. It is not the same as the sadness that comes from the constraints of illness.

Neurologists are looking for the signs of withdrawal that indicate the desire to engage has gone. Depression isn't the same as being too tired to engage.

If you are the patient, almost nothing is more frustrating than being told what you feel or what you think. It will be your mind, not your brain, that dictates how a neurologist sees you. You need to know your own mind, not just accept every suggestion.

Sometimes, your own thoughts are all you have left. Often people gouge and scrape your soul to build a monument out of what they believe matters to you. Invariably you reject this distortion. How you express this is not a sign of depression. It is a rejection of their insult.

Neurologists don't want to medicate normal human emotions. Don't give them an excuse.

There are many antidepressants. I do not use them. They will not cure any form of fatigue.

4) Sleep disorders in MS

Being tired and being sleepy are different things.

"How are you sleeping?" is a reasonable question for a neurologist to ask. Obstructive sleep apnoea, insomnia, and restless leg syndrome are problems in the general population. Some studies suggest these conditions are even more prevalent in the MS population.[12] A study in 2012 showed MS patients with brainstem involvement had a noticeable disposition toward sleep apnoea compared to the controls or MS patients without brainstem damage.[13]

To quote Braley and Boudreau:

"Untreated Obstructive Sleep Apnoea results in a number of cardiovascular physiological changes including decrease in cardiac stroke volume and preload, increased generation of free oxygen radicals, increased

sympathetic tone, and endothelial injury (ischemic/reperfusion). There is mounting evidence that these changes eventually result in increased risk of hypertension, coronary artery disease, stroke, and overall mortality."[12]

You don't have to be a person with MS for these symptoms to develop, but there is a correlation between some types of MS damage and obstructive sleep apnoea.

Management of the symptoms of disturbed sleep may influence fatigue. If disturbed sleep is caused by a breathing difficulty, then machines that provide continuous positive airway pressure (CPAP)[14] may help. If apnoea is not the cause of sleep disorders, then treatment is usually drug-based.

Sleep in MS can also be disturbed by cramps, which are more frequent at night, or by urinary symptoms.

Many drugs are used as sleep aids. (Amitriptyline,[15] Topiramate,[16] Gabapentin,[17] Baclofen,[18] Tizanidine,[19] Clonazepam,[20] Hydrocodone,[21] Tolterodine,[22] etc.). In many cases, the effect on sleep is a secondary consideration when prescribing. Often the drug itself contributes to fatigue.

These drugs aren't rebuilding energy; they are modulating how you use the energy you can draw on.

Lack of sleep is not a good definition of fatigue.

If you demand more ATP than your body can supply, fatigue will always arise. Sleep aids have nothing to do with this.

References

1. Kenner, M., U. Menon and D. Elliott, *Multiple sclerosis as a painful disease.* International Journal of Radiation Oncology, Biology, & Physics, 2007. **79**(5): p. 303–321.

2. Fadil, H., R.E. Kelley and E. Gonzalez Toledo, *Differential diagnosis of multiple sclerosis.* International Review of Neurobiology, 2007. **79**: p. 393–422

3. Elliott, D.G., *Migraine in multiple sclerosis.* International Review of Neurobiology, 2007. **79**: p. 281–302.

4. Villani, V., L. Prosperini, L. De Giglio, C. Pozzilli, M. Salvetti and G. Sette. *The impact of interferon beta and natalizumab on comorbid migraine in multiple sclerosis.* Headache: The Journal of Head and Face Pain, 2012. **52**(7): p. 1130–1135.

5. Putzki, N., A. Pfriem, V. Limmroth, O. Yaldizli, B. Tettenborn, H.C. Diener and Z. Katsarava. *Prevalence of migraine, tension type headache and trigeminal neuralgia in multiple sclerosis.* European Journal of Neurology, 2009. **16**(2): p. 262–267.

6. Davis, S.L., T.C. Frohman, C.G. Crandall, M.J. Brown, D.A. Mills, P.D. Kramer, O. Stüve and E.M. Frohman. *Modeling Uhthoff's phenomenon in MS patients with internuclear ophthalmoparesis.* Neurology, 2008. **70**(13 Part 2): p. 1098.

7. Stuart, M.C., M. Kouimtzi and S.R. Hill, Editors. 2009.*WHO Model Formulary 2008.* World Health Organization: Geneva.

8. Santarnecchi, E., S. Rossi, S. Bartalini, M. Cincotta, F. Giovannelli, E. Tatti and M. Ulivelli. *Neurophysiological correlates of central fatigue in healthy subjects and multiple sclerosis patients before and after treatment with amantadine.* Neural Plasticity. **2015**: p. 616242.

9. Shaygannejad, V., M. Janghorbani, F. Ashtari and H. Zakeri. *Comparison of the effect of aspirin and amantadine for the treatment of fatigue in multiple sclerosis: a randomized, blinded, crossover study.* Neurological Research, 2012. **34**(9): p. 854–858.

10. Rammohan, K.W., J.H. Rosenberg, D.J. Lynn, A.M. Blumenfeld, C.P. Pollak and H.N. Nagaraja. *Efficacy and safety of modafinil (Provigil[R])*

for the treatment of fatigue in multiple sclerosis: A two centre phase 2 study. (Paper). Journal of Neurology, Neurosurgery and Psychiatry, 2002. **72**: p. 179.

11. *Treating MS/Medications/Ampyra Prescribing Information.* Available from: https://ampyra.com/prescribing-information.pdf. Accessed November 2020.

12. Braley, T. and E. Boudreau, *Sleep disorders in multiple sclerosis.* Current Neurology and Neuroscience Reports, 2016. **16**(5): p. 1–8.

13. Braley, T.J., B.M. Segal and R.D. Chervin, *Sleep-disordered breathing in multiple sclerosis.* Neurology, 2012. **79**(9): p. 929.

14. *Continuous Positive Airway Pressure.* Available from: https://www.sleephealthfoundation.org.au/cpap.html. Accessed November 2020.

15. Holmberg, G., *Sedative effects of maprotiline and amitriptyline.* Acta Psychiatrica Scandinavica, 1988. **77**(5): p. 584–586.

16. Bonanni, E., R. Galli, M. Maestri, C. Pizzanelli, M. Fabbrini, M.L. Manca, A. Iudice and L. Murri. *Daytime sleepiness in epilepsy patients receiving topiramate monotherapy.* Epilepsia, 2004. **45**(4): p. 333–337.

17. Foldvary-Schaefer, N., I.D.L. Sanchez, M. Karafa, E. Mascha, D. Dinner, and H.H. Morris. *Gabapentin increases slow-wave sleep in normal adults.* Epilepsia, 2002. **43**(12): p. 1493–1497.

18. Cui, R., B. Li, K. Suemaru and H. Araki. *The effect of baclofen on alterations in the sleep patterns induced by different stressors in rats.* Journal of Pharmacological Sciences, 2009. **109**(4): p. 518–524.

19. Vakhapova, V., E. Auriel and A. Karni, *Nightly sublingual Tizanidine HCl in multiple sclerosis: Clinical efficacy and safety.* Clinical Neuropharmacology, 2010. **33**(3): p. 151–154.

20. *Managing patients with restless legs.* Drug and Therapeutics Bulletin, 2003. **41**(11): p. 81.

21. Silber, M.H., P.M. Becker, M.J. Buchfuhrer, A.S. Walters and J.W. Winkelman. *The appropriate use of opioids in the treatment of refractory restless legs syndrome.* Mayo Clinic Proceedings, 2018. **93**(1): p. 59–67.

22. Pleil, A.M., P.R. Reese, C.J. Kelleher and G.J. Okano. *Health-related quality of life of patients with overactive bladder receiving immediate-release tolterodine.* Health Economics in Prevention and Care, 2001. **2**(2): p. 69–75.

Chapter 13

My Path from Fatigue to High Energy Levels

I didn't overcome my fatigue by following some sacred manuscript I found hidden in a long-forgotten library of wisdom. My success was based on trial and error. I'd read something and follow up on it. Sometimes I'd make mistakes. I'd rather not share those errors.

Most of my thinking came from being intuitive and then finding a reasonable basis to support each step.

As I described much earlier in this book, MS does not drop from the sky. It creeps up on you. The change from being an alert, energetic, and fully functioning person to a low-energy shell is often so subtle that you barely perceive it is happening. This is what occurred with me.

As the decline is often so slow and subtle, a diagnosis can be a shock to many. For others, like me, it is a confirmation that there actually was a reason for why things didn't seem right. You feel absolved of the hypochondriac label.

When you are diagnosed, you have already been running down for some time. Your symptoms have now become apparent, fatigue may already be an issue, and you have already noticed some changes. The medical profession, however, sees you as a brand-new case. For them, a new MS patient did drop from the sky.

As it took years for your symptoms to overwhelm you, it will take time, perhaps years, to reverse that. Thankfully, a general improvement happens sooner.

Dealing with Inflammation

Years on an interferon isn't enough

In late 1994, I started my life as a diagnosed MS patient, a clueless novice. The only treatment offered was three days on a steroid drip and a smile as I was sent away. After a brief hospital stay, I was left to accept that the drip might knock me around. My energy levels were about the same as before treatment, and I had long forgotten what I should really feel like. My treatment finished with a course of oral cortisone that completely flattened me, so any recovery from that felt like a significant resurgence. All I did, post-treatment, was recover to where I had been before diagnosis.

In those days, there was no discussion of disease-modifying therapy. It wasn't offered until I relapsed two years later in 1996. Then I began the injection therapy of interferon-β.

This was a drug that made me wish I had just persisted without medication. Nonetheless, I diligently took it for years because I was constantly reminded that interferon was the treatment of choice. Every avenue pointed to it as the gold standard.

Adding an antiviral

About 18 months after I started the treatment, (i.e., after 72 injections), my local doctor suggested I try an antiviral. He wasn't very interested in how interferon-β affected me, so he didn't offer any suggestions about the headaches or the discomfort. He came from a different angle.

"I've been treating an 18-year-old who has chronic fatigue with an antiviral, and he seems to be much better. It's a low dose treatment, but it seems to work. Do you want to try it and see how you go?" he asked, more as a statement than a question.

By this point, I was ready to try anything, so I agreed.

The doctor had already cleared up several bugs in my system, *Chlamydia pneumoniae* and the ulcer bug, *Helicobacter pylori*, among others. Why wouldn't I give him the benefit of the doubt?

The drug was valaciclovir (or valacyclovir). It wasn't a recognized MS treatment, and as an off-label medication was costly. (Now, 20 years later, I pay a tenth of what I paid then.)

The dose he recommended was 500 mg twice a day.

Up to this point, life on interferon-β had been hell. Migraine-like headaches, fatigue, muscle pain, and overwhelming brain fog were regular events for me.

Three days after I started taking the valaciclovir, my brain fog lifted. Suddenly I could think clearly. My energy levels were still low, but without a foggy brain, I felt re-energized. The thick, whitish coating on my tongue melted away, and, slowly, both taste and smell improved.

My doctor was surprised by my positive comments and seemed torn between encouraging me to go on and cautioning me that the medication wasn't typically used this way.

His wavering led me to experiment on myself. Over time, I noted that it was the combination of interferon-β and valaciclovir that seemed to relieve me. If I took one and not the other, my symptoms would return after five weeks or so. Taken together, they seemed to improve my health. Even my friends and family were starting to notice a change.

I, however, still didn't have a clue how everything worked.

~

The interferon-β I used was interferon-β-1a, a Type 1 interferon. This is from the class of interferons assumed to be a marker of noninflammatory activity. Type 1 interferons are thought to shut down viral activity.[1]

Valaciclovir is an antiviral that works against some herpes family viruses. It interrupts the replication of the virus by inserting an analog of a piece of code into the DNA of the virus, terminating it before it can complete reproducing.[2]

The effect of making valaciclovir a daily regimen was profound. The interferon-β injections stopped producing such violent reactions, and my life felt better. It is only on reflection that I can see that my energy levels were still subdued. At the time, I thought I was as energetic as anyone else.

This dual therapy became part of my life. I continued with both interferon-β and valaciclovir for around ten years.

Eventually, the interferon-β injection started to irk me. I no longer reacted badly after I took it. The headaches were mild but persisted. Without any grand plan in my mind, I discontinued the interferon-β and continued with the valaciclovir.

Without the interferon, I felt better and concluded its benefit had become minimal with time. My energy levels felt fine, and the brain fog was a distant memory. I had started Pilates classes a year or so earlier and just did not tire. Dropping the interferon-β felt like throwing away an uncomfortable crutch, and exercise certainly became easier.

For many years now, I have taken two 500 mg doses of valaciclovir daily. One tablet in the morning and one before bed. The hours between each dose are not quite evenly spaced apart, but it is close enough.

A natural product that boosts non-inflammatory responses

If I told you that a chemist had found a substance that could promote noninflammatory cytokines (cell messengers) over inflammatory types, you would say that I should take it.

If I told you it was called (E,E)-1,7-bis(4-hydroxy-3-methoxyphenyl)-1,6-heptadiene-3,5-dione, you would want to know what that meant and, maybe, how to get it.

If I told you it was also called curcumin, the active ingredient of turmeric, you would probably balk. It sounds too simple.

Researchers have found there are anti-inflammatory, antioxidant, anti-parasitic, anti-viral, and anti-cancer properties in curcumin. A study in the September 2008 edition of *Biochemical and Biophysical Research Communications*[3] attributes its widespread effect to its ability to prevent dendritic cells from maturing. In turn, this makes them incapable of triggering major immune cells, called CD4+ T cells, and starting an inflammatory cascade. The researchers noticed this results in a bias towards Th2 cytokines (cell messengers), which are noninflammatory markers.

There are complex notes later in this book that provide the details, but transcription factors such as NFκB are also inhibited by curcumin (Note 12). This simple foodstuff also inhibits adhesion molecules such as I-CAM, which feature in the traditional inflammatory model of MS.[3, 4]

There are so many studies and academic papers looking at curcumin for numerous illnesses. I invite you to search Pubmed, or similar reference libraries, to review them.

I take two 30 mg doses of curcumin daily.

There are several different formulations with similar efficacies on the market.

So, the lessons of the first part of my recovery from fatigue are clear:

Lesson 1

Remove any underlying infections.

This means a physician has to look. That is not easy to arrange.

As I discuss in my note on cytokines (Note 7), there is an inverse relationship between the non-inflammatory marker, IL-10, and the marker of inflammation, interferon-γ. Infections boost inflammatory markers, pushing your profile towards the setting that MS displays. That doesn't help you.

There is also an antagonistic relationship between the different classes of T helper cells; the inflammatory cytokines from Th1 cells actively suppress non-inflammatory Th2 cells. That means inflammatory messengers can overwhelm the markers of a non-inflammatory setting. You need to reverse this.

If you have an underlying infection, the T cells are doing what they are supposed to do. If this results in a suppression of IL-10 and expression of interferon-γ, then you are shifting towards a state where the types of cytokines that predominate in active MS are more readily expressed.

You will need some help to move from a proinflammatory to a non-inflammatory setting. Looking for and treating any pathogen becomes fundamental to dealing with fatigue. Even now, if any infection makes me ill, my MS symptoms bubble to the surface.

You need to be in a non-inflammatory mode rather than staying primed to fight infection. Curcumin helps you get there. Valaciclovir, taken regularly, stops some viral replication.

Lesson 2

Assume, or check, that you have had a herpes-family viral infection. Start a low dose of antiviral that targets herpes-family viruses (e.g., valaciclovir). The next chapter will focus on this.

Lesson 3

Expect the benefit to take time. It took you a long time to get sick. It will probably take a long time to recover.

~

There is nothing in this first part of recovery that focuses explicitly on energy. It is just cleaning the system of pathogens and shifting your body to a less inflammatory setting. Other MS sufferers may have had the same infections as me or may harbor something else.

What is almost universally understood is people with MS have had exposure to Epstein-Barr virus (EBV).[5] This virus stands like a smoking gun in MS research.[6] EBV is a member of the herpes family of viruses. I found great benefit in taking the herpes antiviral, valaciclovir. It is only the start of a treatment, not a cure.

Making Energy

Although I felt well, I never stopped looking to improve my understanding of what was known about MS. Often I came up against terms I didn't understand. I regularly found snippets of research but could not access the full research article. My knowledge was getting better, but I knew there were huge holes. I needed a more general understanding and something to point me in the right direction.

I don't recall why I had entered the local bookstore. Perhaps I was killing time; maybe I just wanted some space. I don't remember.

As I wandered through the store, I noticed a bargain bin full of books that had never enticed a buyer. Sitting on the top was a book called "The Sinatra Solution." I picked it up and flicked through the pages. Here was something more interesting than the cover implied.

I had never heard of Stephen Sinatra.

By now a well-known author in his field, he had been chief of cardiology for two four-year terms and director of medical education at Manchester Memorial Hospital, Connecticut, for almost 20 years. His book was subtitled "Metabolic Cardiology," but to me, it was a guide into how cells harness energy. I read it several times; each time, his argument became clearer. The terminology was all new to me. If you cannot follow what I am saying, try reading his book.[7]

Sinatra's argument focused on ATP. His intention was the rejuvenation of the heart muscle. Still, I saw it as being just as significant for muscles in general and offering a potential pathway out of fatigue.

~

Using his book as a rough blueprint, three elements became mainstays of my daily regimen:

1) Coenzyme Q10,

2) Acetyl-l-Carnitine, and

3) Magnesium.

(Sinatra also put emphasis on the sugar, D-ribose, but the authorities restricted its use in Australia. It is not something I have used.)

The Supplements I use for Energy

Co-enzyme Q10

There is a note in this book where I discuss how foodstuffs, which have been converted into glucose ($C_6H_{12}O_6$), go through glycolysis to become acetyl CoA and then enter the Krebs cycle (Note 14). The glucose is broken up, driving reactions, and liberating its carbon and oxygen elements. All that is left are the hydrogen molecules, which, in turn, split into ions and electrons that travel inside the electron transport chain.

The complexes in the electron transport chain push the ions into a space between the inner and outer walls of the mitochondria. The ions move through this space until they reach an exit, which delivers them to a metabolic machine called an ATP synthase. Their flow through this cellular machine, like water through a waterwheel, causes part of the ATP synthase to spin and cause its base to writhe. This action helps phosphate and ADP reunite to make ATP. Each hydrogen ion unites with an electron that has been carried from complex to complex in the electron transport chain. They meet and combine with oxygen to make water.

The major carrier of the electrons through this chain is Co-enzyme Q10. It can hold two electrons simultaneously and pass them on one at a time. It regulates the flow of electrons. If an electron does not arrive to bind to the oxygen after leaving the fourth complex of the chain, the hydrogen ions are left trapped in the mitochondria, and acidity levels rise (lower pH). Without oxygen acting as the final acceptor of electrons, the last step, the ATP synthase fails.

Co-enzyme Q10 is fundamental to the whole process. It orchestrates the movement of electrons.

~

Studies of CoQ10 therapy provide mixed results. Sinatra strongly supports its use in patients with heart conditions. In disease, the therapeutic benefit is unproven. However, studies conclude that there is evidence that plasma levels of CoQ10 are decreased in a broad range of critically ill patients.[8]

A study in 2019 looked at 60 patients with remitting-relapsing MS who were already being treated with interferon-β-1a.[10] The patients were split into two groups. Each group took 200 mg of CoQ10 daily for three months. One group took the supplement from the beginning of the study for three months. The other group did not start taking the supplement until three months had elapsed. Both groups took interferon throughout the six-month study.

Both groups were tested at the beginning, after three months and after six months.

Those MS patients with the most significant MS symptoms showed the lowest measures of serum CoQ10 in blood samples.

CoQ10 supplementation seemed to make a difference to the health of the patients. For starters, there was a significant improvement in the levels of uric acid (a natural antioxidant), which had been very low across both groups.

There were also some other notable changes:

Levels of reactive oxygen species (ROS), a marker of oxidative damage, were reduced.

Interferon-γ levels were lowered.

IL-13 levels were increased.

Certified EDSS examiners reported a lower level of disability after supplementation across the groups, which the researchers associated with the lower ROS, lower interferon-γ levels, and higher IL-13, all due to CoQ10 supplementation.

A reduction in reported pain was attributed to lower readings of inflammatory IL-1α and increased non-inflammatory IL-4.

Becks Depression Index scores showed a reduction in depression, attributed to the increase in uric acid.

Inflammatory cytokines, chemokines associated with damage, and molecules that activate lymphocytes (part of the adaptive immune system) all fell after CoQ10 treatment. In other words, all patients moved to a less inflammatory profile.

You could argue that it was the interferon-β-1a that drove the changes, but all 60 patients had been on that treatment for around five years.

During the study, four patients out of 60 had some sort of relapse. This occurrence was equally distributed across all the sample groups.

This study was short, only six months in duration, but it strongly pointed to CoQ10 as a partner in MS therapy.

As we age, irrespective of health, we lose muscle mass and function (a condition called sarcopenia). A study in 2012[9] looked at supplementation of CoQ10 in both aged people and healthy young Olympic athletes. It concluded that the ratio of CoQ10 to cholesterol could be a predictor of the risk of sarcopenia. This ratio was also significantly correlated to muscle mass. The older and more obese study group had higher cholesterol and a lower CoQ10 level, which correlated with sarcopenia.

The sedentary older cohort showed no aerobic benefit from CoQ10 supplementation, but 600 mg daily for six weeks led to significant improvements in endurance for the athletic group.

Diet, formulation, dosage, timing, exercise, and the type of people studied were all noted as variables affecting outcomes. The point to draw from this is that the way studies are put together makes a big difference to the conclusions that can be drawn.

Co-enzyme Q10 is soluble in fats, so it ends up in the membranes of all cells. Its critical feature is that it can both receive and donate electrons. It may pick up two hydrogen ions and be known as ubiquinol ($CoQ_{10}H_2$), it may be fully oxidized as ubiquinone (CoQ_{10}) or be a radical form holding on to one hydrogen ion ($CoQ_{10}H\bullet$). It can flux between all these states, and its dual ability to gather and pass on electrons gives it a unique role. Unlike CoQ10, most molecules either just gain or lose electrons. CoQ10 easily does both.

$CoQ_{10}H_2$ protects cell membranes from oxidation. The damage from oxidation can happen in the mitochondria and other parts of the cell. CoQ10 can also regenerate α-tocopherol (a type of vitamin E) so that this molecule can also go on scavenging free radicals.

The pathway that leads to Co-enzyme Q formation also appears to have a role in insulin resistance.

When some researchers[11] looked for a common pathway to insulin resistance, they found the mevalonate/coenzyme Q pathway was altered in all the models they examined. When they deliberately inhibited the CoQ pathway, insulin resistance developed. This is the same pathway that is blocked by statins. The same researchers found that insulin resistance developed when statins were used, and supplementation of CoQ_9 was sufficient to reverse the effect. This suggests that if you are on a statin, you probably should be taking CoQ10.

As CoQ10 is fat-soluble, it is easily absorbed from our food. Red meat, fish, poultry, eggs, vegetables, and dairy products are amongst a wide range of dietary sources.

Although I eat from all these groups, I still supplement with CoQ10. Sinatra recommends 300 – 360 mg daily for a range of heart-related conditions, chronic fatigue, and fibromyalgia. Through experimentation, I found 750 mg daily seems right for me.

The brand of CoQ10 I take is a major brand. Each soft gel capsule contains150 mg of CoQ10 and 10 mg of d-α-tocopherol (equivalent to 15 IU of vitamin E). Consequently, I am also taking 75 IU of vitamin E daily.

Acetyl-L-Carnitine

Carnitine is derived from two amino acids: lysine and methionine.[7] It is most abundant in older sheep, lamb, beef, other red meat, and pork. Plants provide very little carnitine, if any. Individual plants may provide one amino acid or the other, but plant intake needs to be balanced so that lysine and methionine can form carnitine in a vegetarian diet. There is more than a chance that biosynthesis of carnitine will falter in a meat-free diet. The consequence would be muscle weakness and the risk of osteomalacia (failure in bone development) in children.

There are, of course, supreme athletes who live on exclusively plant-based diets. I presume they are getting adequate sources of carnitine's constituent amino acids. Rather than debate the merits of diets, I am agnostic about how you get sufficient carnitine. You just absolutely need it.

Sinatra insists his vegetarian patients consider CoQ10, B12 and carnitine supplementation.

What carnitine does

All fats are made up of carbon chains called fatty acids. Long-chain fatty acids have 14 or more carbons in their tails. The fats in foods like meat, fish, and most edible fats or oils are generally long-chain fatty acids. Most are considered beneficial.

Fatty acids are metabolized in the mitochondria, primarily through the Krebs cycle, and conclude the process in the electron transport chain. The Krebs cycle liberates the carbon in fatty acids. The process, called β-oxidation, is about burning fats.

To get to the Krebs cycle, those fatty acids bind to a modified form of pyruvate, called Coenzyme A (CoA), making CoA esters. This union readies the fatty acids to enter the mitochondria. The issue is that without assistance, the walls of the mitochondria will resist penetration by the CoA esters.

Carnitine is unique. It can cross the mitochondrial membrane. Carnitine binds to the acyl group (the fatty acid chain) attached to the CoA and, with the help of other enzymes, moves the fatty acid into the mitochondria. Here, β-oxidation occurs. The products of this, NADH and FADH2, can then be formed in the Krebs cycle and passed to the electron transport chain.

Carnitine is the essential shuttle that transports the fatty acids across the mitochondrial membrane. It is crucial to the generation of ATP and, ultimately, the availability of energy.

As it can easily move across the mitochondrial membrane, carnitine ensures the refuse of the cycle is cleared from the mitochondria. When β-oxidation has completed its cycle, carnitine binds to the acyl groups that remain and transports them out through the membrane.

Where glycolysis produces about 36 or so molecules of ATP, β-oxidation of a 16-carbon fatty acid ultimately produces around 129 molecules. Glycolysis occurs without oxygen. β-oxidation and the steps of the electron transport chain are oxygen-dependent. Fatty acids and oxygen together provide the most energy. The entry of long-chain fatty acids into the mitochondria is entirely dependent on carnitine.[7]

~

Enzymes in the cell can easily interconvert carnitine to acetyl-carnitine. Acetyl-carnitine is more readily absorbed by the gut and can easily cross the blood-brain barrier. [12]

I take 1000 mg twice daily in the form acetyl levocarnitine (acetyl-L-carnitine) hydrochloride.

You may see the word levocarnitine on CoQ10 packaging. The FDA approved levocarnitine as a man-made form of CoQ10 in 1985. The notes in pharmacy databases and from the manufacturer indicate the use of valproic acid for epilepsy with carnitine may contraindicate. However, a systematic review in 2016 by the British Epilepsy Association found there is no literature at all supporting that concern.[13]

Magnesium

Sinatra called magnesium an unsung hero.[7] It is the constant companion of ATP. Magnesium binds to the negative charge of the phosphate groups in ATP and ADP. Doing this reduces the negative charge of ATP from –4 to –2.[14]

Of the total magnesium in our bodies, 50% is found in our bones. About half of cytosolic (intracellular) magnesium is bound to ATP, and the other half is bound to the structures responsible for protein synthesis called ribosomes. Less than 0.5% of the total body magnesium is in our plasma.

When it is hydrated, magnesium can increase its volume by 400 times (compared to 25 times for sodium and calcium and only five times for potassium). Without hydration, its ionic radius is quite small. This gives it a high electron density. Many enzymes require magnesium to become active. RNA and DNA both need magnesium to catalyze reactions involving their sugar-phosphate backbone.[15]

Most of the early signs of magnesium deficiency are neurologic or neuromuscular defects that may develop with time into anorexia, nausea, muscular weakness, lethargy, weight loss, hyper-irritability, hyper-excitability, muscular spasms, tetany and finally convulsions.[16]

A decades-old study from 1990 found that patients with MS had significantly lower magnesium concentrations than control subjects.[17] The tissues of their central nervous systems and visceral organs (except the spleen) all displayed this magnesium deficiency. As the organs were depleted, the researchers suggested this pointed to dietary inadequacies.

A study in 2016 compared 26 remitting-relapsing MS patients with controls. It also noted a significant difference in magnesium levels between the two groups, while other trace metals appeared very similar. This study still described the serum magnesium levels of the MS patients as being in the "normal" range but noted that the levels were significantly lower than those of the controls.[18]

In 2000, the European Journal of Neurology published a letter from a rehabilitation center in Oxford, England called "The effect of magnesium oral therapy on spasticity in a patient with multiple sclerosis."[19]

In this case, a 35-year-old woman with secondary progressive MS was referred to the center with a range of symptoms. The most severe was "weakness with ataxia (lack of voluntary coordination)." She also had reduced sensation in her legs, cognitive problems, and difficulty swallowing, and exhibited incontinence from both bowel and bladder. Her EDSS score was 8.5, and she was considered to be totally dependent by other measures. Physiotherapy hadn't helped. The drugs baclofen and tizanidine had been administered to the maximum dosage but were unable to diminish either the spasticity or the spasms in her legs.

The clinicians administered 500 mg of oral magnesium glycerophosphate (equivalent to 100 mg elemental magnesium). Additionally, the diet they provided her with should have contained 300 – 360 mg of elemental magnesium. She was regularly assessed over a month-long stay.

Although she remained profoundly disabled, the patient reported a diminution of spasms in her legs, she regained some voluntary leg movement, and caregivers reported that the reduction in rigidity made her easier to care for. The researchers recorded no adverse effects.

What makes our muscles tighten is a process called excitation-contraction coupling. This is a function that depends on the flow of calcium released from a store in each muscle cell called the sarcoplasmic reticulum. The gateway to this store is called the ryanodine receptor. Calcium and magnesium are conducted almost equally by the ryanodine receptor. This means magnesium can block the receptor pore and limit the release of calcium.[20] This would, in no small degree, explain why the Oxford clinicians observed an improvement. Spasticity will be discussed in much more detail in another chapter.

Magnesium comes in different forms. Some, like Epsom salts, can pass quite vigorously through you. Magnesium glycinate (sometimes called diglycinate or bisglycinate) does not.

Ignore blood tests for magnesium. Blood levels are not a good determinate of magnesium status and do not correlate with tissue pool levels.[21]

~

Magnesium glycinate consists of one magnesium molecule and two glycine molecules. Glycine is the raw material of various essential proteins such as glutathione, porphyrin, purine, heme, and creatine. It has numerous functions as a neurotransmitter and is a small molecule that can migrate to the brain.

The brain is rich in a molecule called taurine, which contributes to the regulation of the volumes of neurons and astrocytes and reduces the excitability of neurons, thus counterbalancing the overactivation of excitatory elements.[22]

Both magnesium glycinate and magnesium taurate can reach the brain. However, higher brain concentrations do not translate to higher muscle concentrations. If the dose is high enough, magnesium citrate can increase the measure in tissues. The issue is absorption and excretion. magnesium glycinate is the most comfortable magnesium supplement to take.

Twice daily, I take a large tablet of magnesium diglycinate as 500 mg of magnesium amino acid chelate. It is mixed with small traces of other magnesium forms. Each tablet is equivelent to 50 mg of elemental magnesium.

All three supplements augment ATP in some way

The three supplements all target ATP or its formation.

1) CoQ10 helps transport electrons,

2) Acetyl-L-carnitine helps move fatty acids into the matrix of the mitochondria to yield the highest number of ATP, and

3) Magnesium binds to ATP to improve its functionality, efficacy, and mobility.

All through our day, we are consuming and making ATP. If supply doesn't match the demand, fatigue will occur within a few heartbeats. It is that fundamental.

Why are You so Tired?

Continually, through the day, some ATP is breaking down and degrading into its purine bases. Usually, the first degradation is rescued as ADP by binding to a phosphate molecule in the ATPase complex. In the muscles, the enzyme creatine kinase releases phosphate from the tissue.

Some ADP molecules can combine in the cytoplasm of the cell. This results in one ATP and one AMP forming from two ADP. [14] Nonetheless, over the day, as we are spending energy, the AMP level will slowly rise.

AMP, in the cytosol of the cell, has little value and continues to degrade, losing its phosphate molecule and becoming adenosine. The cell's mechanisms will salvage some of this, but the balance will be lost and return to the bloodstream. Here, some will continue to degrade, becoming inosine then hypoxanthine, xanthine, and ultimately uric acid.

Other adenosine finds its way to adenosine receptors, which couple to proteins that drive a range of reactions. If oxygen is in short supply, adenosine can open potassium channels in smooth muscle and in endothelial cells to increase vasodilation. The increased blood flow reduces the energy demand on the heart by slowing the heartbeat.

Heart cells (myocytes) can act as a sink to reabsorb the adenosine from the space between them as a base material to rebuild ATP from scratch. If this results in high concentrations in the heart, adenosine can induce arrthymias. [14]

The body has four adenosine receptors; A_1, A_{2A}, A_{2B}, and A_{3A}.

A_1 receptors are distributed in the brain (cortex, hippocampus, and cerebellum). They can be found on astrocytes, oligodendrocytes, and microglia in the brain. Low levels of A_{2A} are also detectable in glia as are A_{3A} receptors. Several studies suggest there is an essential role for the transcription factor NFκB in the regulation of both A_1 and A_{2A} receptors in the brain.[23] The transcription factor NFκB, is covered in a separate note in this book (Note 12). It is important in the pathways of several illnesses.

In an average healthy person, the extracellular concentration of adenosine increases during our wakeful period and declines slowly during recovery sleep.[24] It notably builds up in the region of the basal forebrain.

A region called the cholinergic mesopontine nucleus, which can control the activity of the thalamic reticular nucleus (part of the sleep system)[25] is also heavily influenced by adenosine.[24]

Adenosine levels influence sleep

Scientists tested adenosine levels in cats that were deliberately kept awake by play and interruption. Like us, cats have neurons of the forebrain, controlled by the neurotransmitter acetylcholine, that are important for arousal and wakefulness. Without sufficient rest, these became overwhelmed by adenosine. To lower the concentration of adenosine, the cats had to enter delta slow-wave sleep, which is the deepest phase of non-rapid eye movement sleep.[24]

To clear our build-up of adenosine, we sleep. When we rest, the cholinergic neurons throughout the whole body, which use acetylcholine, are at their quietest. The adenosine decouples from these neurons, to be salvaged or broken down. When it clears, we wake up. If the adenosine does not clear sufficiently, we remain on the edge of sleep.

In MS, from my perspective, there is an apparent problem maintaining an adequate supply of ATP. If it is breaking down, and adenosine levels are increasing, then the binding to the adenosine receptors will tilt in favor of sleep. Endless drowsiness will develop.

CoQ10, acetyl-L-carnitine, and magnesium are crucial inputs to support ATP and prevent fatigue.

As I will describe in the next chapter, uncontrolled EBV infection increases adenosine levels.

I know fatigue. It was with me for years. I do not suffer from it now.

References

1. Schoggins, J.W., D.A. MacDuff, N. Imanaka, M.D. Gainey, B. Shrestha, J.L. Eitson, K.B. Mar, R.B. Richardson, A.V. Ratushny, V. Litvak, R. Dabelic, B. Manicassamy, J.D. Aitchison, A. Aderem, R.M. Elliott, A. García-Sastre, V. Racaniello, E.J. Snijder, W.M. Yokoyama, M.S. Diamond, H.W. Virgin and C.M. Rice. *Pan-viral specificity of IFN-induced genes reveals new roles for cGAS in innate immunity.* Nature, 2013. **505**(7485): p. 691.

2. Beutner, K.R., *Valacyclovir: a review of its antiviral activity, pharmacokinetic properties and clinical efficacy.* Antiviral Research, 1995. **28**(4): p. 281–290.

3. Shirley, S.A., A.J. Montpetit, R.F. Lockey and S.S. Mohapatra. *Curcumin prevents human dendritic cell response to immune stimulants.* Biochemical and Biophysical Research Communications, 2008. **374**(3): p. 431–436.

4. Agrawal, S.M. and V.W. Yong, *Immunopathogenesis of multiple sclerosis.* International Review of Neurobiology, 2007. **79**: p. 99–126.

5. Lindsey, J.W., L.M. Hatfield and T. Vu, *Epstein–Barr virus neutralizing and early antigen antibodies in multiple sclerosis.* European Journal of Neurology, 2010. **17**(10): p. 1263–1269.

6. Pender, M.P., *Epstein–Barr virus in the multiple sclerosis brain – an evasive culprit.* Multiple Sclerosis and Related Disorders, 2012. **1**(2): p. 61–63.

7. Sinatra, S.T., *The Sinatra Solution: Metabolic Cardiology: Easyread Large Bold Edition.* 2009. CREATESPACE PUB.

8. Coppadoro, A., L. Berra, A. Kumar, R. Pinciroli, M. Yamada, U.H. Schmidt, E.A. Bittner and M. Kaneki. *Critical illness is associated with decreased plasma levels of coenzyme Q10: A cross-sectional study.* Journal of Critical Care, 2013. **28**(5): p. 571–576.

9. Fischer, A., S. Onur, P. Niklowitz, T. Menke, M. Laudes, G. Rimbach and F. Döring. *Coenzyme Q_{10} status as a determinant of muscular strength in two independent cohorts.* PLoS ONE, 2016. **11**(12): p. e0167124.

10. Moccia, M., A. Capacchione, R. Lanzillo, F. Carbone, T. Micillo, F. Perna, A. De Rosa, A. Carotenuto, R. Albero, G. Matarese, R. Palladino and V.B. Morra. *Coenzyme Q10 supplementation reduces peripheral*

oxidative stress and inflammation in interferon-β1a-treated multiple sclerosis. Therapeutic Advances in Neurological Disorders, 2019. **12**: p. 1756286418819074.

11. Fazakerley, D., R. Chaudhuri, P. Yang, G.J. Maghzal, K.C. Thomas, J.R. Krycer, S.J. Humphrey, B.L. Parker, K.H. Fisher-Wellman, C.C. Meoli, N.J. Hoffman, C. Diskin, J.G. Burchfield, M.J. Cowley, W. Kaplan, Z. Modrusan, G. Kolumam, J.Y.H. Yang, D.L. Chen, D. Samocha-Bonet, J.R. Greenfield, K.L. Hoehn, R. Stocker and D. E. James. *Mitochondrial CoQ deficiency is a common driver of mitochondrial oxidants and insulin resistance.* eLife, 2018. **7**: p. e32111.

11. https://onlinelibrary.wiley.com/doi/pdf/10.1016/0307-4412(93)90042-X

12. Mendelson, S.D., *Metabolic Syndrome and Psychiatric Illness : Interactions, Pathophysiology, Assessment and Treatment.* 2007. Academic Press: San Diego.

13. Zeiler, F.A., N. Sader, L.M. Gillman and M. West. *Levocarnitine induced seizures in patients on valproic acid: A negative systematic review.* Seizure: European Journal of Epilepsy, 2016. **36**: p. 36–39.

14. Ingwall, J.S., *ATP and the Heart.* 2002. Springer: Boston, MA.

15. Crichton, R.R., *Biological inorganic chemistry a new introduction to molecular structure and function.* 2nd Ed. 2012. Elsevier.

16. *Australian Government National Health and Medical Research Council-Nutrients-Magnesium.* https://www.nrv.gov.au/nutrients/magnesium. Accessed January 2021.

17. Yasui, M., Y. Yase, K. Ando, K. Adachi, M. Mukoyama and K. Ohsugi. *Magnesium concentration in brains from multiple sclerosis patients.* Acta Neurologica Scandinavica, 1990. **81**(3): p. 197–200.

18. Alizadeh, A., O. Mehrpour, K. Nikkhah, B. Golnaz, E. Mahsa, A. Golzari, L. Jarahi and M. Foroughipour. *Comparison of serum concentration of Se, Pb, Mg, Cu, Zn, between MS patients and healthy controls.* Electron Physician, 2016. **8**(8): p. 2759–2764.

19. Rossier, P., S. Van Erven and D.T. Wade, *The effect of magnesium oral therapy on spasticity in a patient with multiple sclerosis.* European Journal of Neurology, 2000. **7**(6): p. 741–744.

20. Gillespie, D., H. Chen and M. Fill, *Is ryanodine receptor a calcium or magnesium channel? Roles of K^+ and Mg^{2+} during Ca^{2+} release.* Cell Calcium, 2012. **51**(6): p. 427–433.

21. Ates, M., S. Kizildag, O. Yukesi, H. Ferda, Z. Yuce, G. Guvendi, S.

Kandis, A. Karakilic, B. Koc and N. Uysal. *Dose-dependent absorption profile of different magnesium compounds.* Biological Trace Element Research, 2019. **192**(2): p. 244–251.

22. Oja, S.S. and P. Saransaari. *Significance of Taurine in the Brain.* in *Taurine 10.* Lee, D-H., Schaffer, S., Park E. and H. W. Kim (Editors.) 2017. pp 89–94. Springer: Netherlands.

23. Sheth, S., R. Brito, D. Mukheriaea, L.P. Rybak and V. Ramkumar. *Adenosine receptors: expression, function and regulation.* International Journal of Molecular Sciences, 2014. **15**(2): p. 2024–2052.

24. Porkka-Heiskanen, T., R.E. Strecker, M. Thakkar, A.A. Bjørkum, R.W. Greene and R.W. McCarley. *Adenosine: a mediator of the sleep-inducing effects of prolonged wakefulness.* Science (New York, N.Y.), 1997. **276**(5316): p. 1265-1268.

25. *The brain structures that wake you up and put you to sleep.* https://thebrain. mcgill.ca/flash/a/a_11/a_11_cr/a_11_cr_cyc/a_11_cr_cyc.html. Accessed January 2021.

Chapter 14

Epstein Barr Virus – a Smoking Gun

My father died in December 1965, a week before my eighth birthday. Up until then, we had lived in a small country town in the state of Victoria. My mother realized there was no future in staying there, so she and my younger brother and I moved to Victoria's capital, Melbourne. It all took time, but by mid-1968, I was a 10-year-old in a new school, in a completely different environment.

Either I brought with me or picked up a virus. My impression was that I missed only a week of school. However, I was much sicker than that. Years later, I learned from my mother that for three months, I was bedridden with glandular fever, an illness caused by the Epstein Barr virus.

I do not recall how my illness was treated. There is a vague memory of a nurse doing a blood test. Mostly, I just slept. It was not an experience that anyone dwelt on, but things did slowly change for me after that time.

I became a mediocre athlete despite my appearance. The "clumsy boy" would best describe me—the slow learner who showed patches of aptitude. I was a trier, not a star. The consensus was that I was a nice boy who wouldn't amount to much.

There were little things I noticed about myself that no one was interested in knowing. The most frequent problem was a racing heart. I could be doing nothing at all, and it would start beating at a fantastic rate. My teeth would tingle when it happened, and I felt like everything around me was still while I was rapidly moving. It felt so odd as I was not moving at all.

My mother had been a nurse, so I'd offer my arm and say, "take my pulse." But by the time she did, the fluttering would have disappeared, and I got the message that I had wasted her time. Eventually, after several years the rapid heartbeat settled down, the attacks became infrequent, and then went away altogether.

When I was about 15, white patches appeared on the sides of my tongue. In a matter of months, the whiteness had spread across the whole surface. I'd try scraping it off with a toothbrush, but nothing moved it. There was always a slight metallic taste in my mouth, and subtle flavors meant nothing to me.

Over the years, I tried many things to get rid of this coating, but nothing worked. Anti-candida diets with copious amounts of Nilstat powder made no difference.

In my thirties, I went to see aged ENT specialists who showed me pictures of tongues in books and pronounced I was healthy. By now, the taste in my mouth was frustrating to me. No one else complained of this. Why was I like this?

~

Not long after I had been diagnosed with MS, I bought my first computer. The internet was a brand new, unexplored library of ideas. I'd always search for "multiple sclerosis." Sometimes, I'd search for "autoimmune." When I did, I always ended up in sites about AIDS, as that was the big item at that time. Randomly following a path of links to articles, I ended up staring at a page full of photos of people living with AIDS presenting their tongues to the camera. I leaned forward and stared at several of them. Their tongues were like mine. The coating on them was given a name. They were not described as normal.

The whiteish coating was a signature of how compromised their immune systems had become. They could no longer prevent underlying infections from erupting.

The coating was described as the only physical manifestation of the Epstein Barr virus. It was named oral hairy leukoplakia. I found the picture of a tongue that was similar to my own and hit "Print."

It was the first time I had ever heard of Epstein Barr virus. Anthony Epstein, Yvonne Barr, and Burt Achong had written about it in 1964.[1] Thirty years later, it was still not really well known.

When I searched for associations of EBV with MS, pages and pages of articles appeared. I picked out a few. Armed with these and a picture of a tongue with white patterns like my own, I went to see my doctor. He was interested but initially had no solution. After a few months, he suggested I try the antiviral valaciclovir.

The impact of this anti-viral drug was profound. My tongue cleared, food tasted better, a beer lost its slimy feel and I could sense its bubbles on my tongue. My ability to smell things dramatically changed. I hadn't realized how poor I had been at noticing odors.

The most significant change, though, was that my brain fog evaporated. Suddenly I could think and remember so much more.

I have continued to take two 500 mg doses of valaciclovir daily for decades. The only period where I ceased was the year before my 2014 MS attack. I cannot tell if it is right to draw a relationship between stopping the medication and my big attack, but it feels that they are connected. The reason I had stopped taking the medication was that I felt so well that I thought I didn't need to continue.

~

Epstein Barr virus is a member of the herpes family. Like all viruses, herpes viridae cannot reproduce themselves. They need to hijack the apparatus of a cell and modify it to replicate. They are strands of nucleic acid surrounded by a shell or armor called a capsid.

Viruses do not generate heat and don't meet the definitions of life. Nonetheless, they are "lifelike" and persistent. By changing how our DNA is expressed, they change us. Stopping the treatment for the virus because I felt well, in my view, was a mistake. EBV doesn't go away.

Viruses

So, what is a virus? Even in the 1890s, there was a suspicion that there was an unseen reproducible poison in organisms, and later the focus was on cells. In Latin, the word virus means a venom, a slime, a pungency, or a toxin. That vague allusion became the accepted name for this elusive class of pathogen.

Suspicions grew that something even smaller than a bacterium was often the unknown virus. Finding what it was proved difficult. Scientists could not culture these pathogens in a dish.

They knew something existed; animal experiments told them a lot about the mysterious infection. The blisters of what we now know is herpes simplex could be transferred from humans to the cornea of rabbits. But what a virus was, still eluded them.

The development of the electron microscope in 1940 provided the first opportunity to peer into the world of the virus. Antibiotics made it possible to eliminate the influence of bacteria in cell cultures and just look at how a tiny virus would influence the cell.

Until 1971, it was assumed that antibodies would eliminate viruses. However, the recurrent blisters from herpes infections still developed despite evidence of antibodies. A leading investigator into viruses, Ernest W. Goodpasture,[2] suggested that there could be "latent" forms of virus that could be expressed from a host cell either intermittently or permanently. Testing over time proved this was correct.

In the 1940s, some viruses were proven to consist of RNA and proteins. In the mid-1950s, evidence showed that viral DNA existed and was replicated in infected cell divisions.

Also, in the 1950s, the concept of "slow virus infections" developed. These principally affected the nervous system. Measles was a viral infection that could mutate. JCV (see Chapter 8) could persist for a very long time without activating.

In 1957, it was shown that a cytokine called interferon could stimulate a nonspecific defense against viral pathogens.

In 1988, the Nobel Prize in Physiology or Medicine was awarded to Gertrude Elion for her work showing that acyclovir was a selective antiviral drug against herpes encephalitis.[3]

~

Unlike bacteria or yeast or other living cells, a virus can't replicate by division. It operates as a parasite, hijacking the components of the cell it has infected. There is no protein synthesis machinery in a virus. Instead, a virus has genes that can activate the regulatory proteins and enzymes in the host cell.

In a host cell, viruses can operate in different ways:

1) They can harness the machinery of the host and produce a large number of copies of themselves called progeny. This process is called lysis or the lytic state. Ultimately the cell dies, but many copies of the virus survive. Or

2) They can integrate their genetic information into the genome of the cell, becoming like an extra, silent, splice of genetic code in the host. In this latent state, as the cell replicates, the altered genome carries the virus code into each newly formed cell.

The systems that allow a virus to "uncoat" and transport its nucleic acids into a host is still unknown. Somehow, they survive the cell defenses. Nonetheless, we do know that viruses have selectivity for specific cells. In the wrong cell, if certain proteins are missing, the virus can't replicate.

Epstein Barr Virus

The Epstein Barr virus is a member of the herpes family. EBV uses B cells as its hosts, replicating its DNA by both lytic and latent cycles.

B cells reside in large numbers in the tonsillar tissue. The EBV infection is passed through saliva to the tonsil. Here naïve B cells are introduced to the virus and become latently infected memory B cells.[4]

After B cells are infected by Epstein Barr virus and are in the latent state, they go on to produce infinite cell divisions and are referred to as immortalized. In this mode, the virus can lead to overexpression of some genes resulting in changes in cell cycles. In particular, they trigger the expression of NFκB dependent genes.

When EBV activates a resting B cell, it leads to the expression of six nuclear proteins. They are called Epstein Barr nuclear antigens (EBNAs) and are numbered 1, 2, 3, 3B and 3C. There is one other protein expressed, denoted as LP.[5] The EBNA-LP is divided into a further group of antigens. All these antigens are critical to sustaining the virus and assisting it in avoiding detection.

A key element of EBV is the expression of Epstein Barr Virus Nuclear Antigen 1 (EBNA1). This antigen consists of repeated glycine–alanine residues that protect the virus from degradation and inhibit other antigen complexes.[3] What this means is, the defenses of the immune system can't see the EBV infection.

Apoptosis is the normal, orderly death of cells. A protein called BHRF1,[6] expressed by the Epstein Barr virus interferes with the B cell host to disrupt its apoptosis so that the host cell doesn't die. Using this protein becomes the mechanism that sustains the host while the virus makes many copies of itself inside the B cell. This protein is expressed in both the lytic and latent cycles. Like a horror movie, the B cell survives to support the parasite that infects it.

When B cells are transformed by EBV, they commence a viral transcriptional program called Latency 111.[7] This state leads to the expression of several new proteins, one of which is called EBNA2.

A sequence in what is called the C terminus of EBNA2 causes the virus to develop into two different strains: Type 1 and Type 2 (sometimes referred to as types A and B). The two types vary in their ability to "immortalize" B cells. The sequences of EBNA2 and the proteins in EBNA3s help determine the type. Ultimately, all varieties can be immortalized by the BHRF1 protein.

Type 1 EBV is found worldwide. Type 2 is mainly confined to sub-Saharan Africa.

There is a lot of variance in EBV strains, Chinese and Korean samples have shown Type1 EBNA2 mixed with Type 2 EBNA3s. There have been other examples of inter-strain recombination that make EBV very difficult to understand.[5]

~

In early infection, only a few latent viral genes are expressed. Later, a different set of viral genes amplifies the DNA expression, changing the structural code of the virus, which then switches to the lytic state and starts expressing progeny.

A key protein in the Epstein Barr virus called BZLF1 acts as an activator of this switch to viral replication.[8] BZLF1 is joined by another viral gene called BRLF1, and together, they encode some transcription factors (called Zta and Rta).

This replication is triggered by the same DNA coding, called CpG, that, in a different setting, triggers Toll-like receptor 9 to stimulate the release of Type 1 interferon from T and B cells. If the viral DNA has the CpG code in it and if that has been put in the "off" position by a process called CpG methylation, then the EBV infected cell switches from the latent setting to the prolific lytic setting.[9]

~

Higher levels of EBV antibodies, in particular those specific for Epstein–Barr nuclear antigen 1 (EBNA1), have been consistently found in the serum of patients with multiple sclerosis compared with control individuals.[10] What is lacking is a definitive answer about whether EBV is the activator of MS or has a role in the steps to trigger some other precursor.

Professor Michael Pender from the School of Medicine at Queensland University has proposed a plausible theory that in the presence of a susceptible genetic background, EBV infection may not be appropriately controlled. He argues that circulating EBV-infected B cells could enter the central nervous system, where the virus might activate, and go on to sustain a chronic inflammatory process that leads to multiple sclerosis.[10–12]

~

In a study published in 2017,[4] Pender and others found that CD8+T cells had a diminished response to Epstein Barr Virus in the lytic state. Their response differed when EBV was in a latent phase.

In the latent phase, they noted there was an increase in the CD4+ and CD8+ T cell populations. The CD8+ T cells became functionally active, expressing the expected cytokines. This didn't happen in the lytic phase.

In his 2017 study, Pender measured the amount of interferon-γ produced by CD8+T cells in response to peptides that were expressed in both the lytic and latent cycles. In his healthy controls, the ratio of the lytic to latent CD8+T cell population was 6.08 times. The average ratio across MS patients at all stages of MS was 1.03 times. In other words, in the lytic cycle, the CD8+T cells of MS patients had an abnormally low response.

His study also noted that when the virus entered a lytic phase, and the multiple sclerosis disease was already well established, there was a progressive decline in both CD4+ and CD8+ T cell numbers. The antibodies to the virus's EBNA1 protein expanded, but the CD8+ T cell population fell. Pender argued that the CD8+ T cells were unable to control the EBV infection because they were either exhausted or defective. The result was that the EBV infected population of B cells expanded. This expansion would include any latent autoreactive B cells. Consequentially, this would lead to a perpetual cycle of infection and reactivation.

His view is that Epstein Barr Virus infection is a prerequisite for the development of multiple sclerosis.

Pender argued that a significant element of the immune system, cytotoxic CD8+ T cells, which have been seen in abundance at the site of lesions,[13] usually keep EBV infection under tight control. If these cells are defective, he postulates that autoreactive B cells will then be unrestrained and accumulate in the brain.

Why EBV Infection Causes MS -
The Third Tier of Pender's Hypothesis

In the first tier of Pender's hypothesis, he argued that EBV was essential for MS to develop.

The second tier focused on EBV infected B cells seeding the target organ to produce autoantibodies.

In the third tier of his 2011 study, Pender explored a crucial conundrum. Although almost all MS people are infected with EBV, only a small number of people harboring the virus go on to develop MS. How can a prerequisite be so selective?

His view partly depended on what form of a genetic mutation occurred at the same spot on a particular chromosome. People with MS tend to have the HLA class 11 gene called HLA-DRB1*1501.

If it were a different genetic mutation, such as a variation on HLA-DR3, then an infected patient would be more likely to develop an autoreactive reaction in a different organ, rather than the central nervous system.

In that particular case, the organ would be the thyroid. That is, people with the HLA-DR3 mutation are disposed to autoimmune thyroid diseases, rather than MS.[14]

However, not all people with the HLA-DRB1*1501 mutation develop MS after EBV exposure, so the strain of EBV (Type 1 or Type 2 or a hybrid) helps dictate the likelihood of MS occurring.

Pender also looked at whether the B cells were abnormal themselves but, by 2011, had concluded that there should have been a T cell that limited the infected B cells.

Pender concluded that CD8+ T cells just didn't occur in sufficient numbers. They were depleted exclusively when EBV was the virus.

As the CD8+ T cells were deficient, infected B cells were free to accumulate in the central nervous system (CNS). These B cells would then communicate with and reactivate the autoreactive CD4+ T cells. These cells start producing IL-2, interferon-γ, and tumor necrosis factors, driving a cycle of destruction. As the EBV load stayed high, the T cells would become exhausted.

As we age, CD8+ T cells typically decline.[15] Pender speculated that T cell exhaustion further aggravated this abatement.

He also speculated that sunlight, the critical component for the synthesis of vitamin D, improved CD8+ T cell numbers. The environment, particularly the distance from the equator, could influence CD8+ T cell numbers. He, like me, doubted vitamin D itself was the missing link.

To quote Pender "if EBV infection of B cells in the CNS underpins the development of MS, effective antiviral drugs have the potential to cure MS."[12]

When I read this, I decided that Pender had validated my haphazard decision making, and I continued to take 500 mg of valaciclovir twice daily. The antiviral is a key part of my regimen.

In his masterful study from 2011, *The essential role of Epstein-Barr virus in the pathogenesis of multiple sclerosis*,[12] Pender outlined the three ways he believed that EBV could be treated to control MS:

1) By B cell depletion with monoclonal antibodies to delete the

Another factor to consider is that B cells that are immortalized by EBV are prolific producers of the free radical superoxide. All B lymphocytes produce superoxide, but this overproduction suggests an abnormal oxygen metabolism.

This molecule is a normal response as part of our defenses, but research from as far back as 1991 has likened the output of superoxide of EBV-infected B cells to that produced by neutrophils from patients with chronic granulomatous disease, a primary immunodeficiency disease.[16] They noted that neutrophils (a type of white blood cell) in that disease could not produce the enzyme to breakdown superoxide, and neither could the EBV-infected B cells.

Another study saw this characteristic of EBV-immortalized B cells as a useful way to study oxygen metabolism in other diseases.[17]

When superoxide combines with nitric oxide, it forms the damaging free radical peroxynitrite.

As I state in the note on free radicals (Note 13), peroxynitrite is most clearly an oxidant. When it reacts with major antioxidant stores such as cysteine and glutathione, it converts them to a disulfide form, increasing the measures of oxidative stress. The sulfur amino acid, methionine, which is found in fish, meat, and dairy products, can be converted by peroxynitrite into a disulfide, which can then be oxidized to formaldehyde. Alternately, the methionine disulfide can be fragmented into ethylene and dimethyldisulfide.[19]

The enzyme, glyceraldehyde-3-phosphate dehydrogenase is critical to the pathway that breaks glucose into smaller components. The job it does is necessary for the formation of the energy molecule, ATP. The enzyme is easily degraded and inactivated by even low levels of peroxynitrite. When the enzyme fails, energy production is disrupted.[18]

In short, peroxynitrite is highly reactive and damaging.[19]

So, to use Pender's argument, if people with MS are infected with EBV, they should be predisposed to overproduce a free radical associated with inflammation.

An Alternative Argument for the Depletion of CD8+ T Cells

In both the lytic and latent infection of B cells by Epstein Barr Virus, there are small RNA transcriptions called EBERs (Epstein Barr virus encoded small RNA). There is some speculation that these RNA molecules play a role in protecting the virus from the immune system.

EBER-1 can bind to the enzyme PKR (a double-stranded RNA-dependent kinase) and block its activation.[20] This may be one form of EBV self-protection.

In 1997, a letter to the editor was published in the journal *Leukemia*. The authors noted that EBER-2 had three very similar regions to the enzyme adenosine deaminase.[21] This enzyme would generally break down adenosine into its purine constituents, which ultimately results in a rise in uric acid. An increase in uric acid is associated with the troublesome disease called gout.

There is a large body of research that has concluded that MS and gout are practically mutually exclusive.[22] To have both is very rare.

The authors argued that EBER-2 competes with adenosine deaminase, decreasing its activity. The result is a rise in adenosine, rather than a rise in uric acid, the final breakdown product of adenosine.

One of the roles of adenosine is to downregulate T cell activity.[23] If adenosine increases, it will inactivate the metabolic activity of T cells.

It will mainly affect CD8+ T cell proliferation.

A paper in 2009 pointed out that adenosine interfered with the efficient CD8+ T cell priming by professional antigen-presenting cells (dendritic cells) and semi-professional antigen-presenting cells.[23]

It may be that a rise in adenosine, triggered by the small RNA transcripts from EBV, not only protects the virus but creates an excessive adenosine load in the basal forebrain that triggers fatigue. This same high load of adenosine downregulates the immune response to the EBV infection by switching off the signaling to CD8+ T cells.

The adenosine deaminase enzyme is not deficient or faulty. The EBER-2 just outcompetes it as a defense mechanism of EBV.

Untreated, EBV enters a cycle of self-preservation.

The 'Inside' and 'Outside' Models of MS

All the hypotheses about what causes MS revolve around two primary arguments:

1) The 'outside' model (the conventional view), which suggests that dysregulated immune cells migrate to the central nervous system and attack myelin, or

2) The 'inside' model, which argues that damage to axons and oligodendrocytes happens early in MS disease, and consequently goes on to trigger an immune response.[24] The issue this argument implies is that something other than immune cell activity starts demyelination. Some studies support this idea and suggest immune cell involvement is preceded by demyelination.[24] In other words, something other than an antigen triggers neurodegeneration.

An emerging area of interest, called purinergic signaling, focuses on receptors called P2X7 and P2X4. ATP and adenosine are purines. If these receptors, and others in the same family, are opened by purines, they permit an influx of calcium into a cell. An overload of calcium results in cell death.[25] Perhaps, too much adenosine due to EBER-2 starts a cascade of damage that fits the 'inside' model.

EBV Continues to Interest MS Researchers

A study released in 2020 by a university in Berlin, compared 901 definite MS patients (either at the clinically isolated syndrome or remitting-relapsing stage) with a large hospital population of 16,163 people who had been tested for EBV between January 2014 and December 2016.[26]

Of the definite MS patients, 100% had antibodies to either a current or past Epstein Barr virus infection. Statistically, this was significant compared to the general population who displayed exposure averaging around 98%. It doesn't sound like much of a discrepancy but, given only a few (309 people in the US per 100,000)[27] get MS, it means something when all of that select little group have an EBV infection.

The control group was spread across all ages up to 80 years. The MS group was aged between 27 and 41, with an average age of 33.

Two different assay methods were used to find the antibodies. The bulk of the MS group revealed antibodies to EBNA-1. Some displayed antibodies to the EBV capsid. Some needed a test called an EBV IgG immunoblot to show the exposure.

The control group included newborns. Some of them displayed EBV antibodies passed on from the placenta. Infants often lost their maternal EBV antibodies. This is normal.

There was a significant increase in EBV exposure between the infant group and those between 15 and 19 years of age. The study showed an increasing exposure as each age group was assessed. The control groups between 45 and 79 years revealed exposure levels as high as 98%, but no part of the control group reached an EBV exposure of 100%. Exposure rates for patients with MS peaked in the 20–24 years age group at 100%. The same age group in the controls was only 95%. As MS is considered a young person's disease, this 5% difference was statistically meaningful.

The study concluded that early life exposure to EBV needed following to see what developed over time. Like Pender, they concluded that EBV infection had a role in MS, perhaps as a late-stage development. Its primary finding was that a negative antibody result should alert doctors to investigate if a sick patient had a problem other than MS. The researchers did not attempt to look at why EBV infection is associated with MS. Just that it is.

How Does Acyclovir Work?

Acyclovir has a structure that is similar to the DNA purine, guanosine, but it has no function. This makes it an analog of guanosine that is inoperative.

When the drug enters the host cell, an enzyme made by the virus, called viral thymidine kinase, is attracted to the acyclovir molecule, and adds a phosphate molecule to it. The human kinase does not recognize the drug.

Then, human cellular enzymes recognize the phosphorylated form, and add a further two phosphate molecules to it. The acyclovir can only enter the nucleus of the cell if it has three phosphates. An uninfected cell can only possibly provide a maximum of two phosphates. This aspect makes the drug highly specific to infected cells.

The acyclovir molecule with three phosphates attached to it, enters the nucleus of the host cell and attaches itself to a chain of viral DNA. As it is only an analog of guanosine, it lacks what that real molecule has to continue replication, namely a group called a hydroxyl group at the 3 prime (3') position. The absence of this group results in the chain of replication terminating, and the EBV fails to reproduce.[28]

Most references look at acyclovir, valaciclovir, and famciclovir as primary treatments for herpes simplex and herpes zoster (shingles) viruses. They acknowledge they can influence EBV.

Famciclovir breaks down into penciclovir in the body. In this form, it has a higher intracellular concentration than acyclovir achieves, but it doesn't cause chain termination. Acyclovir and valaciclovir result in chain termination.[28]

Possible Adverse Effects of Using Acyclovir

Although the journal of the British Pharmacological Society[29] notes valaciclovir and acyclovir as safe and efficacious, there is still the possibility that some people will find the drug difficult to tolerate in its early use.

The FDA prescribing notes,[30] in particular, highlight the risk of adverse events when used in patients who have renal issues, advanced diseases such as HIV, and in the elderly. These events include central nervous system adverse reactions (e.g., agitation, hallucinations, confusion, and encephalopathy).

The reported responses to the original marketed product, called Valtrex, occurred with at least one indication of headache, nausea or abdominal pain by more than 10% of adult patients treated and these arose more commonly than in patients treated with placebo treatments. The only adverse reaction occurring in more than 10% of paediatric patients was headache.

The FDA notes also list the following unquantified adverse types of reactions:

General: Facial edema, hypertension, tachycardia

Allergic: Acute hypersensitivity reactions including anaphylaxis, angioedema, dyspnea, pruritus, rash, and urticaria

CNS symptoms: Aggressive behavior, agitation, ataxia, coma, confusion, decreased consciousness, dysarthria, encephalopathy, mania, and psychosis (including auditory and visual hallucinations), seizures, tremors

Eye: Visual abnormalities.

Gastrointestinal: Diarrhea.

Hepatobiliary tract and pancreas: Liver enzyme abnormalities, hepatitis

Hematologic: Thrombocytopenia, aplastic anemia, leukocytoclastic vasculitis, hemolytic uremic syndrome and thrombotic thrombocytopenia purpura

Skin: Erythema multiforme, rashes including photosensitivity, alopecia

I did not experience any adverse reaction at all. However, I am aware of anecdotal evidence of some people experiencing difficulties using acyclovir. It may be that my existing usage of interferon β1a worked synergistically with acyclovir and the result was I did not experience any negative effect. There is evidence going back to 1981[31] that a synergy exists between type 1 interferons and valaciclovir.

All this means is valaciclovir is a drug that should only be used in consultation with a qualified medical expert.

References

1.   Epstein, M.A., G. Henle, B.G. Achong and Y.M. Barr. *Morphological and biological studies on a virus in cultured lymphoblasts from Burkitt's Lymphoma*. The Journal of Experimental Medicine, 1965. **121**(5): p. 761.

2.   *Dr. Ernest Goodpasture Dead; Developed Vaccine for Mumps; Pathologist's Chicken Embryo Virus Led to Immunization Against Many Diseases*. The New York Times, N.Y. September 22, 1960. p. 27.

3.   Modrow, S., D. Falke, U.L. Truyen and H. Schätzl. *Molecular virology*. 2013. Springer: Heidelberg.

4.   Pender, M.P., P.A. Csurhes, J.M. Burrows and S.R. Burrows. *Defective T-cell control of Epstein-Barr virus infection in multiple sclerosis*. Clinical & Translational Immunology, 2017. **6**(1): p. e126.

5.   Allday, M.J., Q. Bazot and R.E. White, *The EBNA3 family: Two oncoproteins and a tumour suppressor that are central to the biology of EBV in B cells*. Current Topics in Microbiology and Immunology, 2015. **391**: p. 61–117.

6.   *UniProtKB - P03182 (EAR_EBVB9) Apoptosis regulator BHRF1 Organism Epstein-Barr virus (strain B95-8) (HHV-4) (Human herpesvirus 4)*. 2019; Available from: https://www.uniprot.org/uniprot/P03182#miscellaneous. Accessed January, 2021.

7.   Kempkes, B. and P.D. Ling, *EBNA2 and its coactivator EBNA-LP*. Current Topics in Microbiology and Immunology, 2015. **391**: p. 35–59.

8.   The UniProt Consortium. *UniProt: a worldwide hub of protein knowledge*. Nucleic Acids Research, 2018. **47**(D1): p. D506–D515.

9.   Bergbauer, M., M. Kalla, A. Schmeinck, C. Göbel, U. Rothbauer, S. Eck, A. Benet-Pagès, T.M. Strom and W. Hammerschmidt. *CpG-methylation regulates a class of Epstein-Barr virus promoters*. PLoS Pathogens, 2010. **6**(9): p. e1001114–e1001114.

10.   Lassmann, H., G. Niedobitek, F. Aloisi, J.M. Middeldorp and the NeuroproMiSe EBV Working Group. *Epstein–Barr virus in the multiple sclerosis brain: a controversial issue—report on a focused workshop held in the Centre for Brain Research of the Medical University of Vienna, Austria*. Brain, 2011. **134**(9): p. 2772–2786.

11.   Pender, M.P., *Infection of autoreactive B lymphocytes with EBV, causing chronic autoimmune diseases.* Trends in Immunology, 2003. **24**(11): p. 584–588.

12.   Pender, M.P., *The essential role of Epstein-Barr virus in the pathogenesis of multiple sclerosis.* Neuroscientist, 2011. **17**(4): p. 351–367.

13.   Johnson, A.J., G.L. Suidan, J. McDole and I. Pirko. *The CD8 T cell in multiple sclerosis: Suppressor cell or mediator of neuropathology?* International Review of Neurobiology, 2007. **79**: p. 73–97.

14.   Jacobson, E.M., A. Huber and Y. Tomer, *The HLA gene complex in thyroid autoimmunity: from epidemiology to etiology.* Journal of Autoimmunity, 2008. **30**(1-2): p. 58–62.

15.   Hall, M.A., K.R. Ahmadi, P. Norman, H. Snieder, A.J. MacGregor, R.W. Vaughan, T.D. Spector and J.S. Lanchbury. *Genetic influence on peripheral blood T lymphocyte levels.* Genes & Immunity, 2000. **1**(7): p. 423–427.

16.   Cross, A.R. and O.T.G. Jones, *Enzymic mechanisms of superoxide production.* Biochimica Biophisica Acta, 1991. **1057**(3): p. 281–298.

17.   Volkman, D.J., E.S. Buescher, J. Callin and A.S. Fauci. *B cell lines as models for inherited phagocytic diseases: abnormal superoxide generation in chronic granulomatous disease and giant granules in Chediak-Higashi syndrome.* The Journal of Immunology, 1984. **133**(6): p. 3006–3009.

18.   Buchczyk, D.P., T. Grune, H. Sies and L-O. Klotz. *Modifications of Glyceraldehyde-3-Phosphate Dehydrogenase Induced by Increasing Concentrations of Peroxynitrite: Early Recognition by 20S Proteasome.* Biological Chemistry, 2003. **384**(2): p. 237–241.

19.   Szabó, C., *Multiple pathways of peroxynitrite cytotoxicity.* Toxicology Letters, 2003. **140-141**: p. 105-112.

20.   Laing, K.G., A. Elia, I. Jeffrey, V. Matys, V.J. Tilleray, B. Souberbielle and M.J. Clemens. *In vivo effects of the Epstein–Barr virus small RNA EBER-1 on protein synthesis and cell growth regulation.* Virology, 2002. **297**(2): p. 253–269.

21.   Gerlitz, G. and O. Elroy-Stein, *Does EBV RNA modulate ADA mRNA translation.* Leukemia, 1998. **12**(2): p. 249.

22.   Mattle, H.P., C. Lienert and I. Greeve, *Uric acid and multiple sclerosis.* Ther Umsch, 2004. **61**(9): p. 553–555.

23.   Linnemann, C., F.A. Schildberg, A. Schurich, L. Diehl, S.I. Hegenbarth, E. Endl, S. Lacher, C.E. Müller, J. Frey, L. Simeoni, B. Schraven, D. Stabenow and P.A. Knolle. *Adenosine regulates CD8 T-cell priming by*

inhibition of membrane-proximal T-cell receptor signalling. Immunology, 2009. **128**(1pt2): p. e728.

24. Domercq, M., A. Zabala and C. Matute, *Purinergic receptors in multiple sclerosis pathogenesis.* Brain Research Bulletin, 2019. **151**: p. 38-45.

25. Fujikawa, D.G., Introduction, in *Acute Neuronal Injury: The Role of Excitotoxic Programmed Cell Death Mechanisms*, D.G. Fujikawa, Editor. 2010, Springer US: Boston, MA. pp. 1–6.

26. Abrahamyan, S., B. Eberspächer, M-M. Hoshi, L. Aly, F. Luessi, S. Groppa, L. Klotz, S.G. Meuth, C. Schroeder, T. Grüter, B. Tackenberg, F. Paul, F. Then-Bergh, T. Kümpfel, F. Weber, M. Stangel, A. Bayas, B. Wildemann, C. Heesen, U. Zetti, C. Warnke, G. Antony, N. Hessler, H. Wiendl, S. Bittner, B. Hemmer, R. Gold and A. Salmen. *Complete Epstein-Barr virus seropositivity in a large cohort of patients with early multiple sclerosis.* Journal of Neurology, Neurosurgery & Psychiatry, 2020. **91**(7): p.681–686.

27. Wallin, M.T., W.J. Culpepper, J.D. Campbell, L.M. Nelson, A. Langer-Gould, R.A. Marrie, G.R. Cutter, W.E. Kaye, L. Wagner, H. Tremlett, S.L. Buka, P. Dilokthornsakul, B. Topol, L.H. Chen and N.G. LaRocca. *The prevalence of MS in the United States.* Neurology, 2019. **92**(10): p. e1029.

28. Safrin, S., *Antiviral Agents*, in *Basic & Clinical Pharmacology, 14e*, B.G. Katzung, Ed. 2017, McGraw-Hill Education: New York, NY.

29. De Clercq, E. and H.J. Field, *Antiviral prodrugs – the development of successful prodrug strategies for antiviral chemotherapy.* British Journal of Pharmacology, 2006. **147**(1): p. 1–11.

30. Access data- US Food and Drug Administration Highlights of Prescribing Information—Valtrex.

31. Stanwick, T.L., R.F. Schinazi, D.E. Campbell, and A.J. Nahmias, *Combined antiviral effect of interferon and acyclovir on herpes simplex virus types 1 and 2.* Antimicrobial Agents and Chemotherapy, 1981. **19**(4): p. 672–674.

Chapter 15

Does Vitamin D have a Role?

How Vitamins Got Their Names

Vitamins were nearly called ergotropes. The name vitamin is a variation on a suggestion by a Polish-born chemist, Casimir Funk, who worked at the Lister Institute for Preventive Medicine in London.[1] In 1912, Funk published an article looking at the deficiency theory of disease that drew on his earlier training. He thought there must be "vitamines" or vital amines in food that were yet to be discovered.

Some years before, despite being a qualified Ph.D., he worked in a laboratory in Berlin as an animal feeder. His task was to feed nearly starving dogs. They were on pure protein diets. While some died, and Funk was blamed, he found that adding minute quantities of milk and meat led the dogs to thrive. The dogs that only had received pure protein supplements died.

In 1910, Funk left Berlin and took up a position at the Lister Institute in London. He resumed his animal experiments with the specific task of finding a protein that could treat beriberi. This time the test animals were birds. Funk discovered that an extract from polished rice could revive the near-dead creatures. In 1924, he wrote that his experiments had "in effect, proved for the first time and in an irrefutable manner, that a grave illness, leading to death, could be provoked by a diet lacking in one specific vitamine."

In his 1912 article, Funk listed a long series of common diseases that all appeared to relate to "vitamine" deficiency. He postulated that the endemic problem of rickets might also be a deficiency disease.

In 1928, scientists in Wisconsin experimented with feeding dairy herds only one type of cereal, either corn or wheat or oats. They studied the survival rates and concluded that there must be "accessory food factors yet to be discovered."[2] This led to a series of experiments in the United States, mainly involving rats. From these came evidence of a fat-soluble factor and another water-soluble factor. There was a great deal of debate about classifying them as amines. Eventually, the "e" was dropped. By consensus, it was decided to use the terms vitamin A to describe the fat-soluble factor and vitamin B for the water-soluble factor. When another water-soluble factor was found to be the cure for scurvy, it was named vitamin C.[3]

Back in 1919, rickets was known as the English disease. However, it was the Scots who had the highest incidence of this bone softening malady.

A researcher called Edward Mallenby fed a diet of oatmeal, the mainstay of Scottish people, to dogs and they failed to thrive.[4] Another scientist, called Findlay, who performed a similar experiment, found dogs kept indoors developed rickets while those allowed outdoors did not. Mallenby fed cod liver oil to his affected dogs, which seemed to cure them. He eventually thought that what is now called vitamin A may be the solution for rickets. One of the Wisconsin scientists decided to test this conclusion by bubbling oxygen through the cod liver oil to eliminate the vitamin A. This preparation no longer prevented vitamin A deficiency, but it still cured rickets. The implication was that another vitamin existed.

In 1921, scientists noted that sunlight could cure rickets.[5]

It took until the mid-1930s to piece these fragments together. Eventually, it was determined that vitamin D3 was a natural vitamin formed in the skin as a result of irradiation of 7-dehydrocholesterol by sunlight. However, this was not conclusively proved until 1978.[2]

The fourth vitamin found was called vitamin D.

There are other vitamins, but the MS discussion focusses predominately on vitamin D.

Vitamin D, Latitude, Sunlight and MS

In 1960, three scientists in the USA wrote a seminal paper: *"Some comments on the relationship of the distribution of multiple sclerosis to latitude, solar radiation, and other variables."*[6]

In a very well-constructed analysis of 1,782 patients discharged with MS between 1954 and 1958, they noted the striking feature that the birthplace of these US-based MS patients was biased towards the north, and the frequency of later illness diminished toward the south. The report also analyzed what that implied, and concluded that exposure to sunlight protected against MS.

In 1974, a new hypothesis was developed by a scientist called Goldberg. He proposed that when looking at similar regional groups, those who ate a diet rich in vitamin D (predominately fish) and also had more exposure to sunlight were better protected from developing MS.[7,8] He argued that myelin development during puberty was affected in those people who had received inadequate vitamin D early in life.

In 1991, scientists used the vitamin D metabolite, 1,25-dihydroxyvitamin D3, to suppress the MS animal model, EAE disease, in mice.[9] Pender did not dispute the effect that was achieved, but he noted that the dosage required was well above anything that can naturally be produced.[10]

~

What skin type do you have? If you expose your skin to the sun, do you turn red, then peel and go back to a pasty color, like me? Are you an African American who never burns and always tans?

If you are like me, you have skin type 111. If you are an African American, you probably have skin type V.[11]

The index of ultraviolet dosage is called the Erythemal UV Index. One unit equals 25 mW/m^2 of exposure.

If my skin type receives one standard unit of UV light, my blood concentration of vitamin D3 will rise 50-fold in eight hours. If you are my American friend with type V skin, 5–10 times the exposure will only lead to a 30-fold increase in blood D3 concentration.[12]

If you are 77–82 years old, a study in 1985 showed that after exposure to UV, you would make something like 37–42% of the previtamin D3 that an eight-year-old would make from the same dosage.[13]

The time of day, the season, the latitude, or whether you use a sunblock can all affect your skin's ability to produce vitamin D3.

Are the foods you consume, such as milk, fortified with vitamin D? That was how rickets was eliminated in many countries. Do you even know if it's been added?

In 2011, the Committee of the United States Institute of Medicine looked at the population's needs for vitamin D nutrients in North America. They concluded that the recommended daily allowance for vitamin D was 600 IU per day for ages 1–70 years and 800 IU per day for ages 71 and older. That corresponded to a serum 25-hydroxyvitamin D level of at least 20 ng/ml (50 nmol/liter), which met the requirements of at least 97.5% of the population.[14] This was intended for ordinary healthy people.

According to the Vitamin D Council, "your body can produce 10,000 to 25,000 IU of vitamin D in just a little under the time it takes for your skin to begin to burn."[15]

The committee of the Institute of Medicine also considered an extensive range of chronic ailments to assess nutrient adequacy for calcium and vitamin D. They concluded that "bone health" was the sole outcome where a vitamin D measure could be considered an indicator. They could find no data for "non-skeletal outcomes" that could support many of the claims made about other ailments to that time.

Perhaps the most significant comment was reserved for the concluding remarks of their report:

> *"Furthermore, higher levels have not been shown consistently to confer greater benefits, challenging the concept that "more is better." The Committee finds that the prevalence of vitamin D inadequacy in the North American population has been overestimated by some groups due to the use of inappropriate cut-points that greatly exceed the levels identified in this report."[14]*

Are MS and a Vitamin D Deficiency Linked?

The role of latitude in describing the incidence of MS appears quite clear, and numerous research papers repeat the original 1960 study's conclusion. Allowing for a more mobile population, MS appears more frequently as we move away from the equator.

Vitamin D deficiency is often argued to be, at least a partner in MS. Yet, when I look for a history of an association between MS and a disease of obvious vitamin D deficiency, like rickets, I cannot find it. An accusing finger from epidemiological studies points at a vitamin D deficiency as a significant component of the development of MS, yet they do not pair MS and any known vitamin D deficiency disease as two sides of the same coin.

There is no recorded pattern that suggests those unfortunate souls whose limbs were bent by a bone softening malady would then subsequently go on to suffer the symptoms of MS. The spasticity, bowel and bladder problems, or cognitive and speech impairments of a neurological nature that we see in MS do not form part of a standard description of rickets. There is some association between fatigue and rickets but I can find nothing that links the type of fatigue seen in MS with that disease.

The deficiency of vitamin D in rickets results in soft bones that create a gait best known as waddling. That term does not describe an MS gait.

~

The correct term for bone softening is osteomalacia. Bone softening (impaired bone metabolism) is not the same as bone weakening or osteoporosis (a loss of mass in the bone).

People with MS have been recorded as having a higher incidence of osteopaenia and osteoporosis. However, this is not uncommon in the general population and may affect up to 40% of post-menopausal women.[16]

A review in 2012[16] only found one study[17] that looked at the change in bone mineral density in MS patients over time. This study looked at three groups (pre-menopausal women, post-menopausal women and men) but the average expanded disability scale score of the subjects was over 6 and it is impossible to determine how much their immobility contributed to bone loss.

It is a fine line that marks the path of vitamin D deficiency. The observation is all the diseases that are now linked to vitamin D deficiency can present levels above that required to prevent rickets.[18] Yet where is the literature linking numerous cancers, cardiovascular diseases, Type 1 diabetes mellitus, Crohn's disease, as well as MS, to rickets? A greater vitamin D deficiency does not create a clearer path to these diseases.

~

A Danish study[19] of 521 patients with MS was compared with a matched control of 921 healthy people. All had been born in Denmark after May

1981 and each had a small amount of dried neonatal blood, drawn from a heel prick within a week of birth, stored in a national biobank. The assayed dried blood was considered to be strongly correlated to neonatal cord blood. After excluding potential confounding factors (gestational age, birthweight, maternal age at birth, Apgar score, and parental ethnicity), the researchers noted that children born with 25(OH)D levels less than 30 nmol/L were at an increased risk of MS. However, they concluded the additional benefit of higher levels was less clear.[19]

A similar study from Sweden[20] found no association at all between MS and vitamin D levels of newborns; however, that review found a considerable degradation had occurred in the older blood samples, due to inferior storage conditions.

The Danish study also concluded that vitamin D levels in the cord blood may not correlate well with maternal mid-gestation levels. Neither did they have complete profiles on the data concerning sun exposure, including outdoor physical activity, body mass index, diet, and intake of vitamin D supplements in adolescence and adult life of either the control group or the MS patients. They concluded, "*Thus our findings largely reflect the association between neonatal vitamin D levels and MS diagnosis up to age 30, and may not necessarily be applicable to MS onset in older individuals*".[19]

However, their most significant conclusion was -

"We observed an inverse association between neonatal levels of 25(OH) D and risk of MS, thus the higher the level of 25(OH)D among neonates the lower their risk of MS in later life. However, we cannot exclude the possibility that this apparent beneficial effect is mediated by a correlation between 25(OH)D levels at birth and levels later in life, in which case maternal vitamin D supplementation would not reduce MS risk in the offspring. This uncertainty notwithstanding, the high global prevalence of hypovitaminosis D among pregnant women and the fact that increasing maternal vitamin D levels is likely to reduce the mother's risk of MS as well as her offspring's provides a rationale for universal vitamin D supplementation in pregnancy."[19]

One Norwegian study in 2008[21] looked at an extremely rare hereditary disease called vitamin D–dependent rickets type I (VDDR I). This disease first presents symptoms in early childhood. Although the study noted the incidence of MS in Norway as 1.5 persons per 1,000 they could not, because of its rarity, establish a similar ratio for VDDR I. The researchers did manage to find three women, all in their fifties, with the genetic marker of VDDR I who were diagnosed with MS.

As all had been diagnosed with VDDR I in childhood, they had all been given cholecalciferol (vitamin D) supplements since childhood. Blood samples from two of the patients were available and they had normal and above-normal levels of 1,25-dihydroxycholecalciferol. The lack of a simple cause-and-effect relationship between vitamin D levels and subsequent MS led the researchers to conclude that only the period of early childhood and life in the womb could be regarded as the susceptible windows for vitamin D deficiency as a causal link.

The Metabolism of Vitamin D

The precursor to vitamin D is provitamin D. In humans this is a lipid called 7-dehydrocholesterol. It is a relatively rigid 4-ringed structure existing in the lipid bilayer of the plasma membranes of our skin. When exposed to ultraviolet radiation, one of these rings, called the B ring, opens and becomes less rigid. The plasma membrane then becomes more permeable to various ions, including calcium. When the ring opens, the lipid becomes previtamin D3. In this form, it is unstable and keeps transforming into vitamin D3 while being ejected from the plasma membrane. A vitamin-D-binding protein in our capillary beds then draws the vitamin D3 into our circulatory system. This protein transports the D3 to the liver, where it is transformed into 25-hydroxyvitamin D3, the dominant circulating form of the vitamin.

To become hormonally active, the circulating form must then be converted in the kidneys into 1,25-dihydroxyvitamin D3. In this final form, the vitamin can bind to a vitamin D receptor to become involved in gene transcription.[22] However, that receptor is part of a larger group and does not act on its own. The vitamin D receptor must form a complex with another receptor, called the retinoid X receptor (RXR).[23, 24] Is that receptor always functional? Not always.[25–27]

As it is fat-soluble, excess vitamin D3 is stored in body fat. A study published in *The American Journal of Clinical Nutrition* in September 2000 noted that obese individuals who had large stores of body fat sequestered vitamin D3 in their fat rather than having it circulate in the blood.[28] Despite having adequate exposure to both UV and dietary sources of vitamin D3, these obese subjects, as opposed to the non-obese, consistently measured as having vitamin D3 deficiency. Their fat became a one-way sink for the vitamin.

The study concluded that there was a strong correlation between body mass and vitamin D3 deficiency and that obese people needed proportionally higher doses of oral supplementation to compensate.

It is difficult to define a sufficient level of vitamin D. Free vitamin D is only a tiny proportion of circulating vitamin D.[29] The term "bioavailable" might sometimes be used for forms of the vitamin not bound to the vitamin D receptor. However, they may still be bound to albumin and not really be free.[30] What is meant by free or bioavailable vitamin D is not standardized across the various studies.

~

I have read through many studies on vitamin D and MS. Often, I was left wondering if the link was as clear cut as the writers suggested. One paper, from 2016, echoed my thoughts:

"Several analytical epidemiological studies have suggested an association between vitamin D deficiency and multiple sclerosis. The biological basis of this association is unknown."[29]

Perhaps, given differences in latitude, body shape, the activity of RXR receptors, skin type, and general health, vitamin D is just a bystander. It ends up being photographed, fingerprinted, interviewed and studied. It is suspicious because it isn't always there. It may be a suspect simply because MS happens in its neighborhood. It still, however, may just be an innocent party.

~

Previtamin D, or 7-dehydrocholesterol, is involved in 23 metabolite pathways.[31]

It is found inside and outside cells, in the liver, the skin, in the testes, the brain, the adrenal glands, in the unborn fetus, and in the fibroblasts that make up our connective tissue.

We can make it, and we can consume it. Our young can take it in through breast milk. It is integral to lipid transport and metabolism. Cells use it in inflammatory responses and for signaling. Membranes are stabilized by it. Energy pathways utilize it to store substrates. It is both a hormone and a signaling agent to other hormones.

We find it in our blood, our cerebrospinal fluid, and our urine. It is everywhere and it is necessary.

The formation of 7-dehydrocholesterol starts with glucose. This sugar is converted by glycolysis to pyruvate, a three-carbon molecule. A further step removes one more carbon to make acetyl-CoA, the feedstock for the Krebs cycle.

If acetyl-CoA is not used in the Krebs cycle, the surplus molecules combine with each other, becoming acetoacetyl-CoA. This new structure reacts with more of the same molecules and eventually becomes hydroxy-3-methylglutaryl-coenzyme A. This is a mouthful and is better known as HMG CoA. The enzyme that breaks this substance down is called a reductase and is the target of statins as cholesterol-reducing agents. By using statins, the metabolism of the pathway is blocked at this point.

Unchecked, HMG CoA breaks down into mevalonate. From this point, there are many steps, but if we jump between the main ones, mevalonate becomes, through transformation and aggregation, a product called isoprene units. Many of these units are used to create another product called squalene. The creation of squalene doesn't happen easily. There are 21 steps involved in this conversion.

Squalene becomes lanosterol, the precursor of 7-dehydrocholesterol. From this stage, the synthesis of vitamin D begins.

When your doctor looks at your cholesterol levels, he is measuring a 27-carbon molecule that descends from lanosterol.

The problem is, if you use a statin to block the enzyme that allows mevalonate to be formed, you have also blocked the pathway to making the precursors of vitamin D. Additionally, you have blocked CoQ10 formation. So, you are interfering with the energy-making processes. A string of other functions will be interrupted, including the creation of bile acids and steroid formation. Statin side effects include muscle weakness, muscle pain, or aching (myalgia), stiffness, muscle tenderness, cramps and arthralgia (joint pain).[32]

If you take a statin, you should be unsurprised if your doctor tells you that your vitamin D level is low.

~

I lived the first nine years of my life in a country town. I was always outdoors. On the first day that the local swimming pool would reopen at the end of winter, I would pester my mother to let me go swimming. The open paddocks were my playground, and my bicycle was my source of freedom. In those days, sunburn was a way of life. I never lacked the opportunity to soak up the sunlight.

All my life has involved the sun. Skin cancers are regularly being cut from me now. I do not feel the vitamin D argument sits well with my history.

If you are deficient in vitamin D, there are so many variables to assess before considering if this vitamin has played a role in your MS.

I have never taken a vitamin D supplement, but I do spend time each day with the sunshine on my shoulder.

Vitamin D Supplementation

According to the food standards for Australia and New Zealand, two forms of vitamin D are permitted to be added to foods; vitamin D2, derived from certain fungi and yeast, or vitamin D3 which is derived from the greasy substance in sheep wool called lanolin.[33] They are considered to technologically perform identically and have similar stability when included in a food matrix. However, there is debate about their bioequivalence.

Vitamin D activity is lost in foods during the commercial shelf life because it is unstable when exposed to heat, moisture, oxygen, contact with trace minerals and UV light.

The standard states, *"Based on (food) industry experience the average vitamin D loss of typical shelf products is considered to be 10% per month at ambient temperature and humidity. As breakfast cereal products usually have a shelf life of between 9 and 12 months"*. The standard provides a theoretical worked example to indicate *"there is approximately a 70% loss of vitamin D content during storage of a fortified breakfast cereal at the end of its commercial shelf life of 12 months"*.[33]

Hypercalcaemia (elevated calcium in blood) and subsequent hypercalciuria (excessive calcium excretion) are indicators of toxicity linked to high vitamin D intakes. Hypercalcaemia is caused by increased bone resorption (causing more circulating calcium and phosphorus) and impaired bone mineralisation through a mechanism that is not fully understood.

The standard says *"long term health outcomes associated with prolonged hypercalcaemia or hypercalciuria are soft tissue calcification and eventually renal and cardiovascular damage. These outcomes are achieved only through high oral intakes (as in supplements) and not through sun exposure or, because of the relatively low vitamin D content of food, through dietary intakes"*.[33]

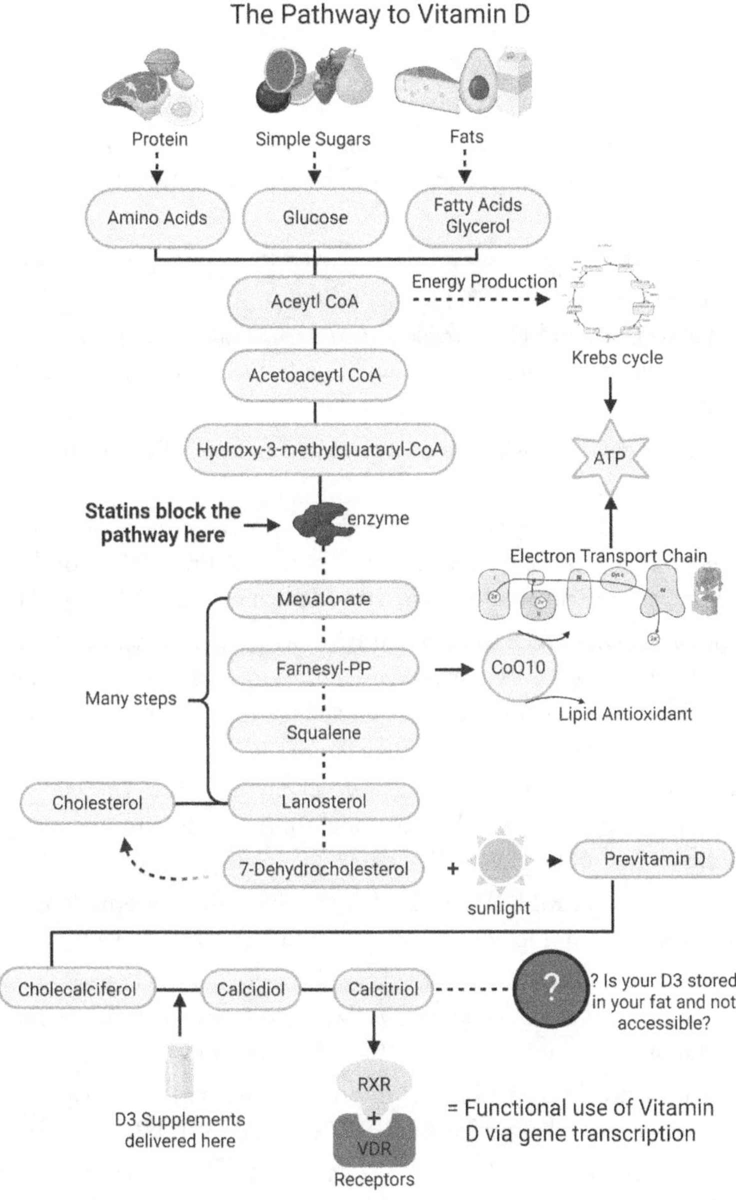

Figure 15.1 The biological pathway to vitamin D.
Created with BioRender.

References

1. Maltz, A., *Casimer Funk, nonconformist nomenclature, and networks surrounding the discovery of vitamins.* The Journal of Nutrition, 2013. **143**(7): p. 1013–1020.

2. Deluca, H.F. *History of the discovery of vitamin D and its active metabolites.* BoneKEy reports, 2014. **3**: p. 479–479.

3. Grzybowski, A. and K. Pietrzak, *Albert Szent-Györgyi (1893-1986): The scientist who discovered vitamin C.* Clinics in Dermatology, 2013. **31**(3): p. 327–331.

4. *An experimental investigation on rickets.* The Lancet, 1919. **193**(4985): p. 407–412.

5. Hess, A.F. and P. Gutman, *The cure of infantile rickets by sunlight as demonstrated by a chemical alteration of the blood.* Proceedings of the Society for Experimental Biology and Medicine, 1921. **19**(1): p. 31–34.

6. Acheson, E.D., C.A. Bachrach and F.M. Wright, *Some comments on the relationship of the distribution of multiple sclerosis to latitude, solar radiation, and other variables.* Acta Psychiatrica Scandinavica, 1960. **35**(S147): p. 132–147.

7. Goldberg, P., *Multiple sclerosis: vitamin D and calcium as environmental determinants of prevalence.* International Journal of Environmental Studies, 1974. **6**(1): p. 19–27.

8. Goldberg, P. and R.H. Walmsley, *Letters to the editor.* International Journal of Environmental Studies, 1974. **6**(2–3): p. 197–199.

9. Lemire, J.M. and D.C. Archer, *1,25-dihydroxyvitamin D3 prevents the in vivo induction of murine experimental autoimmune encephalomyelitis.* The Journal of clinical investigation, 1991. **87**(3): p. 1103–1107.

10. Pender, M.P., *The essential role of Epstein-Barr virus in the pathogenesis of multiple sclerosis.* Neuroscientist, 2011. **17**(4): p. 351–67.

11. Oakley, A. and D., Hamilton, New Zealand, 2012. *Fitzpatrick skin phototype.* 2019; Available from: https://www.dermnetnz.org/topics/skin-phototype/.

12. Clemens, T.L., J.S. Adams, S.L. Henderson and M.F. Holick, *Increased skin pigment reduces the capacity of skin to synthesise vitamin D3.* Lancet, 1982. **1**(8263): p. 74–76.

13.   Maclaughlin, J., M.F. Holick and K. Kasper, *Aging decreases the capacity of human skin to produce vitamin D3.* Nutrition in Clinical Practice, 1986. **1**(1): p. 57-58.

14.   Ross, A.C., J.E. Manson, S.A. Abrams, J.F. Aloia, P.M. Brannon, S.K. Clinton, R.A. Durazo-Arvizu, J.C. Gallagher, R.L. Gallo, G. Jones, C.S. Kovacs, S.T. Mayne, C.J. Rosen and S.A. Shapses, *The 2011 report on dietary reference intakes for calcium and vitamin D from the Institute of Medicine: What clinicians need to know.* The Journal of Clinical Endocrinology & Metabolism, 2011. **96**(1): p. 53–58.

15.   Horlick, M.F., *Environmental factors that influence the cutaneous production of vitamin D^{1–3}.* The Americal Journal of Clinical Nutrition, 1995. **61**(suppl): 638S–645S

16.   Dobson R., S. Ramagopalan and G. Giovannoni, *Bone health and multiple sclerosis.* Multiple Sclerosis Journal, 2012. **18**(11):1522–1528. doi:10.1177/1352458512453362

17.   Cosman, F., J. Nieves and L. Komar, *Fracture history and bone loss in patients with MS.* Neurology 1998; **51**:1161–1165

18.   Sintzel, M.B., M. Rametta and A.T. Reder, *Vitamin D and multiple sclerosis: A comprehensive review.* Neurology and Therapy, 2018. **7**(1), 59–85. https://doi.org/10.1007/s40120-017-0086-4

19.   Nielsen, N.M., K.L. Munger, N. Koch-Henriksen, D.M. Hougaard, M. Magyari, K.T. Jørgensen, M. Lundqvist, J. Simonsen, T. Jess, A. Cohen, E. Stenager and A. Ascherio, *Neonatal vitamin D status and risk of multiple sclerosis: A population-based case-control study.* Neurology, 2017. **88**(1), 44–51. https://doi.org/10.1212/WNL.0000000000003454

20.   Ueda, P., F. Rafatnia, M. Bäärnhielm, R. Fröbom, G. Korzunowicz, R. Lönnerbro, A.K. Hedström, D. Eyles, T. Olsson and L. Alfredsson, *Neonatal vitamin D status and risk of multiple sclerosis.* Annals of Neurology, 2014. **76**:338–346. https://doi.org/10.1002/ana.24210

21.   Torkildsen Ø, P.M. Knappskog, H.I. Nyland and K. Myhr, *Vitamin D-dependent rickets as a possible risk factor for multiple sclerosis.* Archives of Neurology, 2008. **65**(6):809–811. doi:10.1001/archneur.65.6.809

22.   Raghuwanshi, A., S.S. Joshi and S. Christakos, *Vitamin D and multiple sclerosis.* Journal of Cellular Biochemistry, 2008. **105**(2): p. 338–343.

23.   Bettoun, D.J., T.P. Burris, K.A, Houck, D.W. Buck 2nd, K.R. Stayrook, B. Khalifa, J. Lu, W.W. Chin and S. Nagpal, *Retinoid X receptor is a nonsilent major contributor to vitamin D receptor-mediated transcriptional*

activation. Molecular Endocrinology, 2003. **17**(11): p. 2320–2328.

24.   Orlov, I., N. Rochel, D. Moras and B.P. Klaholz, *Structure of the full human RXR/VDR nuclear receptor heterodimer complex with its DR3 target DNA.* The EMBO Journal, 2012. **31**(2): p. 291-300.

25.   Yagishita, N., Y. Yamamoto, T. Yoshizawa, K. Sekine, Y. Uematsu, H. Murayama, Y. Nagai, W. Krezel, P. Chambon, T. Matsumoto and S. Kato, *Aberrant growth plate development in VDR/RXR gamma double null mutant mice.* Endocrinology, 2001. **142**(12): p. 5332–5341.

26.   Brabender, J., K.D. Danenberg, R. Metzger, P.M. Schneider, R.V. Lord, S. Groshen, D.D. Tsao-Wei, J. Park, D. Salonga, A.H. Höischer and P.V. Danenberg, *The role of retinoid X receptor messenger RNA expression in curatively resected non-small cell lung cancer.* Clinical Cancer Research, 2002. **8**(2): p. 438.

27.   Johnson, B.S., R.A.S. Chandraratna, R.A. Heyman, E.A. Allegretto, L. Mueller and S.J. Collins, *Retinoid X receptor (RXR) agonist-induced Aativation of dominant-negative RXR-retinoic acid receptor alpha 403 heterodimers is developmentally regulated during myeloid differentiation.* Molecular and Cellular Biology, 1999. **19**(5): p. 3372.

28.   Wortsman, J., L.Y. Matsuoka, T.C. Chen, Z. Lu and M.F. Holick, *Decreased bioavailability of vitamin D in obesity.* The American Journal of Clinical Nutrition, 2000. **72**(3): p. 690–693.

29.   Matías-Guíu, J., C. Oreja-Guevara, J.A. Matias-Guiu and U. Gomez-Pinedo, *Vitamin D and remyelination in multiple sclerosis.* Neurología, 2018. **33**(3): p. 177–186.

30.   Bikle, D.D., P.K. Siiteri, E. Ryzen and J.G. Haddad, *Serum protein binding of 1,25-dihydroxyvitamin D: a reevaluation by direct measurement of free metabolite levels.* The Journal of Clinical Endocrinology and Metabolism, 1985. **61**(5): p. 969.

31.   National Center for Biotechnology Information. PubChem Compound Summary for CID 439423, 7-Dehydrocholesterol. https://pubchem.ncbi.nlm.nih.gov/compound/7-Dehydrocholesterol. Accessed January 2021.

32.   Pennisi, M., G. Di Bartolo, G. Malaguarnera, R. Bella, G. Lanza and M. Malaguarnera, *Vitamin D serum levels in patients with statin-induced musculoskeletal pain.* Disease markers, 2019. **2019**: p. 3549402–3549402

33.   https://www.foodstandards.gov.au/code/applications/Documents/A1090-VitaminD-CFS-SD1.pdf

Chapter 16

One Step at a Time

Lying in a Bed

In 2014, I was able to walk, with some difficulty, into the hospital. After ten days in the cardiology ward, my gait had reduced to a shuffle.

I could still stand reasonably upright, but needed the IV pole on its rollers, with all the wires and drips hanging from it, to assist me.

The distance from my bed to the toilet in the corner of the wardroom was as far as I could go.

Longer trips involved a wheelchair, but I didn't think too hard about the process. It was just the way the hospital did it. Sometimes they wheeled me to an MRI then left me shivering in a cold corridor. On those occasions, I mulled over the idea of abandoning the chair and marching back to my bed. The obvious problem for me was that I didn't know how far I could go.

I was fed up with being moved like a parcel from one point to the next. My preference was to walk, to challenge myself and find my boundaries.

Days earlier, no one spoke down to me. Now I was treated like a simpleton. If I got out of the wheelchair and found my way back to bed, my concern was that it would be an invitation for the hospital to regard me as a renegade. The possibility that the wrong move might trigger some drug-based retribution "for my own good" hung over me. So, I sat and waited.

Eventually, I was moved from cardiology to a general ward.

Starting Rehab

The hospital had two facilities for rehabilitation. One was a room tucked away beyond a labyrinth of corridors, and the other, a better-equipped main gym, was across a quiet street in a converted two-story mansion. I used both.

My initial introduction to the rehabilitation process was in the main gym. An orderly introduced himself and announced he would wheel me there.

I mulled over the idea of giving in to my weakness. It wasn't that long ago that I had walked out of my office. The last thing I wanted, now, was to surrender that capability.

"Do I have to be wheeled? Can't I just walk there?" I said as I stood.

"Most people prefer the chair, but you can walk if you want. I will go with you to be sure you're OK," he replied. I felt he was just humoring a difficult patient.

"The whole point of going is to help me to walk, so it seems silly to ride," I said, and he gave a good-natured nod.

It was a walk that should have taken five minutes, but it took twenty. We stopped several times, chatting as we went. My little steps and tight torso made it feel like a trudge up a sand dune. Nevertheless, after the sterile hospital, fresh air felt wonderful.

~

When I arrived at the gym, it seemed to be the domain of professionals. Everyone looked busy, and many patients had apparent problems. Some were road trauma victims; others were stroke cases. All patients had some sort of neurological problem.

I would come here for the next year. Initially, I went daily as an inpatient. Then there was a slow taper in visits as I became an outpatient.

Some people were very ill. A few struggled to do simple tasks. I remember watching one poor wheelchair-bound man with bandages wrapped around his head, spitting a lot of bile into a plastic bag held by a physical therapist.

A young girl with lupus came regularly. She had to be hauled from her chair each day and was practically carried like a wounded soldier as they tried to find out how to make her legs work.

Others looked fine, and I wondered why they were there. Perhaps that is what they thought about me.

My initial treatment was to lie face down on a bench while hot gel packs, wrapped in towels, were laid along my spine. As the heat crept into my back muscles, I felt some relief. The gel packs were scorching. Despite the insulating towels, the heat became too intense, and the packs started to burn. I now view their application as amateurish and process-driven. Appropriately done, heat packs are a great relief. In this case, they were only offered for the first few days, and their application lacked integration with any exercise. Why did they bother to warm up my back muscles and then ignore my back for the next hour?

My Muscle Tightness Increases

As I had done Pilates for ten years, I was familiar with how I should move my body. The physical therapists had a different perspective.

Their favorite piece of equipment was a small trampoline-like bouncer that stood about six inches off the ground. They were obsessed with the tightness in my left ankle. By making me prance on this bouncer, the plan was to improve my range of flexion magically. It never happened through doing this exercise. Sometimes they would grab my leg and try to force me to move it a different way. I just found that the yanking of my leg was crude and futile.

My big concern was the tightness that enveloped me from my ribs to my hips. Every step I took felt like I was moving big wooden blocks in my torso. I had become a giant puppet made up of segments that rolled against each other to imitate movement. No one could see this, and no one was interested in what I could feel.

In my Pilates classes, I had gradually learned the names of some muscles. The big muscle that starts near your mid-back and sweeps down toward the front of your hips is called the psoas. This is the muscle that, when contracted, works like a pulley to lift your leg. Drawing your knee towards your chest relies on this muscle shortening. The leg muscles are not strong enough on their own to achieve the movement. I knew my psoas wasn't working correctly.

"My psoas is tight; my psoas is tight," was my endless refrain. The physical therapists didn't care. They only wanted to look at my ankle.

About a week into the process, a young man was put in charge of my session. All the other therapists I had seen were women. I was frustrated by my ever-tightening torso. What were the magic words to get someone to look?

I changed tack.

"My hip flexors are really tight," I said to the man.

"Oh, I can fix that," he said with some certainty.

We went to a bench, and he asked me to sit on the end and then lie down. My legs went over the edge, and I lay along the bench. He then proceeded to push one leg down while I wrapped my hands around the other and pulled it towards me. The action is called a Thomas stretch. As he pushed down on my leg, his expression changed.

"Gee, your psoas is tight," he remarked.

I rolled my eyes. "Finally!" I thought.

To deal with the tightness, he drove his thumb, painfully, into parts of my groin. The leg collapsed. He repeated this several times on both sides. At last, there was a little relief.

"I need this done more regularly," I said as gratefully as I could.

"Then you'll have to see me," he turned his head towards the gaggle of female therapists, "They won't do it."

"Really?" I asked.

In the following year, I never saw him again. Occasionally, a female therapist performed a faux version of the stretch. Their body language betrayed their disdain for getting involved. It is one of the more belittling experiences to be expecting a good stretch and instead be treated like a prop in a pantomime. The overwhelming impression I was left with was that they considered touching a man anywhere to be degrading. They would never willingly relieve my tightness by using a stretching technique. I was used to being slapped gently by Pilates instructors to wake up a particular muscle group. This priggishness was just foreign to me.

Equipment

The equipment in the gym also surprised me. By comparison, my Pilates studio was very well set up. Suddenly, I felt I had taken more than a step backward. Only one therapist had a Pilates background. Her colleagues thought her knowledge was exotic. The solitary piece of Pilates equipment was a locally made reformer. As the physical therapists didn't know how to use it, they locked it in an office on the floor above. I was gobsmacked.

Later, I discovered the smaller facility in the hospital also had a reformer. It was the sort that might be advertised on a late-night advertorial show. I spotted this unbalanced, structurally weak contraption, which had only a passing resemblance to real equipment, tucked aimlessly in a corner. It was the sort of junk that only a bean-counting bookkeeper could approve. In essence, it was functionally useless. I hauled it out of the corner, set it up and tried some simple stretches.

A student physical therapist came over and watched me go through a few basic movements. The concept fascinated him, and it was the first time he had seen one being used. The therapist with a Pilates background came in, and I recognized her. She just left me to play and attended to other patients. Later we had a brief chat. I concluded that Pilates was viewed as something possibly useful, but that the majority of therapists were so enamored with their qualifications that it was beneath them.

~

Most of the hospital equipment belonged in a walk-in, unattended, main street gym. It was equipment that assumed that your muscles could move properly. Mine couldn't.

Finding a Teammate

Sarah, my Pilates instructor, visited me many times when I was in the hospital. At first, she came for evening visits. As time progressed, she asked to come into the gym to understand better what had happened to me.

On her first gym visit, the physical therapists took Sarah aside for 30 minutes. I have no idea what they told her, but she was determined to come again. She observed what they did, and later gave me daily Pilates classes for the first three weeks after I was discharged from the hospital. Each of those classes had no set length. They were as long as we both needed them to be. The hospital, by comparison, worked by set routine and a timetable.

On perhaps Sarah's third visit to the gym, I was told to walk up the large central staircase of the old mansion. The only rule was I could not hold onto a banister.

I stood at the foot of the stairs and contemplated the situation. It was a sizeable climb. My left foot lifted from the ground and landed on the first riser. I could sense the wobble in my body. My right foot left the ground and glided passed its companion. It did not reach the next riser. Instead, I crumpled in a heap on the stairs.

My collapse was so rapid I didn't perceive it as a fall. Suddenly, my chest was on the carpet. The therapist's voice behind me rang out, "keep going." I wobbled back up to standing and tried again, falling twice more.

Finally, I was on the landing and turned to look back. "Can you come down without holding on?" she asked.

The staircase may have had a big red carpet, but to me, looking down, it may as well have been a giant slalom. "I doubt it," was my considered reply.

Holding on to the rail, I descended the stair and repeated the exercise several times. The physical therapists approach was just to order me to do it. There was no guidance. Sarah watched this and formulated a plan.

Over time, Sarah taught me how to balance on one leg. She was the only one who bothered to show me how to move my body through space. Sarah was the one who taught me how to ascend and descend without grabbing for support. The physical therapists taught me nothing.

Becoming an Outpatient

Eventually, I was sent home. There was a plan that I should come back to the hospital each day and continue the rehabilitation work. As soon as this was decided, Sarah told me I should also come to the Pilates studio. The distance between the hospital and the studio could be covered by a tram that ran practically door to door. To reach the hospital from home meant either a walk followed by a thirty-minute tram ride or a train trip with a walk at each end.

Ten days after I was discharged from the hospital, my wife left to stay at a property we owned interstate. She had driven me to the station a few times before she left. More frequently, one of my sons drove me to and from the station.

The hospital banned me from driving until the new year. That was three months away. Although I was sometimes unsure of the wisdom of it I walked to and from the station. The fences of my neighborhood's properties gave me something to lean against if I needed it. A large part of my day was about moving from one place to another. Now, I don't regret any of the walks. They were so obviously what I needed to do.

The first time I left the hospital to go to the studio, I clambered up the steps of the tram. My instinct was that I must be getting better, and I thought I was doing quite well. When I reached the top of the three-step climb and looked down the tram, about thirty people were staring at me. Many rose to offer their seats. The lady nearest me demanded I sit.

The tram driver kept the tram at the stop until I did take a seat.

"Maybe I'm overestimating things," I concluded to myself. Time would prove that my recovery would be more challenging than I expected.

The Real Start of my Rehab

The first few sessions with Sarah weren't actually Pilates classes. In the studio, she wrapped rubber bands, called TheraBands, around my legs, and made me crabwalk around the room. We tried balancing on one leg and did simple exercises to see what I was capable of doing. Everything was difficult, and I was frustrated by my lack of ability.

Nearly every day, we left the studio and walked around the block. The rules were straightforward: I was not allowed to grab anything, and I had to lift my left foot, so it didn't scrape on the ground. It was so much more demanding than the hospital gym.

As we walked, we talked. Every few steps, she scolded me if I touched a wall. To walk around a small city block took at least thirty minutes. Sometimes we stopped halfway for a coffee. Speed was not the objective. Setting the pattern of how I moved was the sole purpose.

After a few days, we again left the studio and found the rear staircase of the building. It was devoid of passing traffic, and every sound echoed through its chamber.

Standing behind me, Sarah made me climb about five steps. Each move required a constant stream of corrective comments. Everything needed to be analyzed: how I stood, how I balanced, what muscles to concentrate on to lift my leg, where to put my foot, how to shift my weight, and there was the constant reinforcement that I could not grab the rail. I kept thinking about how impossible it would be for her to catch me if I fell.

Three months before, I could execute complex transactions, remember a vast array of information, and hold several conversations at once. I never thought about how I moved. I just did it. Now all my concentration was focused on what she asked. That was now my limit.

Floundering in a Pool

The physical therapists suggested that I spend some time in their therapy pool. I had heard that moving against the weight of water helped many people recover from injury. I agreed to give it a try.

Hydrotherapy was probably the most disappointing protocol I attempted. The pool came up to my waist. It gently sloped, so, at its deepest, it came to the top of my chest. Perhaps my expectations were too high. I anticipated a set program that I would follow.

My first visit was much like all the subsequent sessions. I entered an indoor pool facility where I waited until someone spoke to me. Usually, I was asked to change and report back. Each time I found walking across the wet and slippery floor quite challenging. My legs were stiff, there was nothing to hang on to, and the floor looked hard. Sometimes I walked with my arms slightly wide of my body to help me balance. No one ever commented, and I just tried to be a silent, compliant patient. Eventually, someone would tell me to go down the steps into the water. Once in, I was expected to walk around.

The whole process felt aimless. Very occasionally, someone would give me some simple tasks to do. As I had become quite uncoordinated, I don't feel I did a very good job at any of them. Most of the time, I found myself standing in the middle of the pool, wondering why I was there. It might have been a therapy pool for some people, but it increasingly felt like a pond of futility to me.

The therapists sometimes came into the water but often just stayed at the side. They laughed and joked with people who seemed quite content just to stand there. I wanted to do something. Instead, I just felt like a fool who was wasting his time. Nothing useful came out of these sessions. Did they think there was some logical benefit in just standing in water? The therapists often praised each other about how good they were in the pool. In the end, I said I didn't feel I was getting anything out of it, so I was moved to a therapy session they called "running".

Becoming Much Tighter

Me: "I just feel like I want to rip myself apart."

Sarah: "Don't say that! I don't like those words you use. You can't say rip or tear. Just don't!"

Me: "But that's what I feel like. It feels like I'm being compressed. I just want to get out."

Sarah: "Well, don't say tear or rip."

Me: "I'd like to mobilize this group of muscles."

Sarah: "That's better."

Me; "I'd still rather rip them apart."

At this point, Sarah would turn away.

Sarah and I often argued. It was usually good-natured, but we did test each other. I was frustrated by repetition and by the things I couldn't do. She was trying to teach other people who had an equal demand on her time. I would huff and groan in the background and constantly talk.

After the first month, I switched from daily classes to three Pilates classes per week. Sarah was the only person I wanted to teach me. As her private life was unsettled, she kept trying to introduce me to other teachers to free up her day. Managing her staff and business partner hung over her like a great weight. Apart from being regular, I must have been the client from hell.

Nonetheless, I will never forget a time after one evening class. Sarah stood at the sink in the studio, washing used mugs that had built up during the day. She was facing away from me.

"I wish you'd get better," she said softly, her head bowed forward.

"I'm trying," I replied, full of guilt and touched by her tone.

"I know," she said, staring down at her busy hands.

The Therapists Do Some Damage

After the hydro sessions in the pool had proved so fruitless, I was switched to the running class. This seemed to be an aspirational group. I don't know why they called it running. Maybe sometimes people reached that level.

The most common exercise I did in this class was to stand on the balls of my feet and move, in a quick motion, along a corridor and then come back. Occasionally, I had to do a sort of sideways skip along the same length. I couldn't do that without someone holding my hands. It felt like I was learning some medieval dance when that happened. The more I did this exercise, the more painful the side and front of my hips became. Mentioning it was creating discomfort just generated a shrug of the shoulders and a suggestion to do it again.

My leg and foot exercises in my Pilates classes were compromised as the soreness in my hips carried through from the rehab. Externally rotating my legs caused sharp pain. It felt like I had the points of knitting needles jammed in my hips.

"Running" felt like my pelvis was shifted out of position, and it did nothing to fix my increasingly more spastic left leg. I became very quickly heartily sick to death of this program, but kept going despite my better instincts. Often my eyes would well up as the frustration of exercising through pain increased.

As months rolled by and my insurance funding for rehabilitation was coming to an end, I began a series of appointments with the 2IC of the hospital's rehabilitation unit. I told her how sore my hip was. She looked at it and said, "Maybe it's some sort of bursitis of the trochanter." When I told the therapists, the response was almost immediate.

"Well, that's the end of your rehabilitation. There's not much more we can do here. How would you feel about some botox injections? We can arrange for you to go to our spasticity unit. They are very good."

"OK," I said. "Anything is worth a try."

My First Botox Shots

The spasticity clinic was some distance from the hospital. I saw some of the same therapists there who had been in the gym. They all worked with the professor who was ultimately in charge of the whole rehabilitation program.

I liked him. He was smart and relatable without the air of superiority that some academics of his status cultivate.

He explained how the botox worked and that it would release my leg. On this first occasion, I was given three injections of botox into the back of my leg, two into the hamstrings, and one into the calf. The professor was complimentary towards my Pilates classes.

"Keep going," he said.

Finding Relief in Painful Massage

Within two days of leaving the hospital, I had started to develop a noticeable hunch in my back. This was accompanied by my left leg scribing an arc when I walked rather than merely moving back and forth. The tightness in my torso was my overwhelming concern. Although I may not have looked like it, I felt bent over and twisted. The pervasive feeling of being made out of blocks of wood was always with me. The physical therapists never paid any attention to these symptoms. They were only interested in my legs.

Sarah started to introduce exercises to lengthen and strengthen my psoas, but I wasn't very good at them.

My back muscles were starting to hurt. I began to walk like a spider who had survived a hit from a fly swat.

~

After my wife had gone, it was up to me to buy food for the house. I was, justifiably, banned from driving so I had to take a tram to the shops.

Before I had gone to the hospital, I had found a cheap massage shop at a mall. It was staffed by Chinese who barely spoke any English. There was an old man there who used to rub my back. It was not sophisticated, but it helped. Now that was too far away.

In a small arcade off the main street, I found a similar-looking shop. Again, a Chinese man rubbed my back, and it helped.

That was at 11 am. At 2 pm, I went back. An older red-haired man had replaced him, so I asked him to massage my back.

"Oh, my goodness," he said as he put his fingers on my back, "this is going to hurt." He was right. It did.

That was my introduction to Darryl. He owned the studio, which had not been open for long.

The next morning, I went to see Darryl again. As it was a public holiday, it was a day without either rehab or Pilates.

At 2 pm, I struggled to open the shop door but put my twisted left leg inside and pushed my bent body into Darryl's studio. He looked, open-mouthed, at me.

"Do it again," I said.

Despite the work he had done in the morning, I was already back in my twisted, painful shape.

Darryl was amazed. No one had ever reacted like this before. My body was like toughened steel. He confessed, much later, that his fingers hurt after he had worked on me. Over time, I tried each of his employees, and they also had never seen anyone as tight. Surprise was always the initial reaction, then their competitive spirits would kick in. Often, they would go well past the hour just to achieve a result. They all hurt.

I often would say, "It feels so good when you stop." Just to encourage them to keep going.

At this time, I was seeing both Sarah and the hospital rehab people. Occasionally, the massage could bruise me, but I didn't care. I definitely needed Sarah, and I definitely needed Darryl. The rehab people with the formal qualifications just weren't in the same league.

Labels Stick

On my second visit to the spasticity clinic, I told the professor that his 2IC had diagnosed bursitis of the trochanter. Without checking for himself, he accepted the diagnosis. I thought that was strange as the initial opinion was qualified by the words, "some sort of."

He wrote a referral to a surgeon who could inject cortisone into the inflamed area to relieve it.

The process was simple, and the surgeon implied I would gain rapid relief. However, the cortisone made no difference.

Shortly afterward, I dealt with an unrelated problem.

I had a long-standing issue with a frozen shoulder. MS doesn't cause it, but it doesn't help it either. The man who would hydro-dilate my shoulder was called Frank, an extremely well-known surgeon. He would inject a mixture of water and cortisone into the capsule of the shoulder joint and stretch it from the inside. It is a remarkably successful technique, but as we age, it sometimes needs to be repeated.

As Frank prepared to inject me, I asked him if he could do the same thing to my hip.

"No," he replied. "it's a different shape."

As he started the procedure, he said, "What's wrong with your hip?"

I told him about the pain, the cramps in my legs, and the dull ache around my hip.

Without looking up from his job, he said, "That's your piriformis."

As soon as I went home, I looked up the word and found an extensive reference library of articles and videos about a condition called Piriformis Syndrome.

The piriformis is a small muscle tucked behind the gluteus maximus. It is one of a group of muscles that allows your leg to rotate externally. The sciatic nerve runs through or, sometimes, behind it. When the piriformis constricts, it squeezes the nerve, producing pain and cramps down the leg.

I read as much as I could about the syndrome's signs, and they all ticked boxes. When I told the professor of my discovery on my next visit, I could see the penny drop in his expression.

"We're trained to look for one thing at a time," he sighed. He referred me to another surgeon who would again inject cortisone.

~

Over two weeks, this surgeon injected cortisone into both my hips. His technique was to make a careful injection and guide the needle along the surface of the fascia covering the piriformis, then drizzle the cortisone over the area. The process was marginally successful, but I was still sore.

After waiting for a polite period, I made an appointment to see Frank. He was the one who had diagnosed me, so it seemed logical to go back.

His technique was different. He pressed the ultrasound scanner hard against my flesh and asked where it hurt the most. Eventually he said, "Seems to be the lateral portion" and plunged the needle directly into the muscle. Apart from the initial sting, which caused me to swear, I knew immediately he was in the right place. As the needle penetrated my muscle, I could feel a change. As he drove it through muscle and fascia, something released. Walking out of the surgery, I knew this would work.

Even now, my leg no longer cramps. I can stretch out in bed without triggering a massive, painful spasm.

Two years later, I went back to Frank, and he injected my right Piriformis. This time there were no cramps but instead, an endless chronic ache that ran down my leg and under my foot. Frank's technique was identical to the first time. For 24 hours, my right leg felt worse; then, all the discomfort went away. Those muscles on my right hip were just sick of doing more than their fair share and had locked up. Maybe in a few years, I might need repeats, but, for now, both sides are fine.

Piriformis Syndrome can happen to anybody, but if you have MS and the muscle is prone to spasm, it can make life hellish.

I have concluded that the injection technique needs to break the fascia and enter the muscle, as Frank had done. If the needle does not go deep and break the fascia, the treatment won't be successful.

More Visits to the Spasticity Clinic

Three months after my first visit, I returned to the spasticity clinic for a check-up and, apart from the injections for bursitis, they made no changes. At six months it was the same, except for the referral for my first piriformis injections. The leg was still feeling the effect of the first round of botox injections, but I was starting to sense they may have missed a few spots.

Botox works wonders. Within a few days after the first injection, I felt my leg was so much better. Pilates classes became more fruitful. There was a more natural gait in my left leg. As time wore on, the negative side of its effect became slightly noticeable. A leg is quite heavy. When some muscles are "knocked out", you can feel the weight of the limb.

On my fourth visit, nine months after I first presented myself, I wanted to make it clearer to the clinic where my tightness was. I arrived with ink lines drawn all over my legs.

It had become evident to me that the botox shots were somewhat "hit and miss". They had helped, but I kept thinking if they knew exactly where to give the injection, the shots would have been more effective.

Darryl had ceased massaging and passed the day-to-day work over to his employees. It was my good fortune that he introduced me to a girl called Luksy. Not only was she an exceptional masseur, but she was upskilling by doing a year-long course in remedial massage. Working on me became the homework for her classes. When she hit something tight, I would yell, "what's the name of that muscle?" And both of us significantly increased our knowledge of anatomy.

In my mind, I decided if the spasticity clinic could see a map of where I was tight, they would be better armed to select an injection site. I asked Darryl and Luksy to take a pen and draw on my skin along each tight segment. In the end, my legs were covered in lines of scribble.

Initially, the professor said, "You've wasted your time. We're interested in motor neurons, not muscles." Then he started to look at the patterns and could recognize the lines.

~

When I entered his consulting room, his therapists had made me lie on a bench and raise my leg. They measured the angles of my knee and ankle. The top section of my leg was at 90 degrees to my body, and the lower part was bent to be parallel to the bench. The position is sometimes called 90/90.

Physical therapist: "OK, that's done. You can relax now."

Me: "Thanks."

Therapist: "Relax."

A moment passed.

Therapist: "Relax!"

Me: (confused) "But I am relaxed."

Therapist: "No, relax!"

Me: (gesturing with my hands) "I am relaxed."

Somewhat amused Therapist: "No, when I say relax, your leg is supposed to drop to the bench."

"Ahh," I said, "Got it," and I forced my leg to lower.

When it was time to inject, the professor took charge and told the assisting therapists he would do the injections himself. He followed the lines and spread six botox injections down my leg. Never once did he acknowledge the lines had helped, but his actions suggested that my team of artists had been sufficiently accurate.

If there was a medical term that meant "nailed it", then that was the result. The effect of the placement of the injections, as well as their increased number, was that I regained a far more a natural action when I walked. Offsetting that was a noticeable increase in how heavy my leg felt. While my gait became more normal, the price was a heavy limb.

The Pill that Released my Muscles

Three months after my second dose of botox, I returned to the spasticity clinic for a check-up.

"How are you finding the botox?" the Professor asked.

"I love it," was my reply.

He swung his chair away to write up his notes, and I continued, "but my psoas is so tight, can you inject that?"

"No, it's too big. Have you tried baclofen?" he asked.

"Yes, but it made me so bilious I couldn't get past five milligrams." I replied.

He wrote something and swiveled in his chair to face me. In his hand was a prescription.

"This stuff works but has an undeserved reputation for causing problems. Probably because it was used in high doses for too long. Most people hate it because it makes their muscles feel so weak."

I took it from him. "Well, I do Pilates, so I guess I can work through that."

"It's a low dose, but most people hate it," he reiterated.

I looked at his scrawled prescription. It was for dantrolene sodium.

At that point, apart from valaciclovir, I was taking no other prescription medication.

Getting used to Dantrolene Sodium

I quickly learned why most people dislike this drug. In simple terms, it works!

Within a few days, I became aware of my muscles relaxing. As that happened, the tightness that had supported my odd gait melted away, and I was confronted by how weak I was. All the muscles that should have been actively involved in normal movement had abdicated their role. Those that were stiff had taken charge. These weak muscles were simply not used to doing anything. Thankfully, Pilates exercises work the muscles that now needed to fire up.

The professor had warned me to be careful with the steps on stairs. When the muscles relax around the hip, it becomes very challenging to balance on one leg and shift your weight forward to take a step downward. The hip flexors will have become lazy and will barely support your torso.

I could feel my psoas letting go and was very happy with that outcome. My gut told me, correctly, that doing the Pilates classes would strengthen the weak muscles, so the weakness would be transitory.

It did take a while to adjust, and dantrolene, even at a low dose, is very effective. Your muscles are released within days.

Dantrolene sodium remains a mystery drug. There is a long list of possible contraindications with little thorough analysis to justify each call.

Some Chinese research concluded that it blocks nitric oxide formation by inhibiting L-arginine.[1] They argued that it might be a useful treatment when excessive vasodilation causes low blood pressure. Most advice is based on exactly the reverse pattern of cause and effect. The capacity to influence blood pressure may be another reason for people to hate it.

My blood pressure was considered too high by my cardiologist. He knew nothing about dantrolene. The medications he gave me to lower my blood pressure caused so much grief; he eventually took me off them. Maybe this is another reason why people don't like dantrolene. Fluctuating blood pressure and contraindications can be a nightmare.

I recall going with my daughter to watch an Australian Rules football match at an indoor stadium. It was a highly anticipated game, and we were forced to look for seats on the top level. Finally, she spotted two and skipped down the stairs to claim them. I stared down the steps and realized my legs wouldn't hold me to descend.

Very carefully, I turned side-on, grabbed the back of the aisle seat and crab-walked, grasping the backs of seat after seat, down the steps. It is an unusual feeling to have hundreds of people staring at you, holding their breath in case you fall and not yell out how happy you are to be able to go down the steps.

When I reached the row, my daughter was already absorbed by the game. I casually made my way to the seat. She was oblivious to what had just happened, but I could hardly stop grinning. "I can get out of this tightness," I told myself.

Going up the stairs proved to be simple.

Massage and Exercise with Dantrolene

Luksy became my "go-to" person for massage. Her technique involved a lot of stretching, which is precisely what I wanted. Darryl had been more of a pressure point masseur. When you are tight, your muscles tense even more under pressure.

Pressure point massage works, but your body is at war with the masseur. If the masseur pushes, you push back. When that happens, it is painful. As you resist the pressure, your pain receptors are stimulated. Often, I would be in a cold sweat, my mouth agape, and my heart was pounding like I was going to have a heart attack.

Luksy's technique was to stretch the muscle. That meant her force usually balanced the speed of the muscle contraction, so it was easier to give in to her pressure. She did not stimulate the muscle to grip and spasm against her. The dantrolene greatly improved my capacity to go with her pressure, rather than against it. As a result, the pain subsided.

My new-found flexibility gave me a great deal more capacity to exercise in the Pilates studio.

I was still weak and often felt unbalanced. Sarah kept testing my limits by making the exercises more challenging. She took the stability away, so I had to use my body to control my posture, and gradually she added weights and springs to build strength. All the time, I was still sore in my hips, restricted in the length of my stride and easily unbalanced.

Nonetheless, dantrolene had changed both massage and Pilates.

When I was in rehab, I had no weapons. Now I had massage and Pilates. Dantrolene rode over the top of everything. I still had Sarah, but she was increasingly drifting away to her familiar circles. Luksy became the miracle worker. After dantrolene, I was gradually able to reduce my massages from daily to weekly.

A New Weapon

When I had arrived at the spasticity clinic and revealed the lines of scribble that mapped my tightness, most of the physical therapists were mute. The professor had mumbled a bit but was non-committal.

One girl, who I had never seen before, wouldn't shut up when she saw the markings.

"Oh, look what your Pilates has done," she said loudly. "Your teacher has been doing it wrong!"

My eyes flashed with red anger. Who was this idiot I had never seen before making such a judgment?

"No," I said quietly, "I think it's been caused by your running program."

"I have a friend; she does neurological Pilates. You should see her. She can help," she exclaimed over the top of the professor.

"I am happy with my Pilates instructor. It's your running program that has done this. My hips are out of alignment because you make me stand on the balls of my feet. It hurts to do it," I shot back.

After the professor had given me the injections and was trying to explain what I should expect, she again interjected. "Here is her name and number. She is very good. She's a friend of mine and can help."

I had already had a gutful of this woman.

"You need to try something. Try yoga, see my friend, do hypnosis, try something, try dry needling…" she trailed off.

"What's dry needling?" I thought. There was no way I was going to ask this increasingly irritating person.

As the lift doors closed, I rethought my opinion. "She was probably only trying to help. What is dry needling?"

Dry Needling

I looked up dry needling on the internet and read a few articles. I will go into more detail later, but in brief, it involves using the same needles as used in acupuncture to create micro-tears in the fascia that surrounds muscles. Instead of targeting some Chinese medicine meridian point, the practitioner finds a tight spot and inserts the needle directly into it to break up the stiffness.

Intuitively this technique made sense to me. If you can't massage or exercise out the tightness, you need to cut it.

Fortunately, an osteopath sublet some floor space in Sarah's studio. I popped my head through his door and asked, "Do you do dry needling?"

"Yes," was the reply.

Initially, the osteopath tried some dry needling into the backs of my legs, particularly the hamstrings. It helped a little.

I kept going each week while he stuck a few needles in me. There was some benefit, so I persisted. I had already learned to be patient.

This man operated out of two locations, but I only went to one. In time, he stayed at the other site, and his colleague, Cathryn, took over the practice that I attended. She was a better needler than he was. On one occasion, she followed a line of tightness down the front of my leg and stuck a needle into a spot well away from where I thought the pain originated. As soon as she did it, I could feel the muscles relax.

"I like this dry needling," I thought.

Soon I began using Pilates and needling in conjunction. I would be needled then step straight into a Pilates class to open further the tiny tear the needle created. Sometimes I felt weakness where I had been worked on, but I took that as a sign the locked-up muscle could now be retrained.

Eventually, the osteopaths moved on, and a myotherapist moved in. He also did dry needling and was even better than the others.

Tal, the myotherapist, had worked as a chef in an earlier life. He knew how to sew up a piece of meat. His needling went deeper and used more skill than the others. Now when I see him, I walk straight from his room into a Pilates session. I see Luksy weekly on a day that I don't do Pilates.

My ideal therapy arrangement consists of three Pilates classes and one massage per week. As needed, I use dry needling. Every morning and every night I take 25 mg of dantrolene. Just doing one of these things in isolation would be fruitless. I need to do them all.

Cast Out

My final visit to the professor wasn't at the spasticity clinic. It was at his office in the hospital.

He reclined in his chair and spoke with a philosophical tone, "This is a spasticity clinic, and you're not spastic anymore. You won't be coming again."

I waited, expecting to hear who he would write to about me and what I should do from now on. There was no discussion about who would monitor me and provide my dantrolene, which had clearly made a difference. He reiterated that Pilates was a good idea. When massage was discussed, he simply said, "Yes, massage works, but it doesn't last."

This meeting, however, was a dismissal, not a referral.

My hospital life was over. All up, the hospital visits had lasted nearly two years.

There was no "come back and see me in a year," no handover to another authority or even a handshake and best wishes for the future. To him, I was now redundant, not part of his program.

The professor seemed tired. I felt uncomfortable that I was taking up his time.

As I walked down the corridor, I wondered who my doctor would now be. My old GP had distinguished himself by displaying no interest when I called to tell him I was in the hospital. I had not seen him for some time. There was no one waiting for me as I walked on. No cheerful face, no warm arms. Nothing but a list of obligations.

I felt no sense of achievement, no finality, or satisfaction. Only I knew what my body felt like and I also knew that no one else was interested.

The fresh air licked across my face; the noise of local traffic roared around the carpark as I struggled up the ramp. I found my car and sat behind the wheel. The door shut, and I was enclosed, by myself in my little cocoon. I sat for half an hour, thinking about all the things that had happened since I walked into the emergency room. It was my own private, uninteresting story. No one else really wanted to know it.

Life Goes On

Sarah's private life became more complex. I saw less and less of her and gradually went through a cycle of different instructors.

Eventually, Sarah sold the studio to Tal. She lives in a different country now with a family of her own.

No one compares to her. If she had not lifted me out of my low points by being steadfast and kind, I would not be here. When you are balanced on the precipice with no idea which way to go, someone needs to haul you back. Everyone deserves an angel of chance hovering over them. Mine visited me and has now flown away.

~

Life is built on memories. Only sharing them brings them to life.

There is no opportunity to say, "This is where I have come from." It would not be understood.

Each improvement in my physical health has no context for anyone else. I have become a contradiction for those I meet. There is so much I can do now, but I have silent barriers that I can see confuse people.

I do not hide my MS, but it takes a long time for people to understand me. A Pilates instructor once said to me, "At first I took you too seriously. Then I didn't take you seriously enough." It will always be like that.

There was no one at the very beginning. Only Sarah was at the start of this phase. And now, there is no opportunity to say to her, "Remember when we did this?"

There is no shared journey with MS. You appear out of the desert, like some sort of oddity. Then you are expected to return. Your story is your own, but it is a tale no one wants to hear.

Sometimes people visit, but they never stay. There is too much risk they will become trapped in some unhappy ending.

A step is never shared, never becomes a joint memory. It is forgotten.

Every day is a step. One day might be different.

So, on I go.

References

1.   Chou, T.C., C.Y. Li, C.C. Wu, M.H. Yen and Y.A. Ding, *The inhibition by Dantrolene of L-arginine transport and nitric oxide synthase in rat alveolar macrophages.* Anesthesia & Analgesia, 1998. **86**(5): p. 1065–1069.

Chapter 17

"My Neurologist Laughed at Me."

The MS Hug

I live in Victoria. Perhaps 2000 miles away in Queensland, lives a friend of mine I have known since we were twelve years old.

Recently, he called to talk about someone he knew who had MS. The man he described was quite confused by his symptoms. He had trouble convincing his medical advisors that he had pain, difficulty moving, and extreme tightness around his chest.

My friend thought he must be describing something akin to indigestion. Like the medical people, he was also way off track.

I listened to what was described and then said, "That's an MS hug."

The U.K. multiple sclerosis Trust describes an MS hug on its website:[1]

"The MS hug, also known as banding or girdling, is a symptom of multiple sclerosis in which someone feels as if they have chest pain, rib pain or a tight uncomfortable band around their chest. It can be felt anywhere between the neck and the waist and may feel so tight around the chest that it's painful to breathe. For some people, it can be pressure on just one side of their body.

Some people experience a symptom similar to the MS hug but in their hands or feet, where it feels as though you are constantly wearing gloves or boots. For others, the tight feeling is around the head. The feeling can range from annoying to very painful. The feeling is different for everyone and may be described as pressure, an ache, a tickle, a pain or a burning feeling. It may be sharp or dull and can be short or long lasting."

The website doesn't do a great job of explaining what causes it and how to treat it without drugs. The second paragraph of their definition is far too broad. I have had all the experiences described, and they are not alike.

Reading the commentary from afar, it is clear that the committee that agreed to the wording was also struggling to recognize the symptoms of a hug, as opposed to symptoms of something else.

I have had a couple of decent hugs. The worst was part of the event that landed me in hospital in 2014. I have had others that were more painful but less debilitating.

~

Think about how we stand. If we were inanimate objects, rather than people, our shape would soon topple over. Our center of gravity is a little below where our belly button is. We stand on long sticks called legs, and the soles of our feet are insanely small compared to the weight they support. It is our muscles, coordinated by our brain, that let us overcome the enormous force of gravity and move through space without toppling.

A good handspan above our center of gravity is a thin muscle that separates our chest from our abdomen. When that muscle contracts, it flattens, allowing the lungs to expand into a greater space. The greater available volume lowers the pressure inside the lung, so more air is drawn in. That is how we inhale.

When the muscle relaxes, it expands, reducing the space available for the lungs. The air is pushed out. We exhale.

The thin muscle is called the diaphragm. It does not work in isolation. The muscles between each rib, called intercostals, have to allow the rib bones to separate during inhalation and then work with the diaphragm to let us exhale. Wrapped over the ribs, at the front and the back and the sides, are layers of other muscles that must coordinate with the diaphragm.

The diaphragm, at your front, lies just below the bottom of your rib cage. Big muscles on your back, all the way down to the lumbar region, are involved in each breath. The sides of your rib cage are covered in muscles that are integral to the smooth function of breathing.

When the diaphragm and the related muscles can't move through the normal pattern, they fight each other's movement. You lock up. Muscles in conflict create pain.

All these muscles are involved in how your torso rotates. The reason why disabled car parks should allow the driver to drive in and drive out without twisting is to compensate for lack of rotation. (Of course, no one designs car parks that way.)

Drugs won't stop an MS hug. It is a signaling problem. To overcome it requires physical manipulation. If your neurologist just sits in his chair, how can he possibly know which muscles are tight and need releasing? It is a job for a massage therapist.

A good massage therapist is familiar with the techniques that will release your diaphragm. The masseur's fingers will work under the lower portion of the ribcage and sometimes pressure will be applied to the outside to work the intercostal muscles while you inhale and exhale. Then the massage therapist should start working on serratus posterior inferior, iliocostalis, and the erector spinae group. They should employ PNF (proprioceptive neuromuscular facilitation) stretches to improve rotation by stretching the intercostals. For this stretch, it is best if you are in a seated position while they significantly rotate your torso. If that is not enough, then a therapist, very skilled in dry needling, should go over the same muscle groups.

You should keep moving. Don't just sit in a chair.

If you do Pilates, then lying face down on a half-inflated soft exercise ball, with it pushed under your ribs, can create a releasing stretch.

~

If your massage therapist doesn't know where these muscles are or how to do a PNF stretch, then maybe look elsewhere. You are half the team; the massage therapist is the other half. If you have the hug, then the therapist needs to be able to feel the tight muscles and release them. Talk to each other. I don't mean that you have one massage, and then stop. You need several treatments in a week.

~

The man my friend knew contacted me six months later. He had gone to a neurologist and told him that someone had suggested he had an MS hug.

After all that time, the man rang me with one question, "What's an MS hug?"

We spoke for some time about pain and tightness and the issues around the hug.

Eventually, he said, "When I told my neurologist, he just laughed at me."

References

1.   *MS Hug*. Multiple Sclerosis Trust 2020; Available from: https://www.mstrust.org.uk/a-z/ms-hug. Accessed January 2021.

Chapter 18

Pain

Almost 1 in 20 people in the population have to deal with blindness, low vision, or severe hearing loss.[1]

If we could neither see nor hear, how would we know whether we were walking waist-deep in water or across a desert?

Our movements would just be shaped by touch, not by a visual or auditory understanding of where we were.

How our senses and motor reflexes responded to the water and sand, or heat and cold, would instruct us on how we should control balance and react to our environment. This type of sensory interaction is covered under a broad umbrella called somatosensation. It is sensation that covers every aspect of the unconscious actions of the body. In our conscious interactions, it covers every feeling from subtle and pleasurable touch through to response to searing pain.

~

When you are sunburnt and transformed from lily-white to angry-red, you will experience a transient form of pain called allodynia. For you, the pain eventually goes away.

For some people, that pain endures. If the sensation is more constant, even the touch of clothing can be painful. Sometimes it might oscillate and for a moment, the pain might leave, then return to mock you.

A spontaneous pain might be an excruciating headache, a throb, or an ache. It could be as bad as hyperalgesia where normal pain is amplified, so a pain response of 3 becomes a 10. When this happens, a superficial pain often becomes an inescapable, long-lasting chronic burden.

~

The perception, or the absence of pain, is part of our movement process. We usually decide to move in a manner that creates the least pain.

Most medical people work by the maxim "do no harm". They want feedback from you to tell them how to avoid causing pain. When dealing with MS, this can be confusing. We live in such a litigious time that the people treating you tend to stop any activity that produces pain. That's not useful.

They should be able to say, "Because of X, Y, and Z, you will feel pain." You should be able to say, "Yes, I understand what you mean." Together, you should work out how to functionally move to minimize pain. Taking a pill to hide discomfort usually creates other agendas.

Sensory Fibers

The sensory fibers divide into many classes. Some respond to light touch, hair movement, and vibration. They are called mechanoreceptors. Generally, they are big, well-myelinated neurons. They excite the perception of where we are. They often work with a smaller, lightly myelinated fiber called a thermoreceptor. It responds to temperature, particularly cold.

A neurobiologist from the University of Chicago, Professor Peggy Mason, gave a useful illustration of mechanoreceptors and thermoreceptors in her excellent book, *Medical Neurobiology*.[1] She described the situation where competitive swimmers dive into a heated pool. As their bodies are shaved, and the pool is at body temperature, their sensory fibers sometimes perceive neither mechanical nor thermal stimulation. Consequently, as these receptors are not triggered, the swimmers do not feel "wet".

At the other extreme, the mechano and thermoreceptors in the anal canal regularly sample the contents. By working together, they can determine "wetness" to discriminate between solid, liquid, or gas. People with a damaged sensory pathway often suffer from fecal incontinence. The sensory fibers they rely on have failed them.

~

An ascending pathway of the spinal cord, called the dorsal column–medial lemniscus pathway, controls a process called stereognosis. This is the key to how we decide the size, shape, hardness, texture, and characteristics of an object. It is the pathway we use to determine whether we are holding a pin or a chopstick. The pain receptors, called nociceptors, also help us to discriminate.

If the ability of the sensory receptors is impaired, we become clumsy. We can't determine the weight, the size, or how we should grip an object. Incomplete information creates a faulty response. Our movement becomes inappropriate. As an example, I have problems with lesions on my cervical spine. Consequently, my fingers can oscillate between painful sensations and an impaired tactile sensation. I do not get an appropriate feedback from the sensations in my hands to determine the optimal motor movements for my fingers. I struggle to do up buttons on a shirt.

~

Movement and pain are interlinked. All our receptors are supposed to feed information back to our brain so it can determine how we respond.

Pain

The reaction to pain has two elements:

1) The sensory reaction, and

2) the emotional reaction.[1]

There are five types of small diameter fibers involved in the perception of pain:[1]

1) High threshold mechanoreceptors that are lightly myelinated. These are highly localized (e.g., they feel a pinprick).

2) High threshold thermoreceptors that are lightly myelinated. These respond to noxious heat.

3) Polymodal nociceptors that are unmyelinated. These respond to many types of tissue damage.

4) Thermoreceptors that are unmyelinated. These are excited by innocuous temperatures.

5) Pruiceptors that are unmyelinated. These respond to histamine (as would happen with a mosquito bite).

Some pathways overlap. It is the nociceptors that are nonspecific in their response—any tissue damage can activate them. They are the pain receptors that induce protective reactions.

Nociceptor Reactions

When nociceptors are stimulated, they can often trigger an amplification called an axon reflex. The initial stimulus runs down all the branches of the nerve, finding its way to a parent neuron. This can trigger other pain receptors in the surrounding tissue to produce, what Mason called "an inflammatory soup of neuropeptides".[1] This soup can trigger other nociceptors, creating spontaneous and exaggerated pain. This response has two purposes: to fight infection, and reduce the use of the affected body part so it is not reinjured.

Not all pain is the same. Mostly, the pain we think of is superficial. That's the pain we can escape. Then there is deep pain. Our response to deep pain is to become less active and to retreat from social activity. Sometimes the pain is caused by inflammation, sometimes, a nerve is injured, and, on other occasions, the neural pathway is interrupted.

~

MS often comes with pain. The website of the MS Federation, which covers 48 member countries, says two thirds of people with MS report pain as a symptom.[2]

They attempted to describe the types of pain:

Musculoskeletal pain due to muscular weakness, spasticity, and imbalance.

Back pain due to improper seating or incorrect posture while walking.

Contractures caused by weakness and spasticity.

Muscular spasms or cramps.

Facial pain due to trigeminal neuralgia (a nerve pain).

Electric-shock-like sensations that run from the back of the head down the spine.

Neurogenic pain, particularly in the legs, sometimes constant, sometimes burning or tingling intensely.

Pins and needles.

Other tingling, shivering, burning pains, and feelings of pressure.

Heightened sensitivity to touch.

The relentless grip of girdling and gloving.

Painful eye movement.

All of the above, except facial pain, have visited me.

I agree when they say, "the pains associated with these can be aching, throbbing, stabbing, shooting, gnawing, tingling, tightness and numbness".

When fatigue is thrown like a shroud of wet cement over you at the same time as you are experiencing this pain, then life can become difficult.

I am uncomfortable with this website as their first suggestion is to use anticonvulsants and antidepressants. Aside from the risk of contraindications with other medications, they are just palliatives. Using them can be seductive, but the use comes with a price. Think carefully about what you mean by pain.

~

I have found with my MS that I have to look through the pain. Non-steroidal, anti-inflammatory drugs that offer pain relief target the inflammatory soup. They can be useful, but they are not the answer. There often is no injury in my body. Relentless pulling from tight muscles and misguided fascia create most of the problems that need to be addressed.

If the thalamus, or a related structure called the ventrobasal complex, is damaged, then signaling is corrupted and neuropathic pain (sometimes a burning sensation) can result. That is the pain that is not superficial. Drugs that block that pain, like antidepressants or anticonvulsants, may be appropriate for this. They are where you look, after the possibility of superficial pain has been eliminated. They should not be the first thing you try.

Trigeminal neuralgia (the pain in the face) and optic neuritis are pains derived from cranial nerves, so they differ from body pain. Treat them in a way that relieves the pain.

You should treat bladder retention as a medical emergency, not as something where discomfort is ignored. Bladder control requires a signal from the pons, at the base of your brain, as well as unconscious inputs to the detrusor muscle. Your only voluntary control is over the external urethral sphincter muscle. Damage to your spinal pathways can create havoc for your bladder. Always get help.

References

1. Mason, P., *Medical Neurobiology (Second Edition)*. 2017, Oxford University Press: New York.
2. *MS International Federation*. MS symptoms – Pain 2020; Available from: https://www.msif.org/. Accessed January 2021.

Chapter 19

Balance and Posture

Imagine we have walked into a swish hotel. Over at the bar stands Fred, a world-weary salesman in his fifties. In polite circles, we would say he is obese. He is clutching a beer glass that is resting on his substantial distended stomach. His weight is concentrated around his waist.

Talking to him is Sally, the daughter of his best friend. She is very pregnant with twins. The position of the babies pulls her center of gravity forward. To compensate, she extends her upper torso creating a deep concave in her lower back.

Both are standing upright. Although neither thinks about it, they can sense gravity is pulling on them. Their legs are locked in wide stances to spread the load, but their muscles are sore.

Both can feel some back pain. Both are using their muscles to compensate for the force driving down on the soles of their feet.

In walks Sally's mother, Jill. Once upon a time, she was called a supermodel. She is long, lean, and willowy. Old habits die hard, so she is wearing a pair of the highest stilettos money can buy. They lengthen the look of her legs. Despite being pencil-thin and looking fantastic for her age, her legs are sore. The steep angle of her shoes means the full weight of her body is carried on the front of her ankles. Her hips are extended as her center of rotation is being thrust forward. To compensate, she leans slightly back, lengthening the hip flexors.

Jill has brought her three-year-old grandson, Timmy, with her. She lets go of his hand, and he drops to the floor to lie comfortably on his side while he watches how the wheels move on his favorite toy. He makes a few burbling noises. Timmy has the greatest support surface of any of them and is very relaxed and comfortable. He has distributed his weight very broadly and occasionally kicks a leg into the air. His movements are effortless.

Sitting nearby is Jill's husband, Bill.

Like his grandson, Bill has distributed his weight. This time on a chair. Sometimes his trunk is upright, like those who are standing. Most of the time, Bill slouches in the chair. His posture is a half-way house compared to the others.

None of them are still.

Neither is anyone else. All of us are constantly shifting, creating a structural sway. Sometimes we adjust our posture because we have gestured with our arms, and the momentum changes the center of gravity. On other occasions, we just seem to move position for no reason. We do this because the brain is continually thinking about postural stability. When we move, we are unconsciously trying to avoid falling over. If something changes our equilibrium, we need to adjust quickly. Sometimes it is a reflex. On other occasions, we anticipate a disturbance before it happens. If we didn't do this, we would fall over.

~

Bill decides he will go upstairs. He has a lot on his mind. As he strides across the hotel's marble floor and bounds up the stairs, he passes an old lady who is not so steady on her feet. She has several balance issues. Falling for no reason is the signature of posture and balance problems.

Even though he is deep in thought, Bill is not likely to fall. The regions of his forebrain and brainstem are fully functional. His cerebellum is coordinating all the messages and motor functions without a hitch. All his motor tracts work perfectly.

He did not, however, expect that Fred would marry Sally, but that's another story.

Postural Control[1]

Body postures depend on two absolute factors.

1) The location of our center of mass.

In upright humans of average weight, standing on a level surface, this is just below the belly button and just behind the hip.

2) The size of the support surface.

This varies depending on where we put our feet. If we stand with our legs wide apart or sit, the surface becomes large and stable. When standing, as we draw the feet closer together, the support surface becomes smaller.

~

If we stand on one leg, our center of mass shifts, so the center of downward pressure is concentrated on the standing leg. We need to compensate for this by using our muscles to maintain balance. Nonetheless, even a push from three-year-old Timmy could make us fall. To resist his attempts, our abdominal muscles are required to maintain stability when the body's center of mass is moved.

That control over the center of mass is what you see in the movements of ballet dancers, elite sportspeople, acrobats, and gymnasts. Boxers need this control, so that the momentum created by their rapidly moving arms doesn't cause them to topple over as their body follows each punch.

I do Pilates to achieve that sort of control.

Motor Centers and Posture

Movements are either simple (standing up from a seat or waving, etc.) or complex (writing, buttoning a shirt, playing a keyboard, etc.). All the motor tracts coming from your motor centers and down your spinal cord contribute to simple movements. The complex movements are concentrated on your corticospinal and corticobulbar tracts. Neurons can manage the simple movements from your motor control centers by indirect pathways. The signals pass through circuits of connecting neurons called interneurons. The intricate movements develop from direct pathways where neurons run directly from the corticospinal and corticobulbar pathways.

As the simple and complex pathways overlap, there are some things you can do and others you can't. For example, I can walk with you but don't ask me for a dance.

There are other tracts, collectively called the extrapyramidal pathways, that involve actions that we do unconsciously or that are tied to emotion. Professor Mason gives an excellent example of how one person can smile at a joke because it is activating one of these extra pyramidal pathways, but cannot smile symmetrically on command, as a different pathway is lesioned and cannot be activated.[1] The muscles can no longer be voluntarily engaged. In her example, the movement of a voluntary smile is selectively impaired.

~

The signals for what we see and what we hear arrive at sockets in the head and connect to cranial nerves. Most of the nerves involved have mixed functions. They sense the inputs, but they are also involved in motor actions—things like eye movement and facial expression.

Signals are sent down through the base of the brain, where they join a great hub of axons in a structure called the pons. It is like flying into the busiest airport and finding your connecting flight. Signals check-in at the sensory nucleus and find the primary sensory cortices. The midbrain and the cerebellum check and recheck the information. Damage at this level can cause profound problems with both motor and sensory activity.

The somatosensory nerves are more varied than the systems involved in sight and hearing. You can be blind or deaf, but almost no one is completely cut-off from sensation. The nerves involved cover the whole body, inside and out. There are dozens of pathways for some sensations to get through. You would need a catastrophic injury to be utterly anesthetized to any sort of sensation.

Pain is part of the somatosensory pathways. It can be short-lived, spontaneous, or chronic.

All the tactile information, the vibrations, and signals to receptors that indicate where you are in space, hone in on the spinal cord. The information that travels from the most posterior part of our spine hugs the midline. This means the nerves coming from the perineum, between our anus and genitals, will travel along the center of the midline.

As we move further from the midline, out into the torso and then the limbs, the axons carrying signals to and from the spine get longer and thicker. Nonetheless, as they have more exposed surface area, they are at a greater risk of failure or corrupted signals. Long nerves with damage anywhere on their path, can disturb sensation going to the central nervous system and confuse the motor commands coming out. A motor signal that tells a muscle to contract at the wrong time will be picked up by a sensory pathway and start a chain of garbled messages and responses.

Do you need to know where your damage is? The answer is probably a qualified "sort of".

It depends if the damage is at a point where no alternative pathway exists. What we call a nerve is a bundle of axons from many neurons. Losing one neuron is not catastrophic. A General would say, "if you lose one soldier, get another soldier."

If neurons that have consolidated into a nerve or a significant pathway are affected, then a lesion is a big hit to the whole army.

When a neurologist is examining you, he is looking at your motor functions and sensory responses to work out which nerve pathways have been corrupted. He can look at an MRI for confirmation that it is a demyelinating lesion rather than an impingement causing your symptoms. When the cause is MS, the lesion is more likely on a pathway of neurons than a nerve.

~

Many axons feed primary nerves. Your somatosensory, motor, and sensation pathways travel along the spinal cord and consolidate as they meet at the brain stem.

The brain stem is a busy place. It contains the medulla, the pons, the cerebellum, and the midbrain. There is a constant process of sampling and rechecking all the inputs and outputs of your nerve pathways.

The axons of many neurons pass through the central nervous system. They are so bunched up that they are collectively called "white matter." Some travel through specific channels called tracts. They ultimately will funnel to different parts of the body and brain. How this network of nerves is laid out goes back to when our ancestors were little things running on all fours. We are not "wired" the way a computer age technician would design a bi-ped. We are wired up like a four-footed animal.

Your balance and posture are the result of the instructions to motor outputs determined by sensory inputs. If you have a lesion somewhere, the signal is corrupted. If it only affects one or a disparate group of neurons, then you will adapt by using an alternative pathway. If a whole group of neurons involved in one task is damaged, then not only are the messages changed, but so are your actions. How your body moves and where you think you are in space is affected. Your balance and posture are a window through which you can look at your wiring.

Processes Controlled by the Brainstem

Medulla:
- Blood pressure
- Breathing
- Gastrointenstinal motility
- Ingestion
- Equilibrium

Pons:
- Horizontal gaze
- Reflexive eye movements
- Posture
- Rapid eye movement (REM) sleep
- Facial expressions

Cerebellum:
- Motor coordination
- Postural balance, gait, speech, eye movements, reaching, grasping

Midbrain:
- Vertical eye movement
- Near vision
- Pupillary control
- Posture and locomotion
- Non-REM sleep
- Level of arousal

(Reproduced with permission from Mason, P., *Medical Neurobiology 2nd Edition.* Ch 6: The Versatile Brainstem)

References

1. Mason, P., *Medical Neurobiology (Second Edition)*. 2017, Oxford University Press: New York.

Chapter 20

The Effects of Lesions

"Oh, I have MS."

Eventually, I have to say it. Some people politely ignore my limp, and others come straight out and ask. It's their next comment that is telling.

A lot of people say, "I have a friend who has it."

Many people then start to lecture out loud, using me as a platform to bounce their thoughts off. Often, they will say, with an all-knowing tone, "It affects everybody differently, you know."

I usually nod and say little. Sometimes I just say, "Really?"

~

The cardinal features of MS are the lesions in the central nervous system. They are concentrated in the regions of the brain, brain stem, and the upper portion of the spine, particularly the cervical spine. Lesions in the brain produce the fewest debilitating physical symptoms. Fortunately, there is usually more than one region involved in sensory and motor pathways. The very highest levels usually create the least disability, if one input is affected, other pathways can salvage the intended message.

Cranial Nerves

There are 12 cranial nerves, and they can be divided into two groups:[1]

a) Special sensory nerves

There are two special sensory nerves

1) The olfactory nerve, made up of thin unmyelinated axons, which carries the sense of smell straight to the cortex for interpretation, and

2) The optic nerve, which carries all the information from one eye that drives the reflex for luminance. It shares that information with the

corresponding nerve for the other eye. If a physician shines a light into an affected eye, both eyes constrict, but if he shines it into an unaffected eye, neither will constrict. It is not the optic nerve that, when damaged, leads to double vision.

Both nerves are classified as special sensory nerves. They go directly to the forebrain and are also called cranial nerves I and II.

b) Mixed nerves

Cranial nerves III to X and XII exit through the brain stem, so lesions affecting that area may affect their pathways. Of that group, only cranial nerve VIII is purely sensory (the vestibulocochlear nerve). The others are a mixture of sensory and motor functions.

The brain stem encompasses the medulla, the pons, the cerebellum, and the midbrain.

Your symptom is determined by where the lesion is. Damage to the midbrain can impact on muscles that move the eyes. It can affect the sensation on your face, but you can have many more brainstem symptoms.

On your brain stem, it might be that a lesion affects how you chew, speak, swallow, or dribble. It might affect not only how you hear, but your sense of balance. How you move your lips, or the way your upper airway controls coughing or sucking can be changed by an interrupted signal in the brain stem. If this level has a lesion, it can impact how your tongue moves. A lesion can determine your expression, giving you little control over the face you present to the world.

Cranial nerve XI exits in the spinal cord. A lesion on this nerve will affect how the muscles of your neck behave. It can restrict the motion of your head from side to side by interrupting the signal to the trapezius and sternocleidomastoid muscles. In turn, this loss of movement impacts on your scapula, affecting the range of motion of your arm.

Although damage in the brain stem creates a large variety of symptoms, there can be many more, as we have not even looked at the tracts traveling along your spinal cord.

Spinal Cord Anatomy

The spinal cord starts where a segment of the midbrain, called the medulla, ends. That's about the level where you find the base of the skull.[2]

There is a considerable difference between the length of the spinal cord and the length of the spine. The similarly named regions of the spinal cord and spine are adjacent to each other in the upper regions, but the spinal cord ends at the level where the bones of the lumbar area of your spine begin. In an adult, the spinal cord is only about 40 cm in length.[1]

The nerve roots that serve the lower part of your body branch from the spinal cord as a series of long ropey tails. Collectively, they are called the "cauda equina," which is the Latin name for "horse's tail". These roots are all outside the central nervous system. As MS is a demyelinating disease of the central nervous system, the messages going to and from your legs, bowel, and bladder, if they are affected, are disrupted further up the pathways rather than at the cauda equina. Nonetheless, the disruptions to the lower portions of your body can be profound.

The parts of the spinal cord are divided into segments that correspond to the bony vertebral spine. From top to bottom, the regions are denoted as the cervical, thoracic, lumbar, and sacral regions.

Running through these regions are fibers, arranged in pathways. How they are arranged is called lamination. There are no laminated fibers for the head in the spinal cord. The cranial nerves travel directly to and from the brain stem. They do not descend to the spinal cord.[2]

The primary pathways of the motor system are called the corticospinal tracts (sometimes called the pyramidal system). They send information from the cortex to the spinal cord. From there, the signals are relayed on through the connecting nerves that take the message to muscles. Disruption to this relay process is due to a defining characteristic of MS: upper motor neuron damage.

Upper and Lower Motor Neurons

MS is determined by damage to the primary group of neurons (i.e., the ones that are inside the central nervous system). These are carrying the traffic from the cerebral cortex through the brainstem to the spinal cord. Primary neurons are supposed to interact with the second group of neurons that belong to the peripheral nervous system. The cell bodies of the second group are outside the central nervous system, but those closest to the spine have extensions that are connected to the first group.

The second group of neurons, in a sense, are always active. They need very little input to fire them sufficiently to influence a muscle. The first group is pushing an activation signal to the second group, or they are not. They are like an on/off switch. A lesion on a neuron in the first group means an "off" switch is lost for a neuron in the second group. Some primary neurons are purely an off switch.

The motor neurons of the central nervous system are called upper motor neurons. The motor neurons of the peripheral nervous system are called lower motor neurons.

When a lesion appears on an upper motor neuron, the connecting peripheral neuron has lost its on/off switch. The second neuron can become easily excited. Reflexes are a constant source of activation. Muscles contract too much, as reflexes are continually being stimulated. The constant involvement of reflex actions without relief means MS people become hypertonic and exhibit hyperreflexia.

Sometimes this takes time to appear after the first assault on the upper motor neurons. Limbs and muscles can often first appear weak and limp. Over time the constant activation of the lower motor neuron, through reflexes, reverses this, and the classic MS symptoms develop.

Corticobulbar Tracts

Not every motor neuron descends through the spinal cord. The cranial motor nerves that terminate in the brain stem are upper motor neurons. They deliver their messages to a lower motor neuron that could connect to the muscles of the face or tongue or larynx or pharynx. The same on/off switch dynamic is at work.

Flexors and Extensors

Muscles don't plan any action. They do what they are told; they don't think about it.

Our body is a complex balance of muscles that are contracting and muscles that extend to facilitate this. If we lie in the fetal position, the flexors on the front of our body are shortening, curling our torso forward. As we curl up, our hip flexors draw our thighs towards our trunk, the same type of muscle on the back of our legs draws our calves towards our hamstrings. For this to happen, the opposing muscles, called the extensors, need to relax. There is coordination between them; they have to cooperate. How they work together is a reflexive action. There is no signal from the brain to tell a muscle to relax because its antagonist has contracted.

When both the flexors and the corresponding extensors are active at the same time, we are at war with ourselves. We struggle to move.

The same dynamic is at work when we stand, but the roles are reversed. Our extensors hold us upright, and the flexors are relaxed. As we move, the two groups respond to whichever muscle is tightening by relaxing the opposing muscle. This is a basic part of the reflex action that does not involve the brain. The need to relax can be overridden by a reflex that keeps firing. The muscle that should relax will obey a lower motor neuron that is still firing an instruction to contract.

The brain only starts the process by creating the intention to move. If a lesion on an upper motor neuron affects a flexor, it means the muscle is likely to remain active. If our next intended movement means the flexor should relax, it cannot. Both the extensor and the flexor become active. One is active because the brain told it to be, the other never switched off. The muscle that has been instructed to contract has to use greater force to overcome its tense antagonist. As a result, movement becomes difficult, and we seem stiffer.

MS is primarily an upper motor neuron disease. If the lower motor neurons are lesioned, then, generally, muscle tone is decreased, and the muscle becomes flaccid. As it no longer functions, the muscle loses bulk.[2]

Partial Paralysis

Due to the way our bodies are constructed, the flexors are usually dominant in the upper limbs. The arm is stronger when flexing at the elbow than when it extends. The opposite is true when using our legs. The leg is stronger when the knee is extended, than when it is bent. The dominance of the stronger muscle group becomes pronounced with upper motor neuron damage.

If an upper motor neuron lesion affects an arm, then the limb is flexed closer to the body, and the wrist and fingers may be bent.

If a lesion affects the leg, then the knee could be extended, and the ankle may tilt the foot down to a position called plantar flexion. The whole leg may twist inward, across the body so the foot can be placed flat on the floor. The leg no longer moves back and forth. Instead, the gait changes, so the foot scribes an arc as it drags. Balance is affected; falling is more likely.

Stronger flexors usually overcome weaker extensors. This pattern starts to appear even before increased tightness and hyperreflexia finally dominate.[2]

Many people with MS are mobile but stiff. The lesions do not create a complete loss of control, but people with MS often have a constant feeling of unsteadiness as the dominant muscles pull them in the direction that is the opposite of the plan they have in their minds. Sometimes it feels like they are going to be suddenly hurled to one side. They have a sense of loss of control. The mastery of their body has gone.

To overcome this, is another reason I do Pilates.

Somatosensory Nerves

Motor pathways start in the brain and end in the muscles. Somatosensory nerve pathways begin anywhere in our peripheral body and transmit the information (light touch, pressure, pain, temperature, and vibration), either from the skin or from the muscles.

As the peripheral nerves interact with the spinal cord, they sort into two groupings:

1) pain and temperature go to the spinothalamic tracts (also called anterolateral tracts),

2) the sensation of where we are in space (proprioception) and vibration go to the dorsal columns.

All the sensory pathways go through the spinal cord and the brainstem, to a central translation hub called the thalamus. This region turns the signals into a message that can be understood by the cerebral cortex. The thalamus can either relay the message or coordinate a burst of activity.

If the thalamus (or a related structure called the ventrobasal complex) is damaged, then signaling is corrupted and neuropathic pain (sometimes a burning sensation) can result. This condition is where antidepressants or anticonvulsants might have an application as they can block the firing of pain signaling neurons.[1] Think carefully about what you mean by pain if that is a word you use.

Spinal Nerves and Nerve Roots

The simplest way to distinguish between a nerve root and a nerve is to look at where the axons have originated. The central bundles of axons that run up and down the central nervous system and sometimes exit through its tough dural envelope are nerve roots. They are either motor neurons or sensory neurons brought from differing pathways.

The bundles of axons outside the central nervous system make up nerves. They can be a mixture of both motor and sensory axons. Although the axon may enter the central nervous system, if its cell body is outside the CNS, then it is from a lower motor neuron. It will be part of a mixed bundle that makes up a nerve.

If the bundle of axons exiting the dural envelope is mixed, it could contain motor neurons (which we can consciously control), sensory neurons, or autonomic motor neurons (which we do not consciously control). This bundle is a spinal nerve.

A lesion at the root level is not as severe as damage at the nerve level. A motor weakness brought on by a root lesion has only minor motor consequences. However, a sensory lesion at the root level may create a spectrum of results, from minor to significant pain. As many axons traverse the brainstem, a lesion at this crossroads can produce significant effects, as many pathways are then involved.

A lesion at the nerve level may affect the use of a whole muscle, as well as produce the numbness of anesthesia across a large area of tissue. If you can't move a muscle, it is paralyzed. People with MS have more root damage than nerve-level damage, so there is some inhibition of movement, but weakness and pain are common.

The Cerebellum[3]

Our regular, healthy movements are smooth and faultless. This happens because two regions, the basal ganglia and the cerebellum, are providing input pathways back to the cerebral cortex. They present the inputs to the thalamus, which translates the information for the cortex. It is the balance between the pathways that provide us with a smooth, coordinated movement.

The cerebellum looks structurally very similar to the brain. It occupies about 10% of the volume of the entire brain, but this belies its importance. The cerebellum contains 50% of all the neurons found in the whole brain. All the information from the type of sensory nerves that inform how the muscles are moving, called muscle spindles, feeds into the cerebellum. It is the center where the information that tells us where we are in space is processed.

The motor planning from our cortex also feeds into the cerebellum. All the sensory information from our muscles pass through it. There are about 40 times as many input fibers to the cerebellum as there are output fibers. It is ideally structured to compare the motor plans from the cortex with what is actually taking place.

The motor cortex initiates movement, and our muscles respond. The cerebellum does two things:

1) It adjusts our posture if something unexpected happens, and

2) it anticipates, through learning, that a postural disturbance might happen and prepares us.

The result is that we smoothly and unconsciously keep adjusting our balance, so we do not fall.

In effect, the cerebellum can both react and anticipate. A lesion in the cerebellum means our movements can become uncoordinated and erratic. Lesions on the cerebellum can create a significant array of motor problems.

~

There are four types of inhibitory cells in the cerebellum and only one that excites. The key output cell (the Purkinje cell) of the cerebellum is only inhibitory. It produces the inhibitory neurotransmitter, GABA.

~

The cerebellum has several different regions. They control different things.

The vestibulocerebellum

This coordinates the movement of the head and helps maintain balance and posture. It is the part of the brain that lets your eyes keep looking at an object even though your head is moving. A lesion here will affect your ability to focus on an object. Your eyes might jerk (nystagmus).

A lesion in this region can cause balance problems like vertigo or a gait issue called ataxia.

The spinocerebellum

This affects very similar functions to the vestibulocerebellum. A lesion here may cause tremors as well as a coordination problem, called ataxia, which makes you mimic the movements made when you are drunk.

The intermediate spinocerebellum receives information from the limbs. A lesion here can affect your ability to anticipate balance problems, making falling more likely. Reaching for something may result in under or overshooting the target. You may develop an intention tremor, so the closer your arm is to a target, the harder it is to grasp. The intermediate spinocerebellum is involved in the motor function of speech, so a lesion can cause you to slur your words.

The cerebrocerebellum

A lesion here can affect your ability to learn new motor skills. It does not matter how many times you try to catch a ball or learn to drive; you just don't improve.

Sometimes your neurologist might ask you to strike the palm of one hand with the other, then flip the striking hand over and repeat the action with the back of the hand, flipping back and forth. He is testing your cerebrocerebellum for the ability to produce rapid alternating movements. This same region determines how well you can coordinate actions across several joints in your limbs. Recognizing there is an issue here will help determine what sort of exercise program is appropriate for you. It doesn't mean you can't perform an action; it just needs to be broken down into simpler components. Pilates is excellent at doing this.

Bladder Control

Voiding your bladder starts with a signal from the pons, up in the brain stem. That overrides the inhibition in our forebrain at the paracentral lobule of the fronto-parietal cortex. If that lobule has a lesion, then we have lost the social control of our bladder.[4]

If a message passing from the pons to the sacral area of our spinal cord is interrupted by a lesion, then the activation of the detrusor muscle and sphincter in the urethra is disordered. As a result, you might leak but fail to void the contents of the bladder.

Sensory impairment due to a lesion can leave you unaware of when your bladder feels full.

A lesion can affect the bladder control pathway at many different points. More on this in Chapter 21.

Some people have lesions on their brain and/or spine and have few symptoms. Others are unlucky enough to have only a few lesions, but they are located where disruption is the greatest.

Why they are there, in the first place, is the great unknown in MS research.

Your neurologist might work out where you are affected. He will try to find a way to intervene, but don't expect that the next step will be to treat and repair the damage.

The best I can do is suggest that doing what I do for fatigue has coincided with no further deterioration on my MRIs. I can feel the effect of my lesions but don't spend any time thinking about them. My damage is not getting any worse, and I think what I do helps. That, of course, is just a sample of one, not the rigorous double-blinded placebo study that testing requires.

References

1. Mason, P., *Medical Neurobiology (Second Edition)*. 2017, Oxford University Press: New York.

2. Berkowitz, A.L., *Lange Clinical Neurology and Neuroanatomy*. 2017, McGraw Hill: New York.

3. Youssef, F. *Cerebellum 2013*. Available from: https://www.youtube.com/watch?v=1zTsbWcJmK4&t=30s. Accessed January 2021.

4. Gindodia, K. *Neurogenic Bladder*. 2018; Available from: https://www.youtube.com/watch?v=njK6nBmZ_24. Accessed January 2021.

Chapter 21

Bladder Problems

Bladder and bowel problems are, thankfully, minor issues for me. Unfortunately, this is not the situation for many people with MS.

A UK study in 2009 estimated that 75% of all MS patients had a level of troublesome lower urinary tract symptoms.[1] They noted that the degree to which bladder problems affected people with MS correlated with the patient's general level of disability. Those who could walk had more time to consider bladder management than those who were, at the other extreme, bedbound.

Understanding bladder problems can be difficult due to the problem of separating a neurological issue from less specific health issues such as a raised temperature or a urinary tract infection.

Although many people have bladder problems for many reasons, the issues, such as spasms, are more frequent and higher grade in MS patients than the general population.[2]

Even though my bladder control is good, I know that when I "have to go," it is not the time to sit back and hold on.

Urinary leakage is distressing. That same study identified a sample of patients who described its impact on their lives as "high". The paper concluded that patients who could still walk were more distressed by a troublesome bladder than those who used a wheelchair.[2]

~

Neurologists look at bladder issues, but they are more likely going to be managed by urological or specialist nurses. They do a lot of testing, plan management, and provide advice and care.

The neurologists and urologists generally get called in when the issue becomes an advanced problem.

There is a divided opinion on the sort of tests that should be conducted. The consensus of a UK expert panel was that pressure/flow studies (urodynamics) were only valid when surgery or catheterization was being considered. By contrast, the guidelines of a French expert group recommended that all MS patients with lower urinary tract disease should have urodynamic studies.[1] I have read that the tests are unpleasant and intrusive but have never experienced them.

Infection

More than one underlying issue can cause bladder dysfunction, particularly in women. The nurses will look at the alternatives that might be causing the problem. MS may not be the central issue.

The urinary system is classified into two tracts: the upper urinary tract, and the lower urinary tract.

The upper urinary tract consists of the kidneys and the tubes that take the fluid from them to the bladder. Those tubes are called ureters. In an adult, the tubes are about 12 inches long and are thick, fibrous, and mucous coated. They can contract. The upper half of a ureter is in the abdomen and the lower half in the pelvic region.

If urine is retained at the upper level, it can cause an inflammation of the kidney called pyelonephritis. Stents or surgery can keep the tubes open, and, commonly, antibiotics are employed. An upper tract infection can cause pain and tenderness in the back and sides, chills, fever, and nausea. Both sexes can share these common symptoms. An upper urinary tract infection needs immediate attention. If bacteria move from the kidney to the blood, a condition called urosepsis can develop.

The lower urinary tract infections are more common throughout the general community. This tract involves the bladder and the passage for urine to exit the body, called the urethra. Lower tract infections are generally not as severe as upper tract infections. The length and location of the urethra in women in relation to both the vagina and the anus can lead to the transmission of bacterial infections to the urinary tract. As the urethra in females is shorter than in males, bacteria have less distance to travel to reach the bladder. Unfortunately for women, recurrent infections are common.[3]

Bladder problems in MS are regarded as highly amenable to treatment. Checking for urinary tract infections and then monitoring the residual volume in the bladder is described as "relatively non-invasive".[1]

In some countries, but not all, the standard practice for management starts with cystometry. During this procedure, a catheter is inserted through the urethra into the bladder. As a first step, the residual urine in your bladder is measured. Another catheter or probe may be inserted into the vagina or anus to measure pressure in the belly. Any fluid is then drained away.

Next, fluid or gas is passed through the catheter to the bladder, and the patient will be asked when the urge to urinate begins. After this is measured, the bladder continues to be filled. The patient is then placed on a commode chair and asked to empty the bladder while the pressure is recorded.

Sometimes medication will be given to the patient, and the test is then repeated. When the testing is complete, the catheter, any probes or electrodes will be removed, and the patient is hopefully free to leave. Acquiring an infection is one of the risks with this procedure.[4]

Strategies to manage bladder issues in MS include physiotherapy, medications, timing, or injections of botulinum toxin A into the smooth muscle, known as the detrusor muscle, around the bladder.

Neurogenic Bladder

People with MS often have a condition called a neurogenic bladder. This is the broad classification for people who have a lack of bladder control caused by brain, spinal cord, or nerve-related problems. Many unrelated conditions can also create a neurogenic bladder.

Problems can be related to a central nervous system disruption, but the peripheral nervous system can also be the cause.

There are three distinct areas that a medical advisor will consider:

1) The suprapontine region of the brain. This is the home of a center within the brain where parasympathetic signals (that we do not consciously control) originate before they descend through pathways to a lower part of the spinal cord called the sacral region. The originating center is called the pontine micturition center. A common symptom of damage here would be urgency incontinence. You just have to go!

Acquired and progressive illnesses, such as MS, are associated with this sort of damage. Inappropriate voiding, the inability to initiate emptying, incontinence, and lack of control over the smooth and skeletal muscle actions concerned with voiding are common problems originating here.[5]

2) The suprasacral region covers the high thoracic and cervical spine. If a lesion occurs at this level, then the pathway from the suprapontine region to the sacral region of the spinal cord is interrupted. This can be a typical MS problem area. It can create uncoordinated sphincter and bladder responses, impaired sensory effects, and incontinence. If the lesion is high, it can also cause reduced colonic motility. Traumatic injuries, such as car accidents, might cause lower damage to the spinal cord, which can cause a loss of control over motility. MS damage occurs in the higher areas.

Poorly sustained bladder emptying, leading to significant residual fluid and a "high-pressure bladder," is common. This impairment can feed back through the sympathetic spinal center (which we do not control) and impact on a patient's control over blood pressure. A principal international committee on lower urinary tract dysfunction noted lesions above the T6 level increased the risk of a significant blood pressure problem called autonomic dysreflexia, which can display symptoms such as uncontrolled hypertension and bradycardia.[5]

3) The infrasacral or conus region. This is not where you would expect damage in a typical MS patient. Damage at this level creates a bladder that does not function at all. A diabetic problem, rather than MS, may be at the heart of a loss of bladder function at this level.

How the Bladder Works

Motor control of the bladder starts in the brainstem, specifically in the pons. The critical region of the pons is called the pontine micturition center. It works in conjunction with the pontine storage center. The overriding intent of the micturition center is to cause you to void. As we move past infancy, our brain adapts by sending inhibitory signals to the pons, so we learn to not continuously void. Toilet training teaches the brain to inhibit voiding until we are in a socially acceptable setting.

A healthy condition should see the bladder fill with no pressure. The pons should be controlling the urge to continuously void. As the bladder fills, it starts to stretch. The receptors attached to the bladder send a message to the pons to stop inhibiting the urge to empty. Our brain then interprets all the extraneous factors to determine if that is appropriate.

If it gets the approval of the brain, the pons sends a parasympathetic signal (that we do not control) to tell the bladder to contract. At the same time, a signal passes to the inner sphincter and also to a muscle that controls the outer sphincter to relax. The contraction of the bladder squeezes the liquid through the now open sphincters. When receptors signal that the bladder has emptied, the pons signals the muscle actions to reverse.[6]

~

A smooth muscle, called the detrusor muscle, surrounds the bladder. The receptors that control bladder relaxation and sphincter muscle tightness are called adrenergic receptors. The neurotransmitter that activates them is called norepinephrine.[7]

To tighten the bladder so it empties, the neurotransmitter acetylcholine activates a different receptor called a muscarinic receptor. Like we see with skeletal muscle, the muscarinic receptors, when activated, trigger calcium to be released to cause contraction.

The message to tighten arrives via the sacral region of the spinal cord (at the base). Most of the time, it is inhibited. Until stimulated, the urge to squeeze the bladder is weak.

There is a combination of reflex actions, unconscious autonomic actions and conscious actions at work. If we lose normal pathways for the reflex and autonomic activities, the conscious decisions are often not enough to control our bladder.

~

If a suprapontine lesion or a suprasacral lesion leads to significant retention of urine in the bladder, and this causes incontinence, due to an overflow, there are several treatment options.

Your general mobility helps determine the treatment. If you are bedridden, an indwelling catheter is the best option. If you can walk, either aided or unaided, or use a wheelchair, then medications called antimuscarinics become the first suggestion. Sometimes it is necessary to augment this with catheterization. There is also the option of modifying your habits, so you plan your activities to ensure facilities are available when you need them.

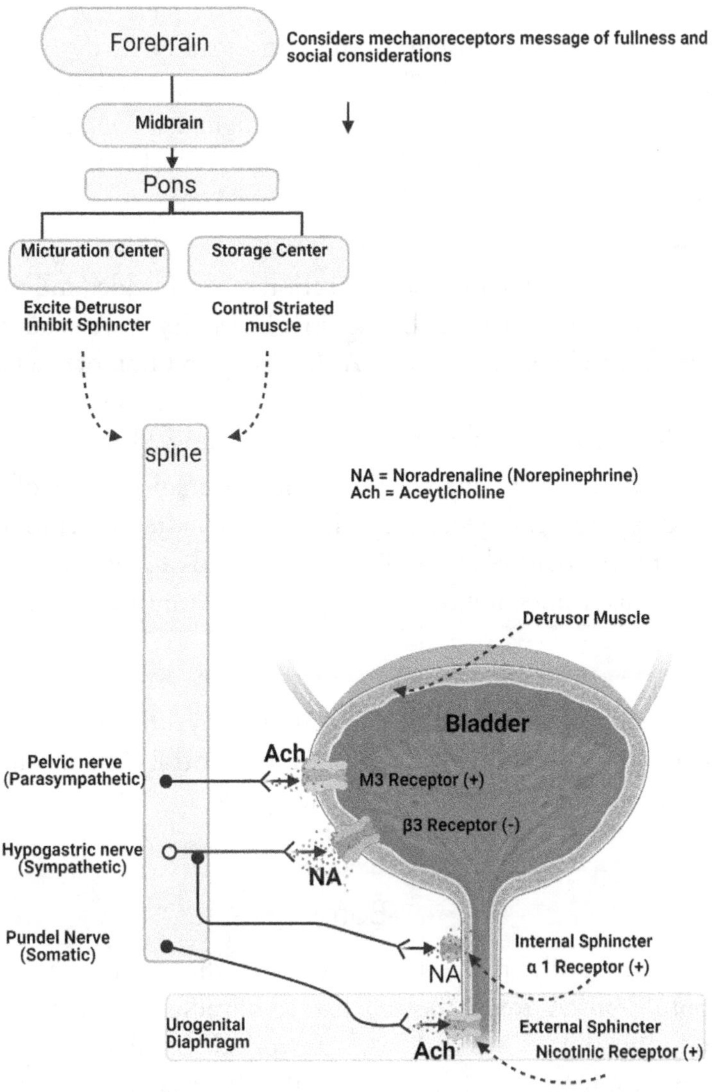

Figure 21.1 How the bladder contracts. We cannot consciously control the parasympathetic and sympathetic pathways. Drugs can modulate them. We can control somatic pathways.

In the bladder involuntary pathways predominate. We only consciously control the external sphincter.

Created with BioRender.

When the detrusor muscle is underactive, and the sphincter is overactive, it creates a condition called detrusor sphincter dyssynergia. The bladder fills, but voiding is difficult. Apart from catheterization, another conservative treatment for this condition might be a medication called an α-1 adrenergic antagonist. This medication blocks the ability of the neurotransmitter norepinephrine to relax the bladder as it simultaneously signals the internal urethral sphincter to tighten.

The nerve responsible for both relaxation of the bladder and tightening of the urethral sphincter is the hypogastric nerve. Its nerve roots arise well outside the central nervous system. As MS is a condition of the CNS, any damage at this level is very unlikely to be attributed to multiple sclerosis. If the nerve is affected, a signal from higher up is more likely to be corrupt.

Some medications might have a use in the management of detrusor sphincter dyssynergia as a secondary effect[8] (i.e., α-adrenoreceptor blockers, benzodiazepines, dantrolene sodium, agonist β-adrenergics, baclofen). Often, antimuscarinics are used in conjunction with these medications.[5]

~

Since I have been on dantrolene sodium, my impression is that my bladder control is excellent. In fact, I feel my control is better than it was before I started using it, but I am not the expert.

Botox

Almost universally, there is an acceptance that using the neurotoxin called botulinum A toxin (botox) has revolutionized the treatment of bladder dysfunction in MS patients.[2, 8] It works by inhibiting the release of the neurotransmitter acetylcholine. Specifically, it targets a protein called SNAP-25.[2]

Injections are not a permanent cure. There are differing opinions on how long botox remains effective and how often it can be used. As well as influencing muscle action, there is some evidence that it improves the sensation of bladder fullness.

A typical healthy person voids about seven times in a twenty-four-hour day.

MS patients, however, can have a range of bladder problems. A presentation from Dr. Gary Lemack of UT South Western Medical Centre in Dallas, Texas listed the occurrence of common bladder problems in their MS patients as follows, *"up to 86% had urgency incontinence, up to 72% had urge incontinence, and 49% had some sort of voiding disturbance"*.[2]

These figures wouldn't be constant. Many of their patients were remitting-relapsing cases, so their symptoms would come and go.

Most of the activity of the bladder occurs without our conscious involvement. We consciously control the external urethral sphincter, part of the urogenital diaphragm, by using the pudendal nerve. Nevertheless, as MS sufferers, we don't have a lot of ability to make our own choices. Management techniques depend on whether you are ambulatory or not, whether you can build your life around the timing of voiding, what medications you take, or whether you need to intervene with catheters or other devices.

References

1. Fowler, C.J., J.N. Panicker, M. Drake, C. Harris, S.C.W. Harrison, M. Kirby, M. Lucas, N. Macleod, J. Mangnall, A. North, B. Porter, S. Reid, N. Russell, K. Watkiss, and M. Wells, *A UK consensus on the management of the bladder in multiple sclerosis.* Journal of Neurology, Neurosurgery and Psychiatry, 2009. **80**(5): p. 470–477.

2. Lemack, G. *Treatment options for refractory neurogenic bladder conditions, Rare Immunologic Disorders Symposium.* 2013; Available from: https://www.youtube.com/watch?v=2AoA0863rFk&t=185s. Accessed January 2021.

3. Verneda Lights, E.B. *Everything You Need to Know About Urinary Tract Infection.* Available from: https://www.healthline.com/health/urinary-tract-infection-adults. Accessed January 2021.

4. *Cystometry.* Available from: https://www.hopkinsmedicine.org/health/treatment-tests-and-therapies/cystometry. Accessed January 2021.

5. Drake, M.J., A. Apostolidis, A. Cocci, A. Emmanuel, J.B. Gajewski, S.C.W. Harrison, J.P.F.A. Heesakkers, G.E. Lemack, H. Madersbacher, J.N. Panicker, P. Radziszewski, R. Sakakibara and J.J. Wyndaele, *Neurogenic lower urinary tract dysfunction: Clinical management recommendations of the Neurologic Incontinence Committee of the Fifth International Consultation on Incontinence 2013.* Neurourology and Urodynamics, 2016. **35**(6): p. 657–665.

6. Murphy, Z. *Renal Micturition Reflex.* Ninja Nerd Science 2017. Available from: https://www.youtube.com/watch?v=RLK9RiotyyQ&t=358s. Accessed January 2021.

7. Michel, M.C., β-*Adrenergic receptor subtypes in the urinary tract.* Handbook of Experimental Pharmacology, **2011**(202): p. 307–318.

8. Pichon, B., F. Bloch, S. Bart, E. Roze, M. Perrigot and M. Vidailhet, *Management of the detrusor sphincter dyssynergia.* Current Bladder Dysfunction Reports, 2013. **8**(2): p. 114-122.

Chapter 22

Bowel Problems

The Australian government is very keen on pre-emptive screening to catch bowel cancer early in its development. All people aged over 50 are encouraged to do some sort of test.

In 2014, about three months before I had my most significant MS attack, I had attended a day-procedure center for a standard bowel screening.

The day before the procedure, I had to fast and consume a large quantity of a liquid that would wash my bowel clean, so the doctors could see the surface clearly while I had a little sleep. A week later, I saw the surgeon who performed the investigation.

To my surprise, he said that I had an area of impacted feces, high in the bowel, that he had to remove.

"The question is, what caused that?" he said but never followed up. Instead, I was given a clean bill of health and told to come back in five years.

~

In the weeks leading up to my attack, my stomach felt bloated, bile would rise into my mouth, and I experienced uncomfortable cramps.

When I been in the hospital for two weeks and had been moved from cardiology to a general ward, a thought crossed my mind, and I buzzed for a nurse.

"I don't think I've been since I got here," I said.

The nurse bought a container of thick whitish fluid. "Take this," she said.

It made no difference.

A few days later, I asked an older nurse.

"Don't take that stuff," she said, rolling her eyes. "You need a fruit-based product. It will work."

Sure enough, after what felt like a profound internal argument and a fair bit of straining, things started to move. What I had produced was hard and relatively small, but it was a promising start.

~

Roughly a year after I left the hospital, I began to experience the opposite effect. Only once was I caught by it. In a public place, I just lost the active management of my bowel. My backside was not even slightly concerned that my brain was screaming at it to hold on. The stuff just flowed from me. It was soft, large, and it just kept coming. I was going as quickly as I could to a toilet, but it wasn't going to wait.

Thankfully, I was able to endure this without anyone noticing. I was humiliated, embarrassed, and above all, angry. My anger was directed at myself. How could I let this happen? What if I had been seen? Is this what I have to look forward to?

I used the toilet facilities to tidy myself as best I could, drove home, showered, and washed out my soiled clothes.

My mind split into two personalities. One was seething. Angry that I could have done such a thing. The other couldn't care less. I could almost hear it sneer, "Well, what do you expect me to do about it?"

I resolved that my first priority each day was to plan that an accident like that would never happen again. So far, so good. A successful day starts with a good movement. If that doesn't happen, my mind does not rest.

~

Constipation has been recorded as a feature of multiple sclerosis for many years.[1] There have been reports where clinicians have pondered whether it may be amongst the earliest of symptoms to appear.[2]

It is not a topic that everyone is comfortable discussing. A review in 2006 noted that a significant proportion of traditionally trained doctors and many members of the public sought a structural or cause-based reason for any illness and often gastrointestinal (GI) problems don't have an apparent basis.[3] The report noted that when medical practitioners did not find a rational explanation for bowel related problems they became dismissive or negative rather than helpful.

Sometimes, in an attempt to find an answer, inappropriate testing would be done, and the patient with a bowel problem was left feeling isolated and delegitimized.

Since the 1980s, there has been a growing recognition that, what are now called functional gastrointestinal diseases are related to motor and sensory disorders, hypersensitivity, inflammatory responses, mucosal function, stress factors, and bacterial flora.[3]

~

The primary organization that assembles information on functional gastrointestinal disorders is called the Rome Foundation. They have redefined the conditions as disorders of gut-brain interactions.

The foundation started as a series of committees in 1988. They went on to initiate a basic classification system in 1990 and then a framework for research in 1993. Although this sounds like they have had plenty of time to develop a database, their first recognized global study didn't happen until 2017. Their fourth seminar, held that same year, focused on the release of a software-based decision-making toolkit (called the GI Genius) to guide clinicians to the right conclusion. Despite how slow this all sounds, the Rome Foundation sets the benchmark.

The foundation tries to remain untainted by commercial industry influences, but its advisory council is full of pharmaceutical companies. Nonetheless, I think they are doing the best they can to managing the inherent conflict. Having pharmaceutical companies involved is not necessarily a bad thing. The work the foundation performed classifying GI problems moved the goalposts so far that the FDA started to pay attention. And as the FDA were interested, that raised the profile of GI problems, so pharmaceuticals began to get involved.[4]

The Rome Foundation's most recent criteria from 2016 is contained in books that draw on over 120 contributors from more than two dozen countries. My impression is they represent outstanding people who really care. They know that gastrointestinal pain exists and that in the clinic, there is a lack of "sophistication, precision, and specificity" in treatment. They concede that no centrally targeted agent can solve GI problems.[5]

In the context of MS, I have never met with a gastroenterologist, but what I have read suggests I should at least have had a conversation with one. As my bowel issues are so mild, a local doctor is not going to let me near one. A neurologist has never mentioned my bowels, ever.

~

The areas of the brain thought to be involved in gut function include the cingulate cortex, insula, thalamus, somatosensory cortex, and the prefrontal cortex.[6] There are a series of psychological disorders often associated with irritable bowel disease (anxiety, depression, panic disorders), and a widely held view exists that more than half the patients diagnosed with IBS have at least one psychiatric disorder. A stressful life (whatever that means) is also often cited.[7]

I can think of nothing more aggravating than knowing my MS may have affected those regions of my brain, and being told, by someone in love with their job, that I must have a psychological disorder.

Ignoring the structural issues, healthy bowel function requires that your bowel has the proper enervation, the right hormonal factors, and adequate nutrition. The consistency of a stool depends on colonic contractions, water reabsorption, and how mucous delivers the waste products to the rectum. Then it depends on the reflexes and sensory nerves to determine when the content is released.[8]

The gastrointestinal tract is governed by the autonomic nervous system (which we do not consciously control). However, unlike most other parts of this system, we can exert some control over the bowel. The nervous division of the gastrointestinal tract is called the enteric nervous system. The number of neurons involved is so large that it is often called "the second brain".[9]

The sympathetic arm of the autonomic nervous system enervates the bowel through the T5 to L3 nerve roots. The parasympathetic division goes to the left colon and rectum via the sacral nerve roots S2 to S4. This means that if you have an injury above the T5 level, then your ability to control your rectum or bowel movements is likely to be compromised.[10]

Those nerve roots are related to the peripheral nervous system. It is damage above those locations that matters in MS. The lumber and sacral roots are not part of the central nervous system, so if they don't receive correct signals from an upper motor neuron, then they are likely to end up producing hypertonic muscles. No quantity of antidepressants is going to change that!

~

A study published in 2014[10] compared 45 patients with MS, plus 19 patients with a spinal cord injury above T5, to 25 healthy subjects without any bowel issues.[10] The MS group was divided into low EDDS scores (below 5) and highly disabled scores (above 5). Both groups had similar constipation and incontinence burdens. Those who were more disabled had more significant urge problems and slightly higher sensitivity.

One interesting comment was that the researchers didn't use a control group of MS patients without bowel problems because "it would have been difficult to recruit an asymptomatic MS group".

They found that the MS patients had alternating patterns of bowel compliance. Antimuscarinic drugs (as used for bladder control) and anti-spasticity drugs were noted to promote constipation.

What this shows is that even if you are diagnosed as having "mild MS," you can still have as significant a bowel problem as someone who is quite disabled. I doubt anybody will discuss that with you.

~

So, what do I do?

There is an old saying, "breakfast like a king, lunch like a prince and dinner like a beggar."

That is a fair summation of my standard mantra. I avoid things that I know do not agree with me. All types of bread and grains (except rice) are things that make me feel bloated, slow, and uncomfortable. Where possible, I substitute with colorful fruits and vegetables. I don't use any dairy products, except a little butter in some cooking and occasional tiny quantities of hard cheese. When I do consume dairy, that arises not by choice, but just from being polite. I bluntly refuse cream as it makes me feel quite unwell.

Breakfast is full of fiber. I eat a banana, two boiled eggs and finish with a whole avocado, halved, with the pip hole filled with pomegranate seeds.

After that, I walk the dog and get a long black coffee. In Australia, that means a long shot of espresso (sometimes two) topped up with boiling water. That is like hitting a detonator!

Overseas, there is something called an Americano. I don't know why anyone would drink that stuff. Frankly, it's awful, and it doesn't do anything for my bowel function.

Lunch is sashimi or rice paper rolls, and dinner is whatever hits the table. The evening meal is done by 7 pm, so I have hours before I lie down to sleep.

I focus on timing my movements, so they are completed early in my day. That removes the uncertainty about what might happen. It is also most comfortable to manage.

Three days a week, I exercise, doing Pilates. I repeatedly twist and massage my stomach through exercise. The COVID-19 lockdown in 2020 showed me how important that is. If I don't use all those muscles in my torso, I become less regular. Pilates helps me stretch the lumbar and sacral region of my back. The exercise unlocks the peripheral nerve pathways that feed, not only my bowel and bladder but all the muscles throughout my hips and glutes that the nerves to my legs pass through.

If nothing seems to be happening by the evening, I resort to a gentle, off-the-shelf stool softening treatment that will draw water into my gut. You shouldn't need to call in the Dam Busters. Sitting doing nothing all day is the chief enemy of regularity.

References

1.   Hinds, J.P., B.H. Eidelman and A. Wald, *Prevalence of bowel dysfunction in multiple sclerosis. A population survey.* Gastroenterology, 1990. **98**(6): p. 1538–1542.

2.   Lawthom, C., P. Durdey and T. Hughes, *Constipation as a presenting symptom.* Lancet, 2003. **362**(9388): p. 958–958.

3.   Drossman, D.A., *The functional gastrointestinal disorders and the Rome III process.* Gastroenterology, 2006. **130**(5): p. 1377–1390.

4.   *Interviews with the President, How has the Rome Foundation changed with Rome IV.* The Rome Foundation 2020; Available from: https://theromefoundation.org/about. Accessed January 2021.

5.   *Meet the Rome Foundation.* Available from: https://theromefoundation.org/wp-content/uploads/Meet-The-Rome-Foundation-2019-web.pdf. Accessed January 2021.

6.   Vogt, B.A., *Inflammatory bowel disease: perspectives from cingulate cortex in the first brain.* Neurogastroenterol Motility, 2013. **25**(2): p. 93–98.

7.   Rapps, N., L. van Oudenhove, P. Enck and Q. Aziz, *Brain imaging of visceral functions in healthy volunteers and IBS patients.* Journal of Psychosomatic Research, 2008. **64**(6): p. 599–604.

8.   Preziosi, G., A. Gordon-Dixon and E. Anton, *Neurogenic bowel dysfunction in patients with multiple sclerosis: prevalence, impact, and management strategies.* Degenerative Neurological and Neuromuscular Disease, 2018. **8**: p. 79–90.

9.   Gershon, M.D., *The Second Brain: The scientific basis of gut instinct and a groundbreaking new understanding of nervous disorders of the stomach and intestine* (First Edition). 1998, HarperCollinsPublishers: New York.

10.   Preziosi, A.G., D.A. Raptis, A. Raeburn, J. Panicker and A. Emmanuel, *Autonomic rectal dysfunction in patients with multiple sclerosis and bowel symptoms is secondary to spinal cord disease.* Diseases of the Colon & Rectum, 2014. **57**(4): p. 514-521.

Chapter 23

Speech

I can speak clearly and make myself understood. Sometimes I strain a little to project the sound. Most of the time, it is not a big issue.

There are numerous suggestions that about half of all MS patients have problems with clarity of speech or how easily people can interpret their words.

Our ease of conversation is determined by how well the words flow and how effectively we can project our voices. It must be difficult for a person who knows she sounds drunk, to ask a stranger for directions to a toilet. How we talk has a significant impact on our quality of life.[1]

~

The primary speech disorder in MS is called dysarthria. It's a very broad term for neurologic movement disorders related to speech. Sometimes it is described as paroxysmal ataxic dysarthria.[2]

In ordinary speech, five processes work together and overlap to make our delivery smooth and rapid.[1]

They are:

Respiration: How quickly we fill our lungs, followed by how we control exhalation for speech.

Phonation: How the airflow changes the pitch and volume of our voice.

Resonance: How the movement of our soft palate changes the quality of our voice.

Articulation: How well we coordinate the lips, tongue, jawbone, and soft palate to create clear speech.

Prosody: How we use conversational speech to create emphasis and meaning.

When lesions create spasticity, weakness, slowness, or a lack of motor coordination in MS speech, any aspect of the volume, the clarity, the control over phrasing, or the pitch can be affected.

In the US, the National Multiple Sclerosis Society's clinical bulletin[1] divided speech problems into three different sorts of dysarthria:

1) Spastic dysarthria

This happens when lesions affect the corticobulbar tracts. These are the pathways that control the voluntary movement of the face, some shoulder and neck movements, the jaw, the tongue, and the upper airways.

Damage here can make your voice sound harsh, affect the inflection in your speech, slow your rate of speech, create sucking and jaw jerk reflexes, and restrict how much your jaw moves. When there is excessive muscle tone, spasticity limits the motion of your jaw and reduces your speed of movement.

2) Ataxic dysarthria

This occurs when lesions affect your cerebellum. The role of this part of the brain is to coordinate the motor control centers. When your cerebellum is affected, your ability to control movements of the tongue, lips, and jaw are changed. You might speak very loudly, have prolonged gaps between words, or draw out a sound longer than usual.

Your bodily movements may accentuate your difficulties with speech. Visually, the lesions on the cerebellum may produce tremors in the head, arm, hands, or trunk. As you reach for something, the closer you get to your target, the more you seem to struggle to reach it—often overshooting what you are reaching for. You may have eye problems or struggle with balance. This combination would be a difficult issue to live with and confronting for someone who did not understand what affected you.

3) Mixed dysarthria

You show any combination of spastic and ataxic dysarthria. The lesions could be anywhere, affecting the pathways.

~

A study in 2003 reported that tongue function was a significantly greater problem than lip function in MS.[3] Dealing with any dysarthria requires individual treatment programs that would encompass learning new skills to control your breath pattern by changing respiration, using cues to choose words, controlling the rate of speaking, pausing between words, and practicing volume control. Some people can find these tasks challenging. Guidance from some sort of speech therapist is ideal, but the referral rate to the right people is low.[1]

Some people with MS suffer from dysphasia (or aphasia). They have difficulty finding the right words or forming sentences. This condition possibly relates to disruptions in the various parts of the brain that control thought, short-term memory, verbal fluency or attention. It is not the same as dysarthria. A speech therapist may be able to help overcome this. When I was fatigued, I experienced similar symptoms.

References

1.   Miller, P., *Dysarthria in multiple sclerosis,* National Multiple Sclerosis Society, Clinical Bulletin, Information for Health Professionals. 2011.

2.   Duffy, J.R., *Functional speech disorders: clinical manifestations, diagnosis, and management,* in Handbook of Clinical Neurology, M. Hallett, J. Stone and A. Carson, Editors. 2016, Elsevier. pp. 379–388.

3.   Hartelius, L. and M. Lillvik, *Lip and tongue function differently affected in individuals with multiple sclerosis.* Folia Phoniatrica et Logopaedica, 2003. **55**(1): p. 1–9.

Chapter 24

Types of Body Tissue

Although I had reached the end of my year as a rehab outpatient of the hospital, I still continued to visit the hospital spasticity unit. They were treating my left leg with botox to reduce its severe rigidity. The doctors in charge were kind enough to complete a report for my insurance provider to prove that I qualified for a payment.

I sat with the 2IC of the rehabilitation unit as she perused the questions. Occasionally, she would curse under her breath, turn to me and say, "these questions are insulting."

Finally, the questionnaire was done.

"How are you?" she asked.

"Not too bad," I said, without giving any details.

Leaning forward, she looked straight at me and said, "Just a bit tight, I guess."

I had no idea if I had to see her again, so I replied, "Yeah, a bit."

I had already relearned how to walk, was constantly being pulled into the wrong shape, hurt all the time, and my brain was thinking like it had been shot out of a cannon. I saw no point in telling her all that. My hunch was I had told her what she wanted to hear.

There was nothing in the hospital's rehabilitation exercises that I felt had helped me. My ability to sit there was only due to all the help my Pilates instructor had given. Not them.

I had seen firsthand that some types of exercises worked, and some were useless. In a big hospital, you cannot change the process. I think it would have helped if they paid some attention to why muscles tighten and the role of connective tissue.

When I first saw the rehabilitation unit in October 2014, the physical therapists said their goal was to keep me out of a wheelchair for six months. They thought I might need one sooner. To them, I was just one of those stubborn types. They admired my efforts, but their body language told me they knew what the conclusion would be.

They only saw the relationship between muscles and nerves. It populated their conversations. They must have been aware of fascia, but it was of no importance to them.

However, if you have tightness caused by MS, you need to understand the role of connective tissue.

~

As our session concluded, the 2IC of the rehabilitation unit showed me the door to her room and admired how I moved. "You're doing really well. I mean *really* well," she said, to emphasize the point.

I walked away from her office and went straight to my next Pilates class. I had a long way to go. It was no time for self-congratulation. There was no point in telling her what I was doing. She was the authority. I was the patient.

~

There are four types of body tissue. We have only touched on some in this book so far.

1) Neural tissue

Neural tissue is where the attention is focused in MS research. It is made up of neurons and the supporting neuroglia.

The neuroglia (or glia) include the astrocytes, the myelin-producing oligodendrocytes, the scavenging cleaners of debris called microglia, and the ependymal cells which form the impenetrable barriers of the brain.

For a long time, it was thought glia exceeded neurons by a ratio as high as 10:1. A new counting method, using an isotropic fractionator, suggests that the ratio varies throughout the nervous system, and the concept of high ratios of glia to neurons was probably due to incorrectly identifying small neurons as glia.[1] This more recent technique puts the numbers of neurons and glia on an equal footing.

In the peripheral nervous system, neuroglia appear as the satellite cells that are similar to the astrocytes of the central nervous system. Schwann cells, not oligodendrocytes, make the myelin in the peripheral nervous system.

2) Connective tissue

Connective tissue is an overlooked category. Blood, which carries nutrients as well as waste products, is sometimes included in this group, but it is not where we should focus. There are more types of connective tissue. Dealing with these other types of connective tissue is a big part of how I address my MS.

3) Epithelial tissue

The cell layer lining the vascular system is known as endothelium. Some members of this cell group can be flat, single layer cells. Others are cube-shaped, and some are arranged in columns. Transitional epithelial cells, often found in the urinary system, can stretch and then regain their original shape. There are also categories of epithelial cells that can be stacked on each other. Epithelial tissue can have problems, but it is not where we should focus.

4) Muscle tissue

The best-known tissue is muscle tissue. This group has three different categories.

If the tissue helps to move the position of the bones, it is skeletal muscle. If it lines the hollow cavities, it is probably smooth muscle. The last sub-type, cardiac muscle, is somewhat structurally like skeletal muscle, but it operates on an involuntary basis. We do not tell our heart to beat, as we don't consciously control it. Skeletal muscle, we can control.

~

When treating MS patients, there is simply not enough attention paid to the function of connective tissue. There is also an overriding assumption that muscle tissue is just the slave of neural tissue.

The interrelationships between skeletal muscle tissue and connective tissue are largely ignored, and the result of that is disastrous for MS patients. All the focus is on neural tissue.

Connective Tissue

For centuries, anatomists learned the structure of the human body by cutting down through the skin to find the muscle. They would scrape aside the fascia, once called sinew, as if it was the unwanted detritus exposed in mining the secrets of the corpse. The cutting moved from top to bottom and around the muscle.

Their interest was in the mechanics of muscle movement. They wanted to know which muscle contracted to lift part of the body and which muscles lengthened to allow this to happen. When the action occurred, they wanted to know what bone was moved. Eventually, they looked at what nerve pathway signaled the contraction and what nerve signaled the other muscles to cooperate, to make movement smooth and controlled.

Each muscle was viewed as a separate unit. The sheets of connective tissue were seen as just a coating to create a lubricated wall to separate the muscles from each other and our skeleton.

It is only very recently that the dissecting knife has been turned on its side and guided along the fascia to explore what that looks like. Rather than being made up of discrete units, like many other systems in our body, the fascia is one continuous sheet. There is no beginning and end. It is only a man-made distinction that separates one area of fascia from another. The plantar fascia, which is often identified in a painful foot condition, is absolutely part of all the other fascia. From top to toe, there is only one network.

While intuitively we may know this, it is not taught to medical practitioners. What medical practice dictates is that connective tissue is of little consequence and deserves only a cursory nod.

Nonetheless, a change in attitude is developing. Full acceptance will take generations. Older points of view don't change. They are taken to the grave as absolute truths. It is the younger students that are being taught about the significance of fascia. What they are taught depends on the tolerance of the people who are teaching them to accept a different concept.

All the therapists I saw in my rehab might have given a tacit green light to a discussion about fascia, but they were muscle people. If I asked where the fascia came from, they would say, "I don't really know".

An origami master can take a flat sheet of paper and fold it into a three-dimensional swan. When it was a flat sheet, we couldn't see the swan, and when we look at the fascia, it is much the same. We can't see the whole net of complex folds.

When we start as the most basic embryo, our tiny collection of cells divides into discrete segments. In the middle of one of these segments is a smaller area called the mesenchyme. This region secretes an immature fibrous form of collagen, which will go on to form a body-wide net.

As our internal programming twists and turns our expanding shape, the net grows with it. Our bones, organs, muscles, and nerves grow through and around this net. It covers everything and is always continuous. At points, the net thickens, and at other places, it becomes so thin it is almost transparent.

As we develop, parts of our structure will fold back on themselves. The fascia goes with it, creating islands of muscles and organs that could be cut out like they are separately bagged items. It is still one fascial net. The bones appear to be bagged in their own net but, when they move, they are pulling on the whole fascia. The lung is made up of hundreds of fascial pockets, but when we breathe, they all pull on the one fascia.

Muscles are viewed as isolated units, but the strain in any muscle is not unique to it. The stress is distributed by the fascia across all the groups of the body. Where the pull is being felt has no consequence to someone who only sees a muscle in isolation. There are slings of pull across the body and lines of force created by movement. You cannot fix tightness without understanding its consequences.

~

Every movement involves strain. The forces are always being distributed. How rigid, or plastic, or elastic are the structures that have absorbed that distributed load? Are some of them compressed, like bone? Or are they stringy ligaments and tendons?

Some structures in our body might push outward against the tension that pushes inward. Sometimes the less rigid structure is more resilient. If a rigid structure, like bone, gives way, then the tension still has to be distributed.

Our skeleton does not hold itself up. We are not built as bone on bone. Remove the soft tissue, and our bones would just pile up on the floor. Our soft tissue determines our structure. The bones are just 'spacers'. A cast on a broken arm is to stop the soft tissue from pulling the bone apart again. Every bone is floating, suspended in a sea of muscles, tendons, and sinew. Bones are not screwed or nailed to each other.

~

If a yacht unfurls all its sails, it is not the mast, the hull, or the cloth that flaps in the breeze that determines how the boat will move. It is the rigging; the arrangement of ropes and pulleys. They distribute the forces of the wind against the tension in the sails. Your fascia works the same way.

If the force of the wind changes, you can add to and subtract from the tension in the sail by adjusting the rigging. Your fascia does not change that quickly. With MS, your muscles are your sails that are pulling in one direction, your body will add to the fascia that balances that force. When your muscle needs to relax, it is still being pulled by the fascia. The rest of your body will resist that pull by relying on another stabilizing fascia. Those two countervailing stresses will change the way your muscle responds to any third force. If your muscle becomes spastic or rigid, you become wrapped in a net of restrictions that limit movement and create pain.

Conceptually, the model of the distribution of force is called tensegrity. This is an engineering model developed by the designer R. Buckmaster Fuller.[2] Everything in our bodies is interrelated, because action creates forces that need to be distributed. This model applies right down to the structure of our cells. Every cell will change according to the mechanics of what surrounds it.

The cover story from Scientific American in May 1998 said:

"...from the molecules to the bones and muscles and tendons of the human body, tensegrity is clearly nature's preferred building system. Only tensegrity, for example, can explain how every time that you move your arm, your skin stretches, your extracellular matrix extends, your cells distort, and the interconnected molecules that form the internal framework of the cell feel the pull—all without any breakage or discontinuity."[3]

If your fascia, influenced by the behavior of your muscles, starts pulling you abnormally, you need to address it.

A brilliant work by Thomas W. Myers called Anatomy Trains builds on this. It is a textbook.[4] If you are a practitioner who looks at muscles, you should read this or you will live in ignorance. If you have MS and no one can tell you why you are so sore and tight in certain places, this book will help you understand.

~

When you have tight muscles, stiffness, postural problems, or loss of movement or balance, or any of the signs of upper motor neuron damage, then you need to understand that your symptoms are not just about nerves and muscles. If that is all you concentrate on, then you are ignoring a significant factor.

In 2007, a film called *Strolling Under the Skin* by the hand surgeon, Dr. Jean-Claude Guimberteau, was shown at the first fascia conference in Boston. It showed images of living connective tissue and revealed the chaotic, yet efficient structures, that formed a continuous tissue. Their architecture permitted movement without breaking. The film provided irrefutable evidence that the prevailing view of functional anatomy, where the elements are unconnected was incomplete. The dialogue accompanying the film is aimed at a technical audience. I have tried to make the topic more approachable in this chapter but the images tell the story more eloquently than I do.[5]

References

1.   von Bartheld, C.S., J. Bahney and S. Herculano-Houzel, *The search for true numbers of neurons and glial cells in the human brain: A review of 150 years of cell counting.* The Journal of Comparative Neurology, 2016. **524**(18): p. 3865–3895.

2.   Ananthasuresh, G.K., *Buckminster Fuller and his fabulous designs.* Resonance, 2015. **20**(2): p. 98–122.

3.   Ingber, D.E., *The Architecture of Life.* Scientific American, 1998. **278**(1): p. 48–57.

4.   Myers, T.W., *Anatomy Trains: Myofascial meridians for manual and movement therapists (Second Edition).* 2009, Elsevier: New York.

5.   https://www.youtube.com/watch?v=eW0lvOVKDxE Accessed September 2021.

Chapter 25

Functional Lines of Fascia

It took me a long time to understand the significance of fascia. Neurologists never discuss it. Most exercise people are just focused on muscles. Intuitively, and perhaps by training, massage therapists have a better idea. They are the real 'hands-on' people.

Thomas W. Myers divides the distribution of fascia into functional lines.[1] Fascia doesn't all run in the same direction. Sometimes your fascia will cross the body like an X across the torso. Other lines run down our sides. Some lines are deep, and others superficial.

Every part of us is covered in lines of fascia. They stabilize our posture, transmitting the strain so we can counterbalance the weight of our limbs. Fascial lines enable us to sit or stand and to have better control over the power and precision of our movements. They link the deep supporting muscles of our body, help synchronize the patterns of movement with breathing, and give order to the placement of our organs.

The Deep Front Line

When I first saw the diagrams in Myers' excellent book, the one that leaped off the page at me covered the most three-dimensional line of fascia. He called this the Deep Front Line. It represents our myofascial core. It could have been a map of where I had felt the most tightness since my 2014 attack. The areas it relates to on the back of the legs had been a source of ongoing problems for me for years.

Myers described the Deep Front Line as starting on the underside of the foot, then passing in front of the hip joint, pelvis, and lumbar spine. As it is a volumetric line, another track passes up the back of the thigh to the pelvic floor and re-joins the first track in the lumbar area. The Deep Front Line connects the psoas muscle (that I had complained to the physical therapists was so tight) to the diaphragm. It continues, up through the rib cage, into the neck.

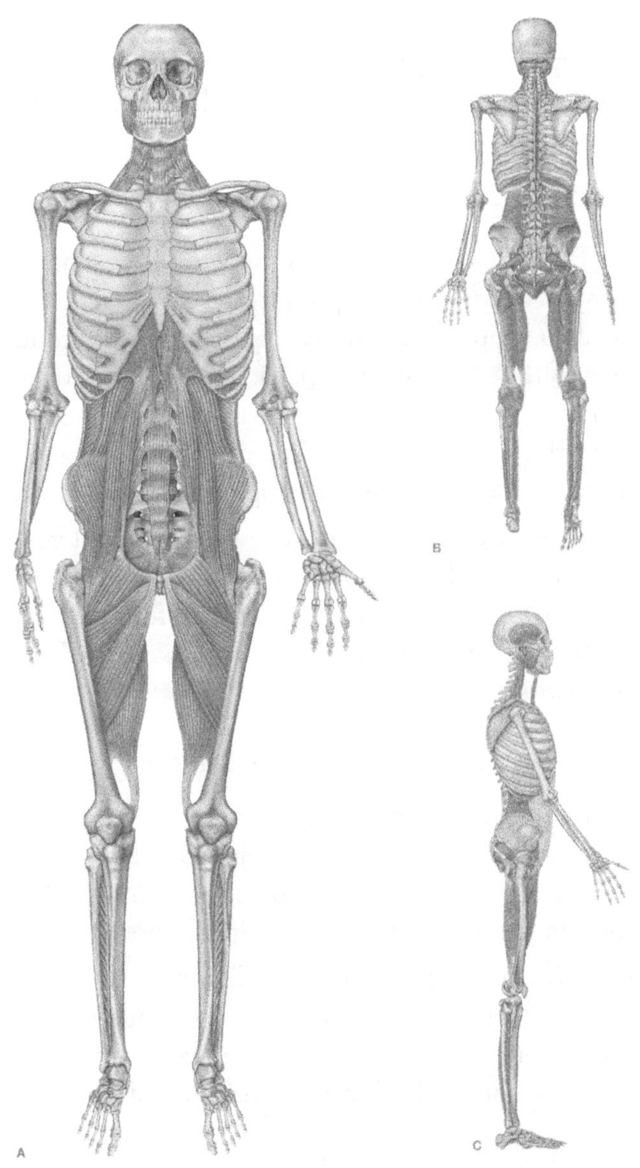

Figure 25.1 The Deep Front Line: When I first saw this figure in Thomas Myers book, Anatomy Trains, the shaded areas were like a map of where I felt tight. They were my blocks of wood and bands of steel. Predominately, the shaded areas relate to flexion. The physical therapists were only interested in my ankle. They had no interest in the tightness in my torso.

Thomas Myers Anatomy Trains p. 184. Reproduced with permission.[1]

In the hospital, no one ever inquired where I felt tight. They were only interested in, very crudely, getting me to walk. How much better would their process have been if I had been offered this picture so I could point at it and say "there"?

~

If the Deep Front Line of fascia cannot move as it was intended to, then the pelvic and spinal cores collapse, producing a shortening in stature. This line is supposed to support the lumbar region from the front. The shape of the balloons of the abdomen and pelvic area depends on it. The hips, and consequently the legs, are stabilized by it. How we breathe, expanding and relaxing our ribcage, relies on this line of fascia moving to support the action. It is fundamental to carrying the weight of the head on the shoulders.

Following my big attack, all these areas were tight and got tighter, but the physical therapists and neurologists had no interest. All they did was sometimes say, "How are you?" They never waited for the answer, and they never showed me a picture like this. These areas were my blocks of wood and bands of steel.

The Superficial Back Line

As I moved through my recovery, I gradually felt more and more tightness in my back. The relentless pulling throughout my Deep Front Line was something Sarah tried to overcome through my Pilates exercises. She helped, but, in truth, the dantrolene helped more.

It was an endless task to get more flexibility into the Deep Front Line. But as I recovered, I became more aware of a countervailing pull in my back. While the front of my torso was dominated by flexors that kept pulling, the extensors on my back became tighter and tighter.

~

When you have MS, it doesn't hit all at once. In your torso, the flexors are stronger than the extensors. The extensors have to overcome the power of the flexors. The weaker extensors can become overworked, but your posture depends on them. You need to be able to find extension, and even hyperextension, in your back.

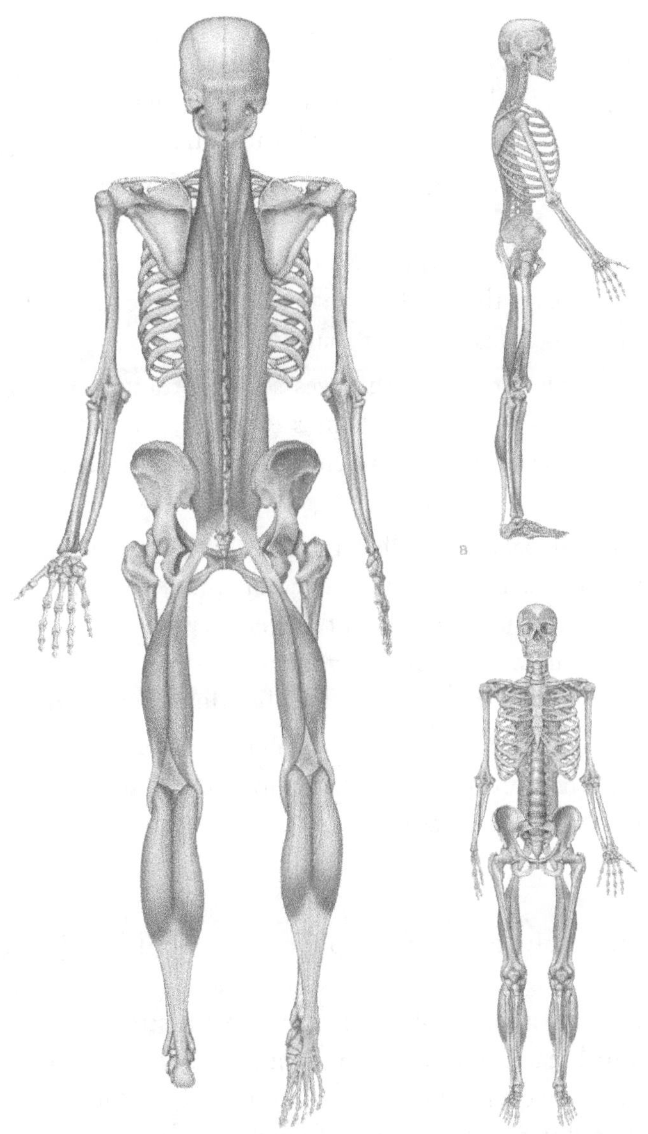

Figure 25.2 The Superficial Back Line: This is the line of fascia involved with the slow twitch extensor muscles that let you stand all day by overcoming the contracting flexors in the deep front line. As they tire, these muscles start to ache. When they fail, your back stoops forward and your legs bend. They hold you erect by contracting, but if the fascia is tight contraction becomes counterproductive, causing pain. Massage, dry needling and PNF stretches relieve this.

Thomas Myers Anatomy Trains p. 74. Reproduced with permission.[1]

The most critical extensors are related to your Superficial Back Line. This line supports the body in an upright extension. Its function is to stop you from curling into a fetal position. The muscles through this line are designed for endurance. They need to do their job through all your waking hours.

There are two major Superficial Back Lines: left and right. They need to be balanced. Each line runs in two segments. Firstly, from the toes, under the foot to the back of the knees. Secondly, from the knees up to the back of the head, then over the skull to the brow. When the knee is locked, these present as one line of fascia rather than two.

The upper segment makes the eyes so important in determining the posture we assume. When I do Pilates exercises, I let my eyes guide my head, rather than leading with my chin. The eyes and the spine should be synchronized for movement.

The superficial backline will determine how your pelvis rotates. If it is shifted, so your sacrum (the base of your spine) is impacted, then your sacroiliac joint will change the load transfer between your spine and lower limbs. In turn, this will impact on your hamstrings. Your knees and your ankles will carry strain if your superficial backline is compromised.

If you do not think you have a problem, try a straightforward test. Stand up, bend forward with your knees locked and touch your toes. That is testing your Superficial Back Line.

~

The most extensive belts of fascia on the Superficial Back Line encompass the groups of muscles collectively known as the erector spinae. If this group tightens up, it will limit the length of your stride, change your gait, influence your breathing, dictate the range of rotation of your torso, and hamper the control over the muscles in your neck. All these movements are continuously pulling on your sheet of fascia.

There is a range of stretches using Pilates equipment that can help offset this tightness, but dry needling this segment, in conjunction with Pilates, gives the greatest relief. If you get into Pilates, there is no movement more joyous and liberating than rolling a released Superficial Back Line over a high barrel. You feel like you are made of water. Often, you need to be dry needled to achieve this.

The Spiral Line

Just like an elite athlete, you need to be balanced no matter where you throw your body in space. A movement by one part of your body always creates an imbalance somewhere else. Even walking does this.

Our bodies use rotation all the time. We aren't windup toys that take off in one direction and never deviate till we topple over. We twist our frame: our hips rotate, our torso turns, our limbs swing through the air to counterbalance a shift in the center of gravity. All these motions use the Spiral Line. Without it, we would fall over.

~

In practical terms, we can treat the Spiral Line as several spirals.

One spiral starts from the base of the skull. It crosses at the neck and feeds down into the rhomboids to wrap around the sides of the ribcage. A further spiral (really an extension of the first) then wraps across the ribs. It travels down the front of the torso, to the opposing hip. A raft of Pilates exercises and massage techniques target these first two turns of the spiral. The exercises keep the spirals supple and elastic to retain flexion in the upper spine, and help the scapula to move sympathetically for arm movement. We can call this series the upper Spiral Line.

The lower Spiral Line passes from the front of the hip to the outside of the knee to the inside of the ankle. You can see its impact by watching how your knee tracks.

Dry needling and Pilates exercises to correct knee tracking will change your gait. When I do Pilates, someone is always watching me. My number one aim of correction is to check how my knee is tracking. Sometimes I concentrate on the angle of my foot to find the ideal path, and sometimes I just focus on my knee. Often it is not easy to fix as my body wants to go on a frolic of its own.

The lower Spiral Line is all about the stability of our gait. There are ligaments and huge muscles all through the pelvic region. They are supposed to allow us to move our legs asymmetrically (i.e., one leg is forward, and one is somewhere else). Dry needling and Pilates are very important in retaining a natural gait.

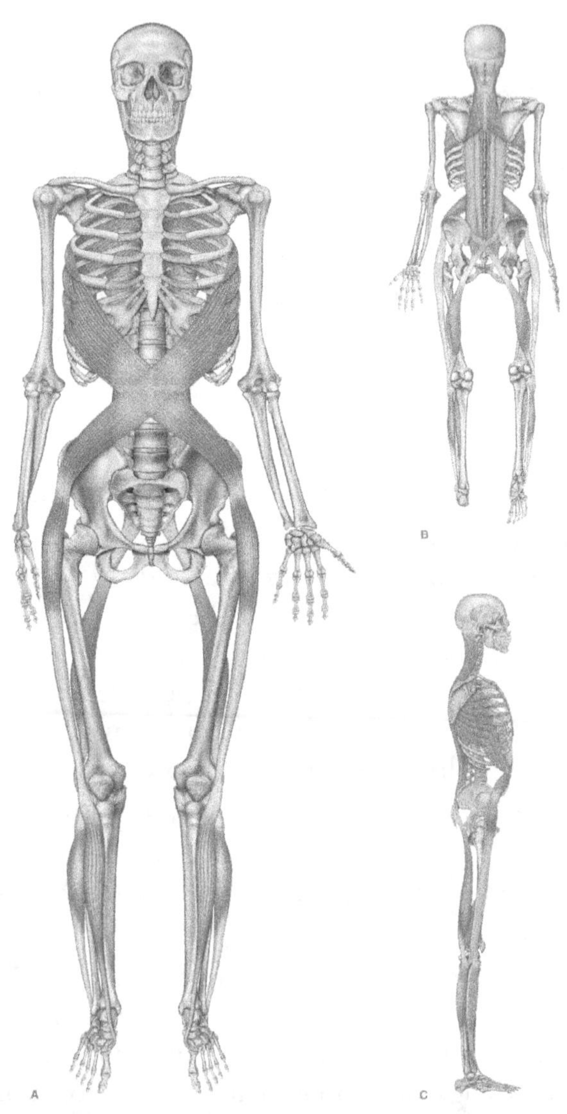

Figure 25.3 The Spiral Line: You cannot rotate and influence the deep front line and your Superficial Back Line unless you engage the Spiral Line. Traditional massage and dry needling have minimal impact but PNF stretches can improve your range of rotation. None of those options are as effective as the eccentric contractions best represented by Pilates exercises. If you cannot rotate freely, the extensive muscles on your back will reinforce the rigidity of your torso, limiting a normal gait. A relaxed Spiral Line is essential to developing a normal gait.

Thomas Myers Anatomy Trains p. 132. Reproduced with permission.[1]

So is massage. Unfortunately, there is an absurd reluctance to work on the complex muscles between the waist and the thigh. Both practitioners and patients need to get over their moral squeamishness. PNF (Proprioceptive Neuromuscular Facilitation, see Chapter 33) stretches can be extremely beneficial for the muscles and ligaments in this area.

~

There are other significant lines of fascia. There is the deep arm line, the superficial arm line, and the deep and superficial back arm lines. There are leg lines and lateral lines. There are superficial front and back lines.

Some lines cross the body so we can do 'athletic' motions. We see these lines in action in a golf swing, a tennis serve and in the leap of a hurdler. All those things are aspirational if our upper motor neurons are damaged.

There is no pill or magical medication to make these lines function as they should. I scratch my head when I read that a 25 m walking test was used as a benchmark for success with a medication. A medication may have some therapeutic consequence that influences the immune system, but it won't change how your fascia works when you attempt to walk. What are they thinking? It doesn't even make sense.

1. Myers, T.W., *Anatomy Trains: Myofascial meridians for manual and movement therapists (Second Edition).* 2009, Elsevier: New York.

Chapter 26

Upper and Lower Motor Neurons

When we send a signal from our brain to a muscle, it is a two-step dance. The intention, and the primary message, travels through our brain and spinal cord along a path that involves a neuron called an upper motor neuron.

This first neuron talks to a second motor neuron. The cell body of the second neuron originates outside the spinal cord. It is called a lower motor neuron. This is the neuron that takes the instruction to the muscle.

More often than not, the brain is trying to quieten the activity of the lower motor neuron.

~

Imagine you have just bought a puppy. You've chosen a completely untrained animal that's about ten months old. It's excited by everything and is clueless about following commands. You put the young dog on a lead and go into the park. Immediately you are confronted by a 'pop-up' farmers market. The dog is thrilled.

You have led the dog to the park, but everything it experiences in the park is making it react. Your only hope of controlling the dog depends on the connection between the two of you—in this case, the lead. If that connection is lost, the dog will happily and haphazardly react to everything. He won't care what you say. The warnings, threats, treats, or tears you use won't mean anything to him. You are a new owner. He barely knows you and is too excited by everything around him. You control the extremely excited dog by using your voice, tugging on the lead, and offering it bribes.

This is very like the relationship between upper and lower motor neurons. The upper motor neuron is a controlling influence on the lower motor neuron, much like the puppy's lead.

However, in MS, the messages from upper to lower motor neurons are likely to have been disrupted. When this happens, the lower motor neuron ignores the upper motor neuron and remains excited by any interaction. It misses any calming signal or any command to rest. Without an instruction to stop, the lower motor neuron will keep signaling a muscle to contract every time movements in your body stimulate it. To your lower motor neuron, reflex actions are like the farmers market is to the dog: they stimulate further activity.

~

In a healthy body, the upper motor neuron can relay messages from the brain to stop the lower motor neuron reacting. It is the same sort of relationship that exists when you make the puppy lie down. Damage in MS removes this connection. You don't have a signal that causes the muscle to rest.

~

A muscle contracts because a lower motor neuron signaled it to do that. If the brain believes that the contraction should end, it sends a signal to the neuron (not the muscle) and the neuron stops the stimulation. That message is called GABA.

If the lower motor neuron does not receive the GABA message, it will continue to stimulate the muscle, driving it to keep contracting. Any further reflex stimulus will make it tighten even more. There will be no rest. Like the hyperexcitable puppy, it will go on and on.

Stiffness and spasticity in MS are due to damage to upper motor neurons. They have lost their control over lower motor neurons. This aspect is not a mystery.

Drugs that modulate your immune system don't repair the damage that has already occurred. The best they can do is stop further damage developing and, perhaps, allow remyelination to outpace demyelination.

A disease-modifying medication can't be your only strategy to solve the symptom of spastic muscles. You have to look elsewhere.

Chapter 27

Excitation-Contraction Coupling

So, why do muscles contract? What is the process called, and how does it happen?

Muscles tighten and relax through a process called excitation-contraction coupling. The force in the muscles as they contract pulls on the rigging of our connective tissue. That tissue helps distribute the force across the body. If nothing signals that the required force has been achieved, then the connective tissue will continue to exert a pull, the muscle will continue to shorten, and the body will gradually twist into a distorted posture to accommodate the ceaseless tightening.

Our muscles contract and relax. They do this constantly. It is why we can move. It determines how we breathe, talk, pump blood, eat, excrete, and carry out all the functions we take for granted. Some actions of muscles are totally involuntary, and others are controlled by our own conscious decisions.

If our muscles only contract, we can't move. The muscle is spastic or rigid or hypertonic.

If our muscles cannot contract, we can't control them. The muscle is limp and useless.

Patients with MS are more likely to have spastic muscles—a sign of upper motor neuron damage. Checking for this is part of what the neurologist is doing when he scrapes the sole of your foot and tests your reflexes.

When your foot is scraped, the neurologist is looking to see what sort of reflex action is stimulated. If you have MS, your big toe is likely to flex in response to the wrong area being stimulated. The stimulus overpowers the normal flexors in the toe. You react like an infant whose nervous system is not yet fully developed.

This reaction is called the Babinski sign,[1] after the Nobel nominee who described it in 1896.

All our senses, actions, and reactions are responses to neurotransmitters released from the end of a nerve cell's axon. The target of the neurotransmitter might be a neuron, or a muscle cell. The steps that come after the neurotransmitter reaches a target muscle are together called excitation-contraction coupling.

Not every reaction relies on a message being sent from the brain to a muscle. If you touch something hot, you pull away very quickly. This reaction is called a reflex. In this case, neurotransmitters send a message from sensory receptors straight to muscles via the spine. A secondary message goes to the brain to reinforce that pulling away was the right thing to do. The reflex was stimulated by an arc that did not involve the brain. Many of our actions are just reflexes.

Other muscle movements are learned responses that we do so often that we don't consciously decide to do them. If you aim to hit the letter "J" on a keyboard, you might look for the letter, but you don't consciously think about moving your arm, then hovering over the button and then striking it with your finger. It's a learned action that we do so often that the pattern is ingrained.

Nonetheless, everything is driven by impulses pushed along our nerves.

All those motions, whether conscious movements, reflexes, or learned patterns, rely on excitation-contraction coupling. Too often, knowledge of this process remains trapped in academia.

Common Features of Muscles

Although there are different types of muscles, they all have some common features:

1) They can be excited by stimulus from neurons.

2) They can contract.

3) They can be stretched (to a point).

4) They can return to a resting state (otherwise known as elasticity).

These characteristics let them do things like move bones, resist gravity (determine our posture), stabilize our joints, and assist in producing heat.

The Babinski sign is not the only reflex test for your foot. There are others.[1] Similar tests are looking for comparable reactions, called plantar reflex reactions.

The main ones are checked by:

Bing's Sign: Pricking of the top of the foot (dorsum) or the first toe with a pin.

Chaddock's Sign: Circular stroking of the skin around an area on the outside of the ankle (lateral malleolus).

Cornell's Sign: Stroking the top of the foot (dorsum) along the extensor tendon of the first toe.

Gonda's Sign: Forceful stretching and snapping of the second or fourth toe downwards.

Gordon's Sign: Applying deep pressure to the calf muscle.

Mendal Bechtrew Sign: Tapping of top of the foot (dorsum) over the outer side at the cuboid bone.

Moniz Sign: The ankle is forcibly and passively plantarflexed.

Oppenheim's Sign: Compressing the thumb and index finger on the front surface of the shin bone (tibia).

Rossolimo's Sign: Tapping the ball of the foot or flicking and snapping the end of the toe below the toenail (distal phalanges) to extend them.

Schaeffer's Sign: Applying deep pressure on the Achilles tendon.

Stransky's Sign: Pulling out and snapping of the fifth toe.

Strumpell's Sign: Applying deep pressure on the outer side (anterior) of the shinbone (tibia.)

Ultimately, these tests are looking for signs that the muscle action is abnormally brisk. This happens if the muscle is over contracted and can't relax.

The Three Types of Muscles

We have three types of muscles. Each has different properties.

1) Cardiac muscle

This muscle contracts slowly and has low levels of maintained tension. The messages from nerves can either excite or inhibit its action. Nerves that control it come from the autonomic nervous system, which operates without our conscious involvement. Its cell membranes have crevices called tubules that play a role in its electrochemical signaling.

Cardiac muscle cells are coupled to each other. By comparison, skeletal muscle cells are electrically isolated from each other.

Calcium from both the cellular stores and the extracellular fluid plays a role in activating heart cells. In the cardiac muscle, calcium binds to a protein called troponin, but only at one site on the protein.

The neuroendocrine system, which incorporates the glands that produce hormones, influences the cardiac muscle to control the behavior of its filaments. This means, unlike skeletal muscle, calcium is not the major influence on cardiac muscle activity.[2]

Every cardiac cell will contract with each beat. As the heart can change its output force, it is far more adaptive than skeletal muscle.

Structurally, heart muscle is called striated muscle as the cellular units that make up the muscle, called sarcomeres, give it a striped appearance due to their arrangement.

One of the unique characteristics of cardiac muscle is that its cells can form branches. This helps with signaling between cells and supports the whole muscle complex to move in three dimensions. Cardiac muscle cells are packed with vast numbers of mitochondria.

2) Smooth muscle

Smooth muscle is not striated and contracts differently to other muscles. It is controlled, like heart muscle, by the autonomic nervous system, so we do not consciously control it. The speed of its contraction is very slow; much slower than cardiac muscle. There are no tubules in smooth muscle membrane. Smooth muscle also needs to be viewed separately from skeletal muscle.

Calcium released from the cellular stores and extracellular fluid activates smooth muscle, similar to what happens with cardiac muscle. Unlike striated muscle, the calcium in smooth muscle interacts with an enzyme called myosin light-chain kinase to activate the muscle contraction.

3) Skeletal muscle

These are the muscles that move our bones. We consciously control them. They can contract at differing speeds, from slowly to quite quickly. Nerve impulses can only excite them; they cannot inhibit skeletal muscle contraction. The nerves themselves, rather than the muscle, need to be inhibited to relax the muscle. In other words, the signal from the nerve needs to be switched off. The nerve itself does not signal the muscle to relax. The nerves act like a switch on a lamp; they are either on or off.

Skeletal muscle is activated by calcium binding to troponin. Unlike cardiac muscle, there are two binding sites on the skeletal muscle troponin, making the response to calcium quicker than in cardiac muscle. The calcium comes from a store in the muscle cell called the sarcoplasmic reticulum. Extracellular calcium plays no role.

Like a cardiac muscle, skeletal muscle is striated. This is the muscle type you need to understand above all, when looking at MS.

The Structure of a Skeletal Muscle Fiber

If we cut down through the skin and, just like most anatomists in the past, scrape away the connective tissue, we come to the outer covering on a muscle. It is a form of connective tissue. This layer has a name, the epimysium. It is regarded as a protective layer that insulates the muscle from bone and other tissue. Mostly, it is viewed as "stuff" of little consequence.

Inside the muscle, there is a net of more connective tissue. This forms an inner covering of the outer layer of the muscle. It has offshoots that deviate throughout the muscle, separating segments (called fibers) from each other. This network is called the perimyseum. Running through the perimyseum are blood vessels and nerve fibers that feed and communicate with the cells of the flesh inside each segment.

The connective tissue carries the conduits that allow transport of red and white blood cells. It is a highway for fibroblasts, mast cells, glial cells, pigment cells, and the cells that carry the very stuff of bone to and from our skeleton. As it is full of fluid, it buffers us. If we use our muscles, the movement circulates fluid throughout our system. When the fluid is free-flowing, it will carry nutrients to, and waste away from our cells. If our muscles don't do their job due to strain, trauma, or lack of use, then the fluid starts to dry out. The system becomes clogged. We can see a consequence of this when our skin shows the hallmarks of aging.[3]

Inside a muscle fiber is a string of muscle cells

A skeletal muscle fiber is called a fascicle. Inside the fascicle are even smaller components, collectively named the endomysium.

Each component of the endomysium is a single muscle cell, known as a myofiber. As each cell is longer than it is wide, the shape dictates that it is described as a fiber. A human hair is gigantic compared to the single muscle cell.

Nonetheless, compared to other cells, a muscle cell is a giant. As it is long, it might contain several nuclei. It is too big for just one nucleus to make all the proteins it needs. Many nuclei are found on the outer membrane of a muscle cell.

Cardiac muscle cells may only have one, two or three nuclei each.[2] Skeletal muscles have a lot more.

Myofibrils and sarcomeres

Tubes called myofibrils, run the length of each muscle cell. The myofibrils are made up of short lengths of smaller filaments, grouped into packets. The packets are arranged end on end, giving the myofibril, when viewed side-on, a striped appearance. Each packet contains the same repeated bands and is called a sarcomere.

Contraction happens in the smallest parts of a muscle cell

At each end of a sarcomere, there is a disk, by convention called a Z-disc. Extending inwards from each Z-disc are tiny fibers called actin filaments.

Between each actin filament is another thicker strand, a myosin filament.

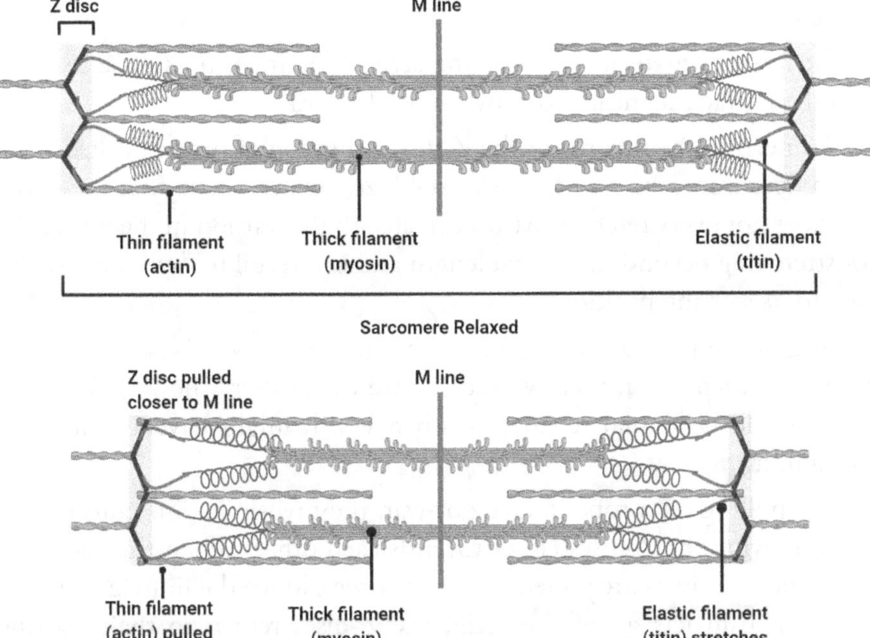

Figure 27.1 The smallest unit of a muscle is called a sarcomere. In a skeletal muscle the ends of the sarcomere are called Z-discs. The Z-discs create common walls between adjacent sarcomeres. One sarcomere will impact on its neighbours.

The thin filament is called actin. It is connected to the Z-discs and has a finite length. Actin has binding sites that are exposed when calcium floods the sarcomere.

The thick filament of a sarcomere in called myosin. It has flexible arms that can adhere to binding sites on actin.

ATP allows the myosin arms to walk along the actin. This will pull the Z-discs closer to each other. When a group of sarcomeres does this in concert, we see muscles contract.

Each myosin filament is connected to a giant protein called titin. This acts like a spring to pull the sarcomere back to its starting position.

Created with BioRender.

This strand also extends inwards from the Z-disc. Each myosin strand has a series of heads on many long arms. These heads can adhere to the actin filament.

The arms of myosin are a moving series. The myosin can use its arms with their attaching heads to crawl along the actin.

Connecting the myosin to the Z-disc is a string of protein called titin, which determines stretch. It acts to stabilize the myosin so that the entire unit does not overstretch. The titin can absorb the tension in the muscle by not stretching beyond its natural length and can recoil to draw the myosin back to its starting position.

Imagine, you and a friend grabbed the ends of a towel. Next, you pulled away from each other, then walked toward each other. The way the towel flexed would be similar to how titin behaves. It might have a little more spring in it.

Like pulling on a rope in a tug-of-war, the myosin action pulls on the actin, drawing the Z-discs closer towards each other. When this happens, simultaneously in many joined sarcomeres, we can see the muscle contract. As the myosin lets go of the actin, the Z-discs return to their starting position. The release lets the sarcomeres lengthen. We call this relaxation.

This activity is often described as the sliding filament theory. It explains concentric muscle contraction (when the muscle is shortened) and is adequate when explaining isometric muscle action (i.e., doing a "plank"). Without including titin as the variable-length spring, the theory can't explain eccentric muscle action. An example of eccentric movement would be how your muscles tighten when you control the lowering of a heavy weight, even though they are lengthening.

<u>You need to understand this step.</u>

What happens when a neurotransmitter signals a skeletal muscle?

We will assume a healthy body to describe what happens in active tension.

~

The dominant neurotransmitter that is released by lower motor neurons to drive skeletal muscle activity is called acetylcholine.

When this neurotransmitter is released from the end of the axon, it crosses a very narrow cleft called a synapse. The axon and the muscle are not touching. A gap exists, so surplus acetylcholine can disperse or be reabsorbed by the neuron. The neurotransmitter that reaches the membrane of the muscle cell binds to receptors. At rest, these receptors, called nicotinic receptors, are closed. Each is made of five proteins that twist away from each other when acetylcholine binds to one of them, creating a pore.

Outside the membrane of the muscle cell, sodium ions are abundant. They are drawn into the opened nicotinic receptor, like water flowing through grains of sand.

The electric charge on a sodium ion is positive. Many sodium ions moving to the inside of the membrane makes the whole-cell less electronegative.

At rest, the inside of the cell is rich in potassium. Sodium and potassium are both positively charged. As a result, the chemicals repel each other. Beyond finding a transitory equilibrium, they do not share the same space. Potassium exchanges with sodium.

Some positively charged potassium ions flow out through receptor channels, but the sodium flowing into the cell is the dominant effect. The result is that the inside of the cell becomes much less negatively charged.

~

As this exchange happens across the whole surface of the muscle cell membrane, a wave of positive electrical energy develops. In muscle cells, this change alters what is known as the motor endplate potential. As the charge on the inside of the membrane becomes more positive, it reaches a threshold that triggers more major sodium receptors to open. When they do, a far more profound inflow of positively charged sodium commences. Sodium surges through these bigger receptors. The extreme voltage change triggers the sodium receptors to close and potassium channels to open. This switch-over by the receptors quickly restores a balance so the cell can return to a resting state.

In the second phase, the wave of positive sodium ions, delivered by the sodium surge, continues to move across the membrane of the muscle cell. This is called the action potential. At various points, some tubules appear like deep crevices in the membrane. They are commonly known as transverse tubules or T-tubules. A receptor, called the dihydropyridine receptor, is scattered down the sides of the T-tubules. It is sensitive to changes in the electrical polarity of the T-tubules.

As the positive sodium ions change the polarity of the T-tubule, the shift triggers the dihydropyridine receptor to move another receptor physically. This last receptor is called the ryanodine receptor.

The ryanodine receptor

On either side of the T-tubule, there are stores of calcium held in the sarcoplasmic reticulum.

The ryanodine receptor usually acts as a plug to stop the calcium from flowing out of the sarcoplasmic reticulum. The action of the wave of positive sodium ions ultimately results in the ryanodine receptor uncoupling from the store, and calcium rushes out.

As calcium floods out of the sarcoplasmic reticulum, its main target is the specialized protein, troponin. Calcium binding to troponin causes the muscle to contract. It does this by exposing sites that permit myosin and actin to bind.

So, the chain reaction is: the neurotransmitter acetylcholine stimulates the entry of sodium, which changes the polarity of the muscle cell membrane, which triggers calcium to be released. The calcium has a significant target in the muscle cell: troponin. When calcium binds to troponin, muscles contract.

It is vital to know this last point. We will come back to it.

The reason I take dantrolene sodium is to block the ryanodine receptor and prevent the release of too much calcium.

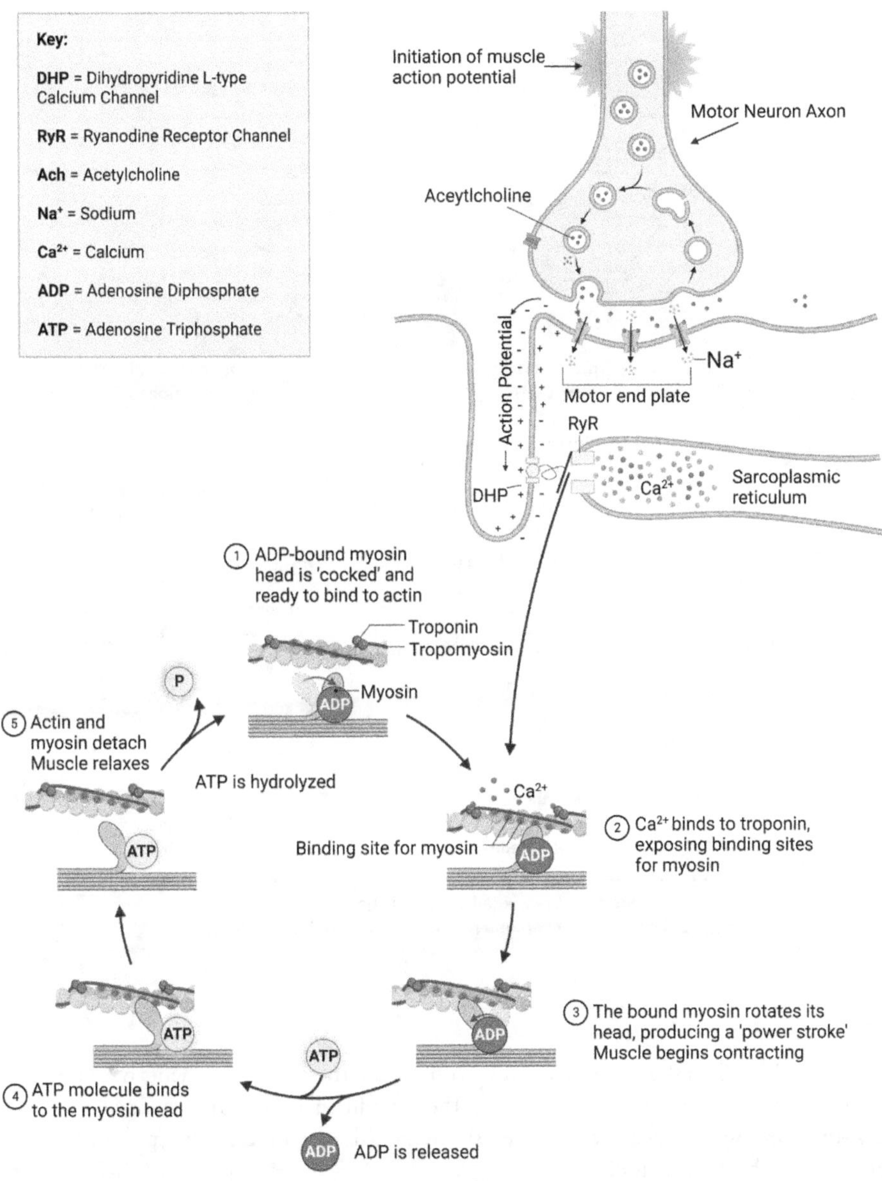

Figure 27.2 of excitation-contraction coupling. Steps 3- 5 of the muscle contraction phase (known as cross-bridge cycling) is completed by the hydrolysis of ATP to ADP. These steps provide the biochemical energy for myosin to change conformation and walk down the thin actin filaments.

Created in Biorender. Based on diagrams in Human Physiology: An integrated approach 8th Ed.[9]

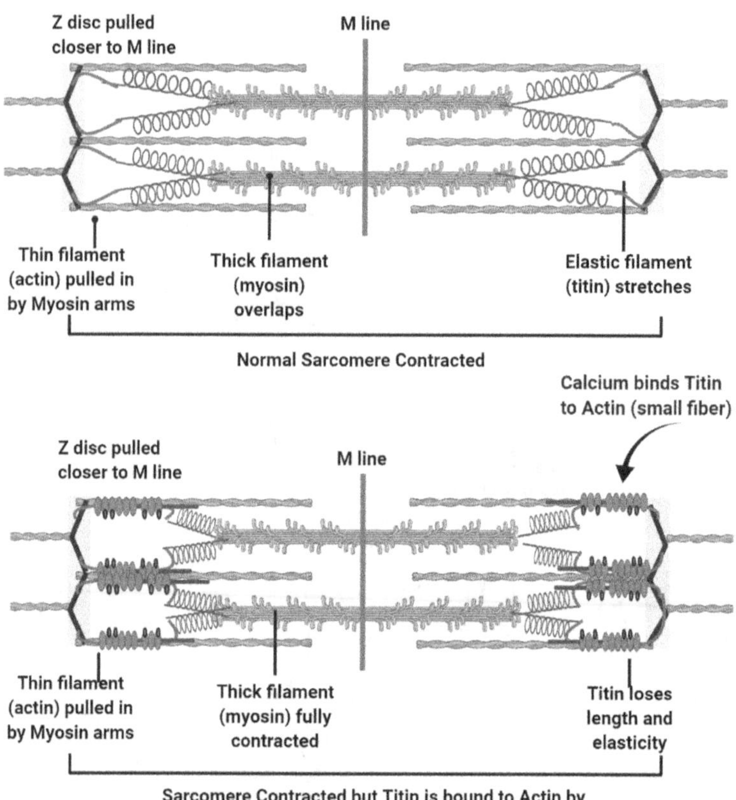

Figure 27.3 When the sarcomere is fully contracted, the myosin filaments have moved towards the M-line by pulling on the actin. The actin filament does not change length so the Z-discs are pulled toward each other, shortening the sarcomere. The spring protein, titin, reverses the contraction.

When calcium has bound actin to titin, the length of the spring is reduced. Myosin has to work harder to lengthen the spring. A shortened titin spring will not draw the myosin back to its original position so the sarcomere stays in a shortened state, increasing passive muscle tension.

Created with BioRender.

Muscle Tension

Two different actions are happening in the sarcomere. The overlap between the myosin and the actin is called 'active tension.' At the end of the myosin, the tension in the titin 'spring' is called 'passive tension.'

The wrapping of connective tissue all through the muscle can add stabilizing strength to passive tension but is not part of excitation-contraction coupling.

The titin protein has a finite length. An example would be to look at two boats tied to a pier. If one boat were tied with a meter-long rope, it would not move far. If the other had a one-hundred meter rope, it would drift in a big arc away from the pier. Both ropes can be 'stretched' to a similar maximum strain between the pier and the boat. One boat is tightly bound to the pier, but the other is not. The boat lashed to the pier reaches its 'passive tension' limit in the first meter. It barely moves. The other boat has a more flexible range. Whatever determines the total length of the titin determines the passive tension in the fiber.

The absolute length of titin determines your flexibility

Since its discovery, titin has been considered a stable part of both the structure and the mechanics of the sarcomere. More recent research has shown that the length of the titin can be changed.[4] On the one hand, the sequences within it can be elastic, and, on the other, calcium can bind lengths of it to the actin fiber, shortening the titin. This action would be similar to wrapping the rope attached to the boat around and around the pilings of the pier, reducing the length of the rope.

If the titin is shortened, then so is the possible muscle length and the capacity of the muscle to absorb force is lowered. We seem to be stiffer.

If too much calcium is released in our muscle cells, some will end up binding titin to actin. This will reduce our flexibility.

Calcium has a powerful influence on its binding sites. If its release were uncontrolled, we would be very stiff. Some proteins and specialized pumps move calcium into the sarcoplasmic reticulum, so there is always an abundant store, but its influence is controlled. Unregulated calcium can become a real problem, affecting protein folding and a range of functions.[5] If calcium becomes unregulated, it can set up a self-perpetuating stimulus as it would be continuously overexpressed.[6]

Calcium overload can also trigger pores in the mitochondrial membrane, the mitochondrial permeability transition pores, to open. This can lead to cell death.[7]

Calcium lets tropomyosin unlock from actin. Myosin can then bind to actin.

When calcium binds to troponin, it causes a ribbon of protein, called tropomyosin, to slide to a new position on actin. As this moves, it exposes a set of sites on the actin filament to myosin. The actin sites become the binding targets for the heads of the arms of myosin.

These hinged arms become the molecular motor that powers muscle contraction.[2] Myosin arms appear to walk along the actin filament. This action pulls the ends of the fibers closer toward each other, creating contraction. Each time a myosin arm moves along the actin, it comes at the cost of one molecule of ATP. You spend a lot of ATP every time you move a muscle.

How myosin moves on actin

When myosin binds to actin, it triggers a chemical process called hydrolysis.[8] The myosin arms have an ATP molecule bound to the head of them. The binding of the two filaments disassociates one phosphate molecule from ATP, reducing it to ADP. The ADP then also cleaves from the myosin head. There is then an opportunity for a new ATP molecule to fill the vacant site. As the ADP leaves and is replaced by ATP, the head of the myosin disassociates from the actin filament, and a lever-action returns it to a resting position. Provided calcium is still causing the troponin to

252

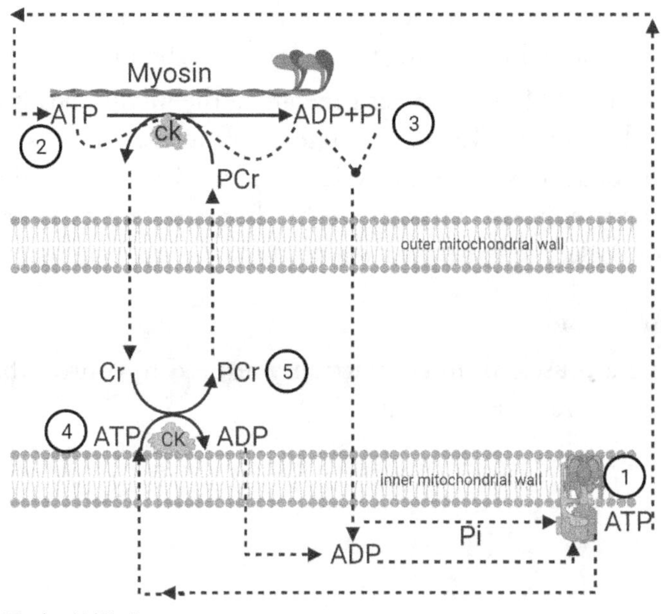

Figure 27.4

Normal muscle movement relies on ATP

1. Nearly all ATP is made inside the mitochondria by a specialised protein called ATP synthase.

2. Newly created ATP leaves the mitochondria and a great deal of it is used to drive muscle contraction by binding to myosin filaments in each sarcomere. Each movement of a myosin arm expends ATP which then breaks down into ADP and a phosphate molecule (Pi).

3. Both ADP and phosphate return to the mitochondria to be reunited as ATP. This is a slow pathway as 1) the molecules are large and 2) they must pass through two membranes.

4. Some ATP (but not much) leaves the mitochondrial matrix through a different pathway. Between the two walls of the mitrochondria an enzyme, called creatine kinase, harvests a phosphate from ATP and donates it to creatine (Cr), creating phosphocreatine (PCr).

5. The Phosphocreatine migrates from the mitochondria and is stored in our muscle tissue. When we exert ourselves, another creatine kinase liberates the phosphate and another enzyme (not shown) uses it to restore ADP to ATP. This is a very fast process and is quickly exhausted. It only lasts a few seconds. Ten seconds for a 100 meter dash would exhaust the fast pathway in even the most elite athlete. The slow pathway can't sustain that rate of ATP use.

In MS, the uncontrolled release of calcium means our sarcomeres are often contracted and our ATP is overutilised by Myosin arms fruitlessly trying to adhere to Actin. We cannot keep up with that demand and the result is muscle fatigue and exhaustion.

expose the binding sites; the action will repeat. The effect is that myosin will pull along the actin, bringing the ends of the sarcomere closer together.

When we die, ATP no longer is generated. The myosin heads and actin filaments lock together. We call this state rigor mortis.[8] There is no ATP to continue the binding and release cycle. Although less extreme than death, when you have a spastic muscle, the binding sites are exposed and the filaments are locked together in a similar way.

What is the lesson?

To release a muscle from contraction you need to control the flow of calcium and ensure ATP is available.

References

1. Ambesh, P., V.K. Paliwal, V. Shetty and S. Kamholz, *The Babinski Sign: A comprehensive review.* Journal of the Neurological Sciences, 2017. **372**: p. 477–481.

2. Sweeney, H. and D. Hammers, *Muscle contraction.* Cold Spring Harbor Perspectives in Biology, 2018. **10**(2) p. a023200.

3. Myers, T.W., *Anatomy Trains: Myofascial meridians for manual and movement therapists (Second Edition).* 2009, Elsevier: New York.

4. Granzier, H.L. and S. Labeit, *The giant protein titin.* Circulation Research, 2004. **94**(3): p. 284–295.

5. Paredes, R.M., M. Bollo, D. Holstein and J.D. Lechleiter, *Luminal Ca2+ depletion during the unfolded protein response in Xenopus oocytes: cause and consequence.* Cell Calcium, 2013. **53**(4): p. 286–296.

6. Laver, D.R., *Ca^{2+} stores regulate ryanodine receptor Ca^{2+} release channels via luminal and cytosolic Ca^{2+} sites.* Biophysical Journal, 2007. **92**(10): p. 3541–3555.

7. Halestrap, A.P. and P. Pasdois, *The role of the mitochondrial permeability transition pore in heart disease.* Biochimica Biophysica Acta, 2009. **1787**(11): p. 1402–1415.

8. Sweeney, H.L. and E.L.F. Holzbaur, *Motor proteins.* Cold Spring Harbor Perspectives in Biology, 2018. **10**(5) p. a021931.

9. Silverthorn, D.U., *Human Physiology: An Integrated Approach. 8th Edition.* Pearson Education Australia.

Chapter 28

The Targets when Dealing with Spasticity

Spasticity in MS arises because the damage to upper motor neurons (the ones associated with the brain and spinal cord) interrupts a message that ultimately tells a muscle to relax. Meanwhile the lower motor neuron, which connects to our skeletal muscle, remains active, driving muscle contraction.

As well as reacting to signals from upper motor neurons, the brain responds to reflex actions. Reflexes, though, don't rely on a command from the brain. The brain, instead, needs to see the effect of a reflex. It is continually sampling information from the body to control balance and posture. Sometimes though, a lesion prevents this information reaching the brain.

Our voluntary movements start in the brain. We think about them, but we don't think about the corresponding movements that make our actions smooth and relaxed. At best, our brain is informed about a reflex activity and sends a command to stop it. Without that command, the reflex is sustained.

If the ability to stop a muscle tightening is lost or diminished, then we are hypertonic, hyperreflexic, or spastic.

There are different targets to deal with MS muscle contractions:

1) Dampen the excitatory signal.

Muscle relaxants aim to do this. Typical examples of their use are seen in operations when a muscle needs to be temporarily immobilized, such as when medication is used to stop the gag reflex while a tube is passed down the throat. The drug of choice for this situation is a neuromuscular blocker. This class of drug works outside the central nervous system.

The other group of drugs used to dampen excitatory signals are spasmolytics. They work in the central nervous system and are what most people think of as muscle relaxants. Using either and doing nothing else isn't as effective as combining them with physical therapy. There is not much point relaxing a muscle and leaving it alone. It still needs to be re-educated.

Excitatory upper motor neurons can send a signal, like norepinephrine or glutamate, to activate a lower motor neuron, but these signals may be too much when other pathways are corrupted. Alternatively, when a balancing inhibitory neuron that sends the calming chemical GABA is damaged and the message doesn't arrive, the excitation of the muscle isn't relieved.

The drug tizanidine binds to a receptor in an upper motor neuron called an α-2 receptor and dampens the excitatory impulse. Typically, this drug is used in MS for spasms.

Targeting the excitatory signal isn't very effective in helping with spasticity.

The advantage of not targeting the central nervous system is that the side effects of euphoria, light-headedness, fatigue, and muscle weakness are reduced. The drugs that target the central nervous system are depressing it. That makes other drugs like alcohol much more potent. There are all sorts of risks arising from that.

Directly targeting a muscle causes transitory weakness but exercise can rebuild that strength. It is far better to exercise along with treatment, than to use direct-acting treatments and do nothing else.

2) Replace the inhibitory signal that is lost

If the inhibitory neuron impulse is lost, the neurotransmitter, GABA, just doesn't arrive. There is nothing to trigger a muscle to relax. There are two different GABA receptors. You may be familiar with the drug Valium (diazepam), which opens a GABA-α receptor. When this opens, chloride floods into a cell and dampens the frequency of reactions.

For spasticity in MS, the more critical target is a GABA-β receptor. When this opens, it allows potassium to enter the cell body of a neuron. The potassium displaces the sodium and dampens the excitatory signal. The most common drug that targets GABA-β receptors is baclofen. This drug also binds to the same receptors on upper motor neurons, reducing their stimulatory

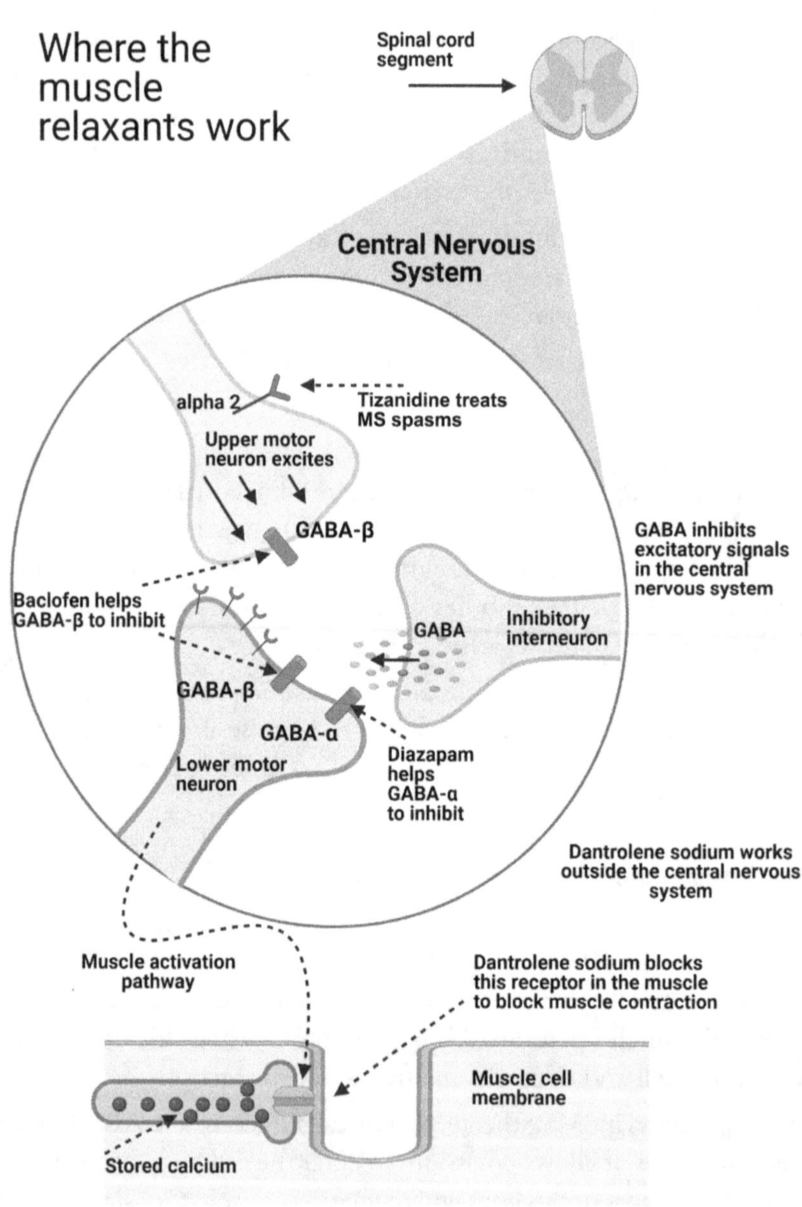

Figure 28.1 Where muscle relaxants work.
Created with BioRender.

Diazepam vs. Baclofen

The drug, diazepam, originally marketed as Valium, can bind to the GABA-α receptor. Binding to this receptor allows more chloride into the nerve pathways related to anxiety, some seizures, and drug dependence (such as alcohol). The result is a calming effect.

Baclofen[1] activates GABA-β receptors. It modulates muscle contraction pathways by allowing more potassium into the cell. The potassium displaces the sodium that triggers muscle contraction.

The GABA-β receptors in upper motor neurons are also affected by baclofen. This can have the effect of making a patient feel weaker and unable to stand up. Baclofen dosing needs to take account of this.

Tizanidine[2]

This drug is also used in MS spasticity treatment. It binds to the upper motor neuron α-2 adrenergic receptors and, like baclofen, can reduce the influence of excitatory neurotransmitters. It might only be used for a short-term purpose.

Tizanidine has no significant effect on spinal reflexes, although its mechanism of action is mostly in the spine. This drug is not very specifically targeted. It can also decrease the heart rate and blood pressure. As a result, if it is suddenly discontinued, there is a risk of rebound hypertension and tachycardia accompanied by increased spasticity.

Pregnant women should not use it. Animal tests have shown it causes fetal harm.[7]

Muscle relaxers

There is a range of other muscle relaxers such as carisoprodol, cyclobenzaprine, metaxalone, chlorzoxazone, and orphenadrine. They appear to work in the brain stem, but how they work is not well understood. If these were being suggested, if I was already on baclofen, tizanidine, or dantrium, I would demand a lot of information about the risks of contraindications. If I was using centrally acting muscle relaxers, I would stay away from alcohol.

firing. Less active signaling means less muscle tightening. Baclofen needs to get to the spine to find these receptors. It loves fat, so most of it doesn't complete the journey. Oral dosing needs to be high to compensate.

3) Diffusely target the tight muscle

Using dantrolene sodium works best for me. This drug doesn't act in the central nervous system. Instead, it blocks the receptor in the muscle that opens to allow calcium to start triggering a muscle contraction. Dantrolene sodium is highly selective for skeletal muscle. The receptors it targets are practically unique to skeletal muscles. They are rare in some parts of the body. That characteristic means your heart and respiratory system are unaffected by this medication.

4) Narrowly, directly target a tight muscle

Direct targeting is usually done by injecting botulinum toxin A, often called botox. Usually, when a neurotransmitter is released, it first fuses with the membrane at the end of the axon. When they lock together, the proteins involved are called a SNARE complex, and look like two halves coupled together. The botox breaks a protein, called SNAP-25, on the axon membrane, leaving nothing for the neurotransmitter to attach to. The SNARE complex can't be formed, and the neurotransmitter can't be released. I have had botox injections in my legs. It works. Often botox is injected in the smooth muscle surrounding the bladder to release a spastic bladder.

References

1.   *Drugbank Baclofen*. 2020; Available from: https://www.drugbank.ca/drugs/DB00181#label-reference. Accessed January 2021.

2.   *Drugbank Tizanidine*. 2020; Available from: https://www.drugbank.ca/drugs/DB00697. Accessed January 2021.

Chapter 29

Dantrolene Sodium

The head of the spasticity clinic repeated it over and over, "Most people hate this."

I, most clearly, don't mind dantrolene sodium at all.

Dantrolene was only prescribed because I complained that my torso was very tight and that baclofen made me feel bilious. It was an afterthought, not a first-line treatment. When I watch video presentations about treating MS, this drug is sometimes not even mentioned. Whenever it is named, it is usually at the bottom of the list, and the presenters concede that they have never used it. It is hard to find a doctor who even knows what it is. Neurologists know it, and so do anesthetists.

The History of Dantrolene

Dantrolene sodium (Dantrium) was discovered by researchers working for Norwich Eaton Pharmaceuticals in the U.S. in 1967.[1, 2]

It was an experimental compound that did not appear to influence the nerves or neurotransmitters but did cause muscle relaxation. Original animal experiments used an intravenous delivery system and created a highly effective response. At that stage, it was a drug without a purpose. Norwich Eaton was looking for anti-infective agents. What became Dantrium was not a significant part of their library.

The intriguing characteristic of Dantrium was that it did not wipe out respiration but made skeletal muscles in the animal models almost flaccid. This attribute made it a possible candidate for treating the rare condition called malignant hyperthermia, which was first described in the early 1960s. This condition most commonly arises, when a patient has a severe adverse reaction to an anesthetic, resulting in spasms and death. This reaction is due to the uncontrolled release of calcium within the cell.

Other muscle relaxants cannot halt the seizure as they only work on the neurotransmitter. Once calcium is already released in the cell, it is too late to block the signaling at the neurotransmitter.

The original thought was to use the drug as a muscle relaxant for animal surgery, but did not take long for the chief researcher, Keith Ellis, to realize that the compound would be an ideal candidate for the treatment of malignant hyperthermia. A South African anesthetist, Gainsford Harrison, successfully experimented on pigs before any testing on humans. These pigs had a condition that mimicked malignant hyperthermia, and that made them unsuitable for any form of shipping.

Toxicity problems and a minimal market saw Norwich Eaton make a commercial decision not to focus on Dantrium development heavily. Still, Ellis published his results in the early 1970s in a somewhat obscure magazine. His article had the effect of creating a great deal of interest. Work continued, slowly, on various formulations of dantrolene.

A high pH and poor solubility were significant hurdles. When they were overcome, the formulation was still a drug without a disease. Trials drove acceptance of its use for malignant hyperthermia by clinicians who, in turn, prompted the FDA to approve its use.

The FDA notes on Dantrium are full of warnings

The FDA placed a warning against oral Dantrium. The cases they reviewed were using high doses of 800 mg for extended periods. Mostly, Dantrium is used as an intravenous preparation for malignant hyperthermia where the doses are anywhere from 1–10 mg/kg for a short period.

I take a 25 mg tablet of oral Dantrium twice a day. When the head of the spasticity unit realized that I didn't mind using it, he said, "you'll be on this for a very long time."

It is the one thing I never want to run out of.

~

The FDA black box warning on Dantrium highlights the potential for hepatotoxicity (chemical driven liver damage). It notes there are instances of fatal and nonfatal symptomatic hepatitis. The report qualifies the incidence of problems by saying doses up to 400 mg have far fewer issues than doses of 800 mg or more per day.

In capsule form, Dantrium is supplied in 25, 50 or 100-mg capsules. From personal experience, 25 mg, twice a day, produces a pretty significant reduction in muscle tightness.

On rare occasions, I will add an extra tablet in the middle of the day. For whatever reason, I have a few days when I am tighter than I want to be. I find it better to spread the dose rather than double a dose to have a little more. That seems to fix the problem.

~

The FDA warning highlights explicitly that the risk of injury is higher in females, patients older than 35, and patients taking other medications. Again, from personal experience, I found blood pressure medications, taken after I had started using Dantrium, were a nightmare and often produced the reverse of the intended effect. The Dantrium created a contraindication.

The FDA report also notes the majority of hepatotoxic events occurred in geriatric patients, who were already on medications that had similar warnings regarding liver damage. They described these cases as "complicated with confounding factors such as intercurrent illnesses and/or potentially hepatotoxic medications." The FDA note concludes that there is a lack of sufficient cases to draw a definitive conclusion about its use in aged patients.

The recommendation of the FDA is to use the lowest possible effective dose. They advise that therapy should be discontinued after a total of 45 days if there was no discernible benefit. My own experience is I was well aware of a change within a week.

~

Dantrium is slightly soluble in water. It is slightly acidic and is more soluble in an alkaline solution. The FDA release suggests it is probably metabolized by "hepatic microsomal enzymes." As this is the likely pathway, other drugs may enhance its metabolism. Nonetheless, the FDA notes that neither phenobarbital nor diazepam affects its metabolism.

After use, the key compound, dantrolene, can be found in measurable quantities in our blood and urine. A 100-mg dose has a biologic half-life of 8.7 hours. We don't completely absorb it, and it is metabolized slowly and consistently. Ultimately, both the duration and intensity of muscle relaxation are dose-dependent.

This drug is indicated for use when spasticity is caused by upper motor neuron disorders (spinal cord injury, stroke, cerebral palsy, and multiple sclerosis). It is not intended to be used where muscle spasms arise from rheumatic disorders.

~

The FDA note says, "*Occasionally, subtle but meaningful improvement in spasticity may occur with Dantrium therapy. In such instances, information regarding improvement should be solicited from the patient and those who are in constant daily contact and attendance with him*".[3]

The reality is nothing like that. Almost no one knows what it is. The prescribing doctor never checks the liver function. In my case, he was surprised that I quite enjoyed the release it provided. Until he dismissed me as no longer spastic, I felt he was just waiting to say, "I told you no one likes it."

Once, I mentioned Dantrium to my cardiologist before he prescribed a blood pressure medication.

His response was. "Oh, there's about 600 contraindications. You can look them up."

No one deserves that.

~

Although I have been using Dantrium for five years now, the FDA report says its long-term safety in humans has not been established.[3] Animal studies, at much higher doses than mine, show a range of side effects that reversed when treatment was stopped.

Studies in a female common laboratory animal, called a Sprague-Dawley rat, showed an increased incidence of both benign and malignant tumors. The doses were very much higher than I use (30, 60, and 90 mg/kg for 18 months).

There are no animal reproduction studies, but the FDA is cautious about using the drug with pregnant women. They did note that one nonrandomized, open-label study of 21 pregnant patients dosed at 100 mg per day for two to 10 days before delivery, revealed that Dantrium crossed the placenta. Subsequently, the levels observed in the newborn babies rapidly diminished. The study wasn't definitive enough to form a conclusion, but the FDA says nursing mothers should not use Dantrium.

~

There are some, but not many studies into the consequences of combining calcium channel blockers, such as verapamil, with Dantrium. In particular, there is a concern that when the anesthetic, halothane, is added to that combination, it may result in cardiovascular collapse and an excess of potassium, called hyperkalemia, may develop.[3]

Dantrium and halothane should have opposing effects. Some studies, looking at susceptible patients, indicate that, when halothane is used, the ryanodine receptor opens notably even if the anesthetic dose is far below a typically effective concentration.[4] It results in extreme calcium release causing malignant hyperthermia. The muscle relaxant, succinylcholine, can produce a similar effect.[5]

Dantrium and the Ryanodine Receptor

Dantrium works in skeletal muscles by blocking a receptor called a ryanodine receptor. The receptor gets its name from the active ingredient of a South American plant, *Ryania speciosa*, called ryanodine.[6] The plant is well known for controlling insect infestations.

Ryanodine receptors are the largest ion channels known to date and occur in a wide variety of cell types. Mostly, they are known for regulating calcium release during the process of excitation-contraction coupling, which drives muscle contraction.

The original receptor discovered was known as RyR1 and occurs mainly in skeletal muscle. A second type, RyR2, was primarily found in the heart, and RyR3 was first identified in the brain. Each is a little different, and the action of neighboring receptors can physically influence a ryanodine receptor. There are at least 300 mutations in the ryanodine receptor group that are associated with skeletal muscle disorders and cardiac arrhythmias.[6] Maybe that is why people don't like Dantrium.

RyR3 is somewhat different than the first two types. It is rarer than the other types. RyR3 occurs primarily in the diaphragm muscle as well as a muscle on the back of the calf called the soleus.

Only RyR1 works in a complex with the dihydropyridine receptor to control calcium release. RyR3 acts more like a booster for RyR1 and is structurally entirely separate. Research suggests RyR3 is not essential for muscle function and isn't a substitute for RyR1 in muscle contraction.[7]

RyR2 is unaffected by Dantrium. As it is mainly found in the heart, dosing with Dantrium has no myocardial effect. However, if the blood pressure medication verapamil is added then a cardiac collapse is likely.[8]

Exactly why the diaphragm muscle is spared from becoming flaccid when Dantrium is used is unknown.

Dantrium and Exercise

One of the reasons that I didn't mind Dantrium is because I exercise eccentrically by using Pilates movements. The most onerous parts of my spasticity affected the areas that Thomas Myers calls the Deep Front Line and the Superficial Back Line. The flexor muscles on the front of my torso and the extensor muscles on my back were always pulling me out of shape.

Within days of using Dantrium, I could feel all these muscles letting go. There were other muscles that I hadn't used for some time because stiffness changes the way you move, and they were very weak. The Pilates exercises helped me to isolate those muscles and concentrate on them to regain functional use.

As the muscles became generally softer, massage was less painful. Before Dantrium, I increasingly felt as though I was always recovering from being bashed in a dark alley. When I was massaged, it felt like I was being hit with hammers. After Dantrium, those sensations went away. I stopped tensing my muscles to fight the masseur, and as I strengthened the ones I hadn't used, my gait and posture became more relaxed.

My firm view is you should not take Dantrium if you intend just to sit and do nothing. The benefit of Dantrium reveals itself if you exercise. The right type of exercise is eccentric, rather than concentric, movement. You need to strengthen muscles in their elongated state, just like a dancer would. That helps you to find proper posture and balance. The overwhelmingly eccentric nature of Pilates exercises is enhanced by using Dantrium.

Interactions

The database DrugBank,[9] is widely used by the drug industry, medicinal chemists, pharmacists, physicians, students, and the general public. In June 2020, it listed 1,134 entries for drug interactions with Dantrium.

My experience is when I tell a doctor that I am on Dantrium, he will sagely nod his head in agreement.

As we sit opposite each other, I will say, "You don't know what that is, do you?"

To date, only neurologists or anesthetists know it. When I ask, all the others look at me, shake their heads, and say, "No."

Dantrium and calcium channel blockers

When blood pressure is too high, there is a range of medications that can be used. One class is known as calcium channel blockers.

The immediate association with calcium that you should think of should be muscle contraction. Given MS upper motor neuron damage results in excessive muscle contraction, you would think that anyone prescribing antihypertensives (high blood pressure medications) would think carefully about what medication an MS patient is already using. In my experience, the risk of contraindication doesn't get a lot of thought.

~

When calcium targets the calcium channels in our blood vessels it causes the blood vessel to constrict, raising blood pressure. If the calcium targets the calcium channels in our heart it depolarizes the heart muscle, causing it to contract. This results in a faster heart rate.

The calcium channel blocker medications are either targeting dihydropyridine channels or non-dihydropyridine channels. The dihydropyridine channels and the medications that affect them are supposed to be focused on our arteries. If you recall the description of excitation-contraction coupling you may remember that these channels are the same type of receptors as those that are linked to the ryanodine receptor which controls calcium release in skeletal muscle cells.

The non-dihydropyridine medications block calcium in both the arteries and the heart muscle.

There are two primary types of calcium channels: T-type channels and L-type channels. In an adult cardiac muscle, they fulfill two different roles. The L-type calcium channel plays a significant role in providing external calcium to heart muscles. It plays a vital part in their specific excitation-contraction coupling process. The T-type channels have a more significant role in the heart's pacemaker cells, but they still depend, to a lesser extent, on adequate extracellular calcium delivery.

In skeletal muscle, ryanodine receptors physically couple to L-type receptors called dihydropyridine receptors. These L-type receptors are responsible for unlocking the ryanodine receptor so that calcium can be released.

In the heart, L-type receptors allow extracellular calcium to enter through the membranes, enabling heart muscles to contract. If you inhibit L-type channels, while the limited number of RyR1 receptors in the heart are being affected by Dantrium, it might be challenging for heart muscles to receive enough calcium to contract adequately. Still, this is not the major problem.

This is the more significant issue:

All arterial blood vessels have a layer of smooth muscle surrounding them that predominately makes up a region called the tunica media. L-type channels predominate here.

L-type channel blockers are very effective at blocking vascular calcium channels (i.e., in our blood vessels). Using them means the smooth muscle layer of the small arteries can't contract. The consequence is the blood vessels dilate rapidly and drop arterial blood pressure. This sudden change can trigger the cardiac nerves to make the heart muscle beat rapidly to raise blood pressure (a condition called reflex tachycardia). This can be very dangerous.

You don't need to combine calcium channel blockers with Dantrium for reflex tachycardia to occur, but there are numerous warnings not to combine them.

L-type channels are inhibited by pharmacologic agents known as dihydropyridines, phenylalkylamines, and benzothiazepines.[10] Check your medications for contraindications with Dantrium.

ACE inhibitors made me cough, which is a common side effect. The adverse outcomes started when I switched to other classes of antihypertensives while on Dantrium. Generally, these drugs did not help my blood pressure at all. Often, it shot much higher. My heartbeat became noticeably erratic, and I felt awful. One of them turned my urine the color of black tea.

The calcium channel blocker medications that affect L-type receptors have 'dipine' as part of their name.

Reaching my cardiologist to tell him what was happening meant I had to deal with his receptionist. She was like a lion at the gate, who relayed to me his advice to continue. I had no control over what she told him. In the end, I read the packaging and followed its advice on how to taper my dose down and discontinued using the antihypertensive.

Ultimately, my cardiologist gave up. Without medication, my blood pressure is only slightly elevated. Sometimes it's quite reasonable. 'Erratic' is probably the word that describes the readings.

A 2013 expert review concluded a spinal cord injury above T6 could cause a blood pressure problem called autonomic dysreflexia.[11] Maybe my problem is just a touch of that.

The FDA warns against Dantrium's use where a patient has impaired pulmonary function, impaired cardiac function, or a history of liver disease.

My experience is that other things you take might contraindicate with Dantrium. Look it up.

Be careful.

References

1. *Origins of Dantrium IV Discussions with Keith Ellis and Henry Rosenberg Parts 1 –20.* 2014; Available from: https://www.youtube.com/watch?v=4rFyEbIpkmc. Accessed January 2021.

2. Snyder, H.R., C.S. Davis, R.K. Bickerton and R.P. Halliday, *1-[5-Arylfurfurylidene)amino]hydantoins. A new class of muscle relaxants.* Journal of Medicinal Chemistry, 1967. **10**(5): p. 807–810.

3. *Dantrium JHP Pharmaceuticals, LLC. Rochester, MI, 48307 U.S. Food and Drug Administration.* 2020.

4. Nelson, T.E., *Effect of Halothane on Human Skeletal Muscle Sarcoplasmic Reticulum Calcium-Release Channel*, in *Mechanisms of Anesthetic Action in Skeletal, Cardiac, and Smooth Muscle*, T.J.J. Blanck and D.M. Wheeler, Editors. 1991, Springer US: Boston, MA. pp. 21–30.

5. Rosenberg, H., N. Pollock, A. Schiemann, T. Bulger and K. Stowell, *Malignant hyperthermia: a review.* Orphanet Journal of Rare Diseases, 2015. **10**: p. 93–93.

6. Van Petegem, F., *Ryanodine receptors: structure and function.* The Journal of Biological Chemistry, 2012. **287**(38): p. 31624.

7. Flucher, B.E., A. Conti, H. Takeshima and V. Sorrentino, *Type 3 and type 1 ryanodine receptors are localized in triads of the same mammalian skeletal muscle fibers.* Journal of Cell Biology, 1999. **146**(3): p. 621–630.

8. Saltzman, S.L., R.A. Kates, B.C. Corke, E.A. Norfleet and K.R. Heath, *Hyperkalemia and cardiovascular collapse after Verapamil and Dantrolene administration in swine.* Anesthesia & Analgesia, 1984. **63**(5): p. 473–478.

9. Wishart, D.S., Y.D. Feunang, A.C. Guo, E.J. Lo, A. Marcu, J.R. Grant, T. Sajed, D. Johnson, C. Li, Z. Sayeeda, N. Assempour, I. Lynkkaran, Y. Liu, A. Maciejewski, N. Gale, A. Wilson, L. Chin, R. Cummings, D. Le, A. Pon, C. Knox and M. Wilson, *DrugBank 5.0: a major update to the DrugBank database for 2018.* Nucleic Acids Res, 2018. **46**(D1): p. D1074-d1082.https://www.drugbank.ca/ Accessed January 2021.

10. Camara, A.K., Z. Begic, W.M. Kwok and Z.J. Bosnjak, *Differential modulation of the cardiac L- and T-type calcium channel currents by isoflurane.* Anesthesiology: The Journal of the American Society of Anesthesiologists, 2001. **95**(2): p. 515–524.

11.   Drake, M.J., A. Apostolidis, A. Cocci, A. Emmanuel, J.B. Gajewski, S.C.Q. Harrison, J.P.F.A. Heesakkers, G.E. Lemack, H. Madersbacher, J.N. Panicker, P. Radziszewski, R. Sakakibara and J.J. Wyndaele, *Neurogenic lower urinary tract dysfunction: Clinical management recommendations of the Neurologic Incontinence Committee of the Fifth International Consultation on Incontinence 2013.* Neurourology and urodynamics, 2016. **35**(6): p. 657–665.

Chapter 30

Baclofen

I didn't try baclofen until after my 2014 attack. There was no need. Until then, spasticity wasn't a big issue. I moved quite freely. In a matter of weeks, that changed forever. Being stiff and sore became the new normal. My neurologist didn't even need to spend a great deal of time working out what had happened. It was obvious.

Apart from one unfortunate dose of an anti-depressant, which I refused to take again, the first medication he put me on was baclofen.

The advice was to begin at a minimal dose and then increase it. I was started at 5 mg, three times a day. After a few days, I was supposed to increase that to 10 mg per dose and gradually step it up to around 25 mg. That never happened.

I didn't feel any change when I used the 5 mg dose. When I increased the dose to 10 mg, I rapidly started to feel bilious. After a few weeks, I pulled back to 5 mg. It had been made clear that I needed to adjust to each dose level before any increase. I tried for several more months on 5 mg, but all that happened is that I felt increasingly tender in my stomach, started belching, experienced reflux, and didn't quite feel myself.

The same physical therapist who ignored my high blood pressure in the gym, derided me for still being on such a small amount.

"That's not even a therapeutic dose," she said in a very condescending manner.

I felt like a fool with no one I could confide in.

Eventually, I was so fed up with belching that I experimented with avoiding baclofen.

I concluded that it wasn't for me.

The Professor who put me on dantrolene sodium suggested I use both medications. I was content not to follow his advice.

Baclofen is not something I use.

If the use of baclofen is suggested to you, perhaps your best option is to watch the many online videos of people who use it and report on their use. Look at their reactions, their levels of concentration, and listen to their reviews.

I was intolerant of baclofen, even at a tiny dose, so I am unable to give a valid firsthand account.

~

Baclofen's classification is as a GABA-ergic agonist. It is an analog (similar but not quite the same) to the neurotransmitter γ-aminobutyric acid (GABA). It is so similar in structure to GABA that it will stimulate the receptors that allow chloride and potassium to enter, stopping activity in a neuron.

Where dantrolene ends the muscle contraction by blocking the release of calcium, baclofen works far earlier and stops the nerve impulse that initiates the first step in muscle contraction.

~

The FDA originally approved baclofen as an oral solution in 1977, and as an injection in 1992.[1, 2] For the year 2017, in the US, there were over 4.5 million prescriptions (in 2016 there were over 5.7 million). That made it the 140th most commonly prescribed medication in the United States.[3]

The injectable form is the next step if the oral form seems ineffective.

The target of baclofen is one type of GABA receptor in the spinal cord, but it may influence others. Baclofen does not readily cross the blood-brain barrier, but its target is in the central nervous system. How it is delivered is always going to be the issue.

Swallowing baclofen means some of it is lost in your saliva, and your stomach acids destroy some more. What is left finds its way to your bloodstream, but your liver then filters it. That step alone can eliminate half of the original dose taken.

Baclofen binds readily to fat. Consequently, the blood-brain barrier, which protects our central nervous system from outside influences, acts as another powerful impediment to the baclofen reaching its target.

Only around 4% of oral baclofen arrives at the spinal cord.[4] This means, to be effective, the oral dose needs to be quite high. The chance of side effects is increased as the dosage goes up.

According to the FDA notes, 63% of patients taking oral baclofen have problems with drowsiness and sedation. About 15% experience dizziness and weakness. Patients who have psychotic disorders, such as schizophrenia or confusion, can become worse on baclofen. People who have the erratic blood pressure problem autonomic dysreflexia, which can be caused by spinal injuries above vertebrae T5 or T6, can have a severe episode of that condition if they miss their baclofen dose.

Baclofen can trigger seizures in people with epilepsy. Stroke patients aren't helped by it and can struggle to tolerate it.[1] Newborn babies whose mothers have been on baclofen start showing withdrawal symptoms (increased muscle tone, tremor, jitteriness, and seizure) a few hours after birth.[1]

As it is dampening the activity of the central nervous system, it can make other drugs (such as alcohol) more potent.

~

Our spinal cord rests in a bath of liquid called cerebrospinal fluid (CSF). That liquid is contained inside protective membranes, collectively known as meninges. The space between two of these layers is called the intrathecal space.

By directly delivering an injection of baclofen into the CSF via the intrathecal space, the required dose can be reduced, so concentrations are 100 times lower than are needed for the oral form. Each small dose, delivered this way, can have an effect for four to eight hours after administration. To control the timing and the dosage, a small, refillable pump can be implanted in the patient.

Even though the dose is lower for intrathecal baclofen, the FDA notes continue to refer to risks such as sedation, somnolence (sleepiness

If you are interested in using Baclofen, there is an informative video online by Dr. Aaron Booster called *Beating multiple sclerosis Severe Spasticity: Baclofen Pumps*.[4]

and drowsiness), ataxia (loss of motor control that mimics being drunk), respiratory problems and cardiovascular depression.

Implanting a pump is only recommended for severe spasticity and spasms due to spinal cord injury or MS. There have been studies that showed that the use of the pump produced some statistically meaningful improvement in cerebral palsy patients.

Therapists need to be adequately trained to administer these pumps. There is a real risk of CNS depression, cardiovascular collapse, and/or respiratory failure. Dosing needs to be closely watched in the initial phase. Any sign of an overdose requires immediate hospitalization. Acute overdose may present as a coma. Refilling the pump needs expert training. Missing the pump and injecting baclofen directly into the tissue can cause a life-threatening overdose.

The FDA notes say, "Abruptly withdrawing intrathecal baclofen, regardless of the cause, has resulted in sequelae that included high fever, altered mental state, exaggerated rebound spasticity and muscle rigidity that in rare cases progressed to rhabdomyolysis, multiple organ-system failure and death".[5] Common reasons for sudden withdrawal include malfunction of the catheter, low volume in the pump reservoir, end of battery life, or human error. Some analgesics have been reported to cause a mass to develop at the tip of the implanted catheter that can cause symptoms similar to sudden withdrawal.[5] Hopefully; a treating physician is awake to the possibility.

Many studies indicate that baclofen works by influencing a particular GABA receptor called GABA-β. There is no conclusive evidence that this is what happens.[6]

The reference library, Drugbank, notes that baclofen may provide neuroprotective effects, and it possesses anti-inflammatory characteristics that could help with drug addiction. They also note that it may produce antinociceptive effects, which means it may dampen the sensation of pain.[6]

Baclofen is generally thought of as a muscle relaxant. As its target is in the central nervous system, it is more correctly grouped as a spasmolytic.

Most muscle relaxants can cause side effects like euphoria, light-headedness, fatigue, and muscle weakness. They can exaggerate the effects of alcohol and distort our skills when driving.[7]

Baclofen is practically the 'drug of choice' for spasticity. As with dantrolene sodium, be careful about what else you are doing while you're taking it.

References

1. *OZOBAX(baclofen)oral solution highlights of prescribing information.* Available from https://www.accessdata.fda.gov/drugsatfda_docs/label/2019/208193s000lbl.pdf. Accessed January 2021.

2. *GABLOFEN highlights of prescribing information.* Available from https://www.accessdata.fda.gov/drugsatfda_docs/label/2010/022462s000lbl.pdf. Accessed January 2021.

3. *Baclofen ClinCalc DrugStats Database, Version 20.0. ClinCalc.* 2020. Available from https://clincalc.com/DrugStats/Drugs/Baclofen. Accessed January 2021.

4. Boster, A. *Beating Multiple Sclerosis Severe Spasticity: Baclofen Pumps.* 2018; Available from: https://www.youtube.com/watch?v=3qxgDeAEaUc. Accessed January 2021.

5. *LIORESAL INTRATHECAL (baclofen injection).* Available from https://www.accessdata.fda.gov/drugsatfda_docs/label/2011/020075s021lbl.pdf. Accessed January 2021.

6. *Drugbank Baclofen.* 2020; Available from: https://www.drugbank.ca/drugs/DB00181#label-reference. Accessed January 2021.

7. PhysioPathoPharmaco, *Muscle Relaxers - Mechanisms, Indications, Side Effects.* 2018. Available from https://www.youtube.com/watch?v=6noV8AHcM6E. Accessed January 2021.

Chapter 31

Botulinum Toxin A

My sessions in the hospital gym came to an abrupt end. They stopped when I told the physical therapists that their 2IC had diagnosed the pain in my hip as bursitis of the greater trochanter.

I can't tell if their exercise program was nearing its conclusion or not. I didn't see any sense of a cohesive plan in anything they did. I'd turn up, do what I was told, and leave feeling more and more dissatisfied that they understood what they were trying to achieve. This frustrating situation had gone on for so long.

Giving my discomfort a name ended my last session in the gym before it began. Labelling it triggered a change in the conversation. Although they had instructed me to put on my gym gear, there was no exercise. Instead, I was told they had gone as far as they could go, and the proposition was put to me that I should go to their spasticity clinic. I had no idea what that meant but agreed anyway.

~

The spasticity clinic was run by a professor who I had rarely seen in the hospital itself. Sometimes, maybe twice, he had appeared at my bedside, and I had assumed that he was the top man. In this setting, however, he was definitely in charge.

The professor worked in a reasonably small room. Before he did anything, I was instructed to walk up and down a corridor while he and his assistants watched how I moved. They discussed my gait amongst themselves, counted my steps, and guided me back to his room. There I removed my trousers and lay face up on a table. The physical therapists assisting him measured the angles of my leg and ankle. They looked at how far I could move or bend my leg.

After a while, the professor stood near the door and held up a small vial.

"Inside this bottle is probably the deadliest poison known to man. However, it has been highly refined, and this stuff has been used for many years. You may have heard of it as botox, but this is a different brand. Same stuff but a different manufacturer", he said as though it was a well-practiced speech. "If you are happy, we will inject a few sites on the back of your leg and see how we go. It will relax your muscles and hopefully improve your gait."

I looked up at him and said, "OK, why not?"

The professor then stood back and watched the therapists while they selected three sites and injected tiny quantities. It was remarkably painless. I barely felt them do it.

"We will see how you are in three months," he said. That was it. No plan, no advice. Just the very generic words to come back if there was a problem.

~

Botox, or its similar competitors, works reasonably quickly. Within a few days, I enjoyed a sense of freedom in my leg that made life so much easier. It was almost as though I had lost the tightness.

The standard view is that the useful life of each botox shot is about three months. As time goes on, you become more aware that your injected limb is heavy. The muscles that are unaffected by the injection now have to carry the weight of the limb and operate its movement.

Muscles influenced by the injection just cease to operate. Where you usually were spastic, with restricted movement, the injection now shifts you to the other end of the spectrum. The toxin causes flaccid paralysis. The muscle is limp. It is cut off from active stimulation. At best, it only moves because it is dragged around by unaffected muscles.

Although all the notes about these injections suggest that each dose lasts three months, I think the effect lasts for longer than that. Maybe after that time, the effect is significantly reduced, but if you exercise correctly, there is still a residual weakness up to a year later.

Having a muscle "knocked out" by this process feels a little weird. It's not painful, but it makes you aware of how often you slightly tense your body in anticipation of a movement. Suddenly, that awareness is gone.

If a drill sergeant yelled, "Squad! Quick! March!", you could call the first two words precautionary commands and the word "March" the executive command. On hearing the first word, you might pull yourself more upright, and your ears would be waiting for the next words. The word "Quick" would lead you to brace your posture in anticipation of kicking your leg forward after the next command arrived. When this style of injection has knocked out a muscle, it doesn't respond to the brain's precautionary commands. Your mind says, "Get ready," but your body doesn't prepare. That whole complex array of sensory signals, small muscle movements and reflexes seems to be missing. You don't notice it with normal movement, but it shows up if you exercise. Consequently, all exercises need to be done slowly and accurately to ensure the muscles follow the correct pattern. Pilates is perfect for this.

A few months after I had been injected with botox, Sarah told me to do a particular exercise on a reformer. It meant I had to stand to the side and lift my injected leg on to the apparatus. I stood next to the reformer and sent the command to my leg to rise up. My body didn't tense, the foot didn't move, and absolutely nothing happened. In the end, I put my right hand under my left leg and lifted it into position. Somehow, I was able to get the rest of me moving as long as my focus was not on the injected leg.

Botulinum toxin is very effective at stopping muscle contraction. Using it provides an opportunity to use exercise to lengthen and correct a spastic muscle. Eventually, the toxin wears off. Not exercising turns the injection into a wasted opportunity.

What is Botox, and How Does it Work?

A class of bacteria, called *Clostridium botulinum*, exists widely in the environment. They thrive in oxygen-deprived conditions and can survive quite high temperatures. These bacteria can produce seven different types of toxins. The World Health Organization regards four of these (A, B, E, and rarely F) as the major contributors to a potentially fatal disease known as botulism. These toxins affect the nervous system. Early signs are fatigue, weakness, and vertigo. Then symptoms of blurred vision, a dry mouth, and difficulty swallowing or speaking become a segue into weakness in the neck, arms, and respiratory system. Then the muscles of the lower body are affected. Vomiting, diarrhea, or constipation and swelling of the abdomen can accompany this. There is no fever or loss of consciousness, but untreated, botulism can prove fatal. Ready-to-eat foods packed in a low oxygen container, or poorly prepared home preserving techniques are often the source of food-borne botulism.

The botulism neurotoxin type A is used to produce the product commonly known as botox. It is a highly purified, diluted version of the toxin that needs to be tailored to a specific requirement in the hands of experts.[1]

Botulinum toxin A inhibits the neurotransmitter acetylcholine from being released from a neuron. In normal activity, the neurotransmitter binds to the membrane at the end of the axon of the neuron using proteins called SNAREs. As their name suggests, they trap the neurotransmitter within small membrane-bound sacks, called vesicles, right at the very end of the axon. The small electrical pulses that signify activity along the neurons trigger a series of steps that result in the vesicles disgorging their contents as they rupture the membrane. That breaching of the membrane releases the neurotransmitter so it can influence a target receptor. The SNARE proteins are required to ensure the sacks are near the membrane.

Botulinum toxin A cuts a SNARE protein, called SNAP-25, so it cannot lock the neurotransmitter in position. Unbound, the vesicles move away from the membrane, and the neurotransmitter is not released. Muscles that do not receive acetylcholine do not commence the cycle of excitation-contraction coupling. They remain flaccid. That is how botox works.

~

You can find the prescribing information for botox by searching for "FDA" and "botox". The highlights version is 35 pages long.[1] The indications and usage sections of the highlights don't even mention the common cosmetic applications.

The notes describe it as a neuromuscular blocker that inhibits acetylcholine. The first mentioned use is focused on the bladder. Both overactive bladder and detrusor muscle overactivity get separate references, although a patient may struggle to tell the difference.

Botox is also used for long-lasting (as opposed to episodic) migraines, a type of sweating problem (called axillary hyperhidrosis), and a range of issues associated with dystonia (involuntary muscle contraction) and spasticity in adults.

In the FDA notes, spasticity is divided into upper and lower limbs. Every suggested site for injection is either a flexor or in a group that acts in flexion. As I have stated earlier, flexors are stronger than extensors. Botox changes that equilibrium.

When botox has reduced the influence of the flexors, the correct approach with MS is to use eccentric muscle movement to lengthen and strengthen all the muscles. If you sit in a chair and do nothing, the effects of the toxin will gradually disappear, and you will be back where you started.

~

It will take a year before the effects of the injections are entirely gone. For a time, you will be acutely aware that some muscles are affected. If you practice the right exercise patterns, the benefits will be apparent. For this reason, as hard as it sometimes was, I continued to use Pilates all through the stages of botox-induced muscle relaxation.

~

There is a black box warning on the FDA approved highlights of a risk that the toxin may not stay localized where it was injected and may cause asthenia (abnormal weakness).[2] A bad reaction might include breathing difficulties. If the toxin spreads, the effects can be dire. It is not approved for use in children with spasticity.

While it is not for everybody, botox can open a window that allows better movement and a chance to create more sustainable mobility.

However, there are other ways to release muscles that do not have the same toxicity risks.

References

1. World Health Organisation Fact sheets/Detail/Botulism 2020. Available from: https://www.who.int/news-room/fact-sheets/detail/botulism. Accessed January 2021.

2. https://www.accessdata.fda.gov/drugsatfda_docs/label/2011/103000s5232lbl.pdf. Accessed January 2021.

Chapter 32

Dry Needling

Dry needling is sometimes known as intramuscular manual stimulation or intramuscular needling.[1]

According to the American Physical Therapists Association, dry needling is a technique where a dry needle (without medication or actual injection) is inserted into an area of muscle called a trigger point.[2] Typically, in the literature, these areas are associated with pain. My experience is that pain is a relative concept and, if you have MS, I prefer to think of these areas as points where the muscle is unnaturally bunched, resulting in restriction of free movement, unnatural posture and sometimes, discomfort.

There is no clear global adoption of dry needling into entry-level physical therapy courses. In some places, therapists are offered a course as a post-doctoral certificate option, and in other areas, the offering looks more like it's been served up by a cottage industry. Acupuncture groups are often highly critical of the level of training involved in dry needling.

Acupuncture also has standards that are all over the place. The World Health Organization has released papers on acupuncture.[3] The primary concern was the adequate training of practitioners.

The World Health Organization proposed formal examinations and statutory regulations to ensure it would,

> *"... bring under control the situation, current in certain industrialized and developing countries, where commercial exploitation of acupuncture training and practice is not uncommon, with all the harmful consequences that may ensue"* [3]

Although the needles are the same, the dry needling technique is entirely different from acupuncture.

In a range of countries (such as the US, Canada, and Australia), acupuncturists need a minimum of three years of full-time training (about

2000 hours). In some countries, they only need 200 hours.[3] Some countries permit doctors to add acupuncture to their qualifications by completing a minimum of 200 hours of training. Physical therapists in the UK are qualified at needling after completing 300 hours, and in New Zealand, the same applies after 150 training hours.

In 2006, an Australian physical therapist needed 150 hours of additional training in acupuncture and could then do a two-day course in dry needling. In 2019, the US Federation of State Boards of Physical Therapy had no set minimum but said dry needling was not an entry-level technique.[3]

All up, it's a dog's breakfast, and you should only go to practitioners with a deep level of anatomical understanding. They are going to needle areas that encase your lungs. You don't need unskilled fools pretending that they know anatomy.

~

Many years before I knew of dry needling, I went to a Chinese acupuncturist. He had a good reputation and many clients. I had found him by the old 'word of mouth' method. His understanding of English wasn't ideal. I told him I had MS and a sore back. It took a little while for him to understand what my condition was. He pulled out a dictionary that translated western medical conditions into Chinese. After studying his book for a while, he looked at me and said, "OK."

I lay face down while he inserted needles along my spine. He left them in for some time and then came back to twist them.

As he played with turning the needles, he said, "can you feel this?"

"No," I replied.

He turned them again, "can you feel this?"

Again, I said, "no."

When the session ended, he looked at me and shook his head, "You got a problem."

I left, feeling no different than when I walked in.

The first area I had dry needling done was on my legs. An osteopath did the treatment. Now I have the benefit of hindsight; I would say he was a little cautious.

He tended to pick targets the same way that the acupuncturist had done years before. Mostly, he needled my hamstrings. It was painless, and I assumed that I needed more sessions.

A few weeks later, his colleague, Cathryn, needled me instead. Her approach was different. She ran her hands across my legs, looking for the tight spots. Then she stuck the needle directly into the bunched area. It was so much more effective. Almost immediately, the muscle relaxed.

Eventually, Cathryn left, and I returned to the original osteopath. By now, I was looking for needling into the tight muscles on my back. He was more comfortable with my legs, but he did put a few needles into my back. I didn't feel that I was getting as much release as I had gained with Cathryn. The osteopath then moved his business further from the Pilates studio, so I asked the Myotherapist, Tal if he did dry needling.

~

Tal's technique was vastly superior to the others. He had done more study than they had into using dry needling but, due to client resistance, hadn't used it in practice a lot.

He needled hamstrings in the same places as the FDA notes would suggest that botox should be applied. Tal was reading the action of my flexors and targeting them far better than the others had.

His real skill shone when I asked him to needle my back. I wanted to release the stiffness in the muscles that oppose the flexors, called extensors. The main target on my back was that ridge on either side of your backbone called the erector spinae group. These are slow-twitch muscles that have to hold you upright all day. They were constantly at war with the flexors on the front of my torso. The fascia that runs through them and around them was locking my trunk in a rigid, robotic, painful stance. Tal placed the needles into the fleshy part between the vertebrae, and the effect was amazing.

He knew what he was doing, he was well trained, and he knew his anatomy very well.

My muscles still tighten, because the signal to relax a reflex does not efficiently arrive. The solution is to be needled by Tal as required. I walk out of his room and do an hour of Pilates, specifically focusing on where I have been needled. Sometimes, I arrive like the Tin Man, but after needling and Pilates, my torso flows like it is made of water.

Dry needling works, but you won't get much out of it if you don't exercise the muscles. They need to be moved around to help exaggerate and prolong the change the needle has made to the fascia. When the needle has released the tension, the muscle needs to be exercised. If you don't do that, then all you have done is make some tiny bloodless holes in your torso. There is no point in doing that as they will quickly heal.

So, what is dry needling doing?

When a lower motor neuron sends activating signals to a muscle, it will make the muscle contract. The more often the message is sent, the more tension will build in the muscle. Any muscle will tighten till the maximum tension possible is reached.[4] Then it is stiff.

Every reflex signal further encourages the tightening to continue. If the loss of myelin means a message for the muscle to relax doesn't arrive, then the muscle stays tight. When the signals to tighten arrive almost on top of each other, it is called a doublet effect. The separate attempts to tighten become fused together, and there is no respite.

When the muscle has reached maximum tightness, it is called tetanus. In a normal situation, there is still a little gap between messages to tighten. That is called unfused tetanus.

When each new signal to tighten does not further tighten the muscle because it is at its maximum tension and the gaps have disappeared, it is called fused tetanus.

Needling the tight muscle interrupts that constant tightening. It slows the development of unfused tetanus and increases the time until fused tetanus arrives.

Compared to a single muscle cell, the needles used are enormous. They hit the tight area just like an object from outer space would flatten a heavily treed forest. A needle disperses the tension, changing the structure of the muscle around it.

Needling releases the muscle, allowing it to move. Don't waste the chance to move when you have it.

The muscle will ultimately tighten because the signal to relax is faulty, but you can needle again.

Dry needling and exercise go together.

References

1. Unverzagt, C., K. Berglund and J.J. Thomas, *Dry needling for myofascial trigger point pain: A clinical commentary.* International Journal of Sports Physical Therapy, 2015. **10**(3): p. 402–418.

2. *Physical Therapists & the Performance of Dry Needling An Educational Resource Paper.* 2012. Available from: https://www.mptalliance.com/wp-content/uploads/2015/12/APTA-PTs-and-Dry-Needling-Resource-Paper.pdf. Accessed February 2021.

3. Ijaz, N. and H. Boon, *Evaluating the international standards gap for the use of acupuncture needles by physiotherapists and chiropractors: A policy analysis.* PloS One, 2019. **14**(12): p. e0226601–e0226601.

4. Mason, P., *Medical Neurobiology (Second Edition).* 2017. Oxford University Press: New York.

Chapter 33

Massage

Long before I had my big 2014 attack, I had realized that I needed massage to relax me. Often my back would tighten. Sometimes my legs would throb as the muscles pulled tighter and tighter. My feet would ache whether I was sitting or standing. I never mentioned this to people as I had already learned that no one likes to hear complaints.

On one occasion, a decade earlier, I made the mistake of mentioning that my legs were tight to a doctor who I was sitting next to at a barbeque. She was so disparaging and condescending about what she perceived as my "self-pity" that I never mentioned it to anyone ever again. It was a social setting. I wasn't asking for advice, just making an observation because I was sore. A glass or two of wine had loosened her lips, and she launched into a speech that could have been titled "You Know Nothing, I am a Doctor". Perhaps she had experienced a bad week, but now I have some insight into the view from the other side of the table.

Silence and patience became my chief weapons. If cramps struck me in the middle of the night, the answer was to slide out of bed and silently walk or stretch for half an hour and pull the contraction out. Absolutely no one wants to hear about a cramp or a spasm or an ache.

As time passed and I became tighter, I would regularly book appointments for a massage. Sometimes it was a physical therapist, sometimes a myotherapist. On other occasions, mainly if I were on holiday, it would be just some alternative therapist with no qualifications at all. More often than not, they were better than the highly-trained providers (and a lot cheaper).

The most useless massages were the ones where the masseur found a tight segment and gently used fingertips to rub the area. On these occasions the masseur would keep doing that until it either seemed to have loosened the muscle or it wouldn't release any further. That technique doesn't change a thing. The best techniques looked at the tight segment as part of a larger group and worked the whole group of interrelated muscles to create a healthy pain-free movement.

Often when you are massaged, the masseur applies pressure to a tight area. Almost as a reflex, you tighten the muscle and push back against the pressure. This creates pain. It is better if you go with the pressure than against it. Sometimes that seems impossible, but it does relieve the pain.

When masseurs land on a troublesome area, let them know but ask one question, "What's the name of that muscle?" If they don't know, they are not your long-term solution. You want someone who, at the end of the massage, can point at a chart on the wall or in a book nearby and tell you what they think the issue is. You want a masseur who can see the interconnected group of muscles.

When I was in hospital in 2014, I was never offered a massage. The head of the entire rehabilitation program said when he dismissed me, "Massage works, but it doesn't last." As they didn't have any sort of system involving massage, I felt like saying, "How would you know? You don't have any masseurs."

~

Massage is a significant part of how I treat my tight muscles. I am fortunate beyond all reasonable chance to be able to see my masseur, Luksy, each week. When I met her, early in my recovery, I was a very tight client.

~

For about a year after I left the hospital, I needed a massage, often daily. During that phase, I went to Darryl's studio and saw a range of masseurs. Every one of them gasped when they touched me and realized the task in front of them. Sometimes, it hurt so much to release a tight muscle that I thought I would have a heart attack.

Their massages worked best if I had hot rocks, wrapped in a towel, placed on me for ten minutes before they started. My tightness was legendary. When I walked in, the masseurs looked at me like mountain climbers would regard Mt Everest. I was the ultimate test of their skill.

PNF stretches—the secret to useful massage

Luksy and I experienced the effectiveness of botox to relax muscles. When she massaged the spots where I had been injected, it was like she was running her fingers over a marshmallow. There was no resistance. However, untreated areas were pretty tight.

I was a combination of tightness, weakness, and stiffness. When you are like that, your range of movement is limited. Doing simple things, like putting on a sock or raising an arm above your head, are almost achievable, but they are accompanied by pain. Big motions, like lifting your leg so that your thigh almost touches your torso, are extremely difficult because numerous muscle groups fight against your will. After Luksy had become my primary masseur, I started using dantrolene sodium and massage became far more tolerable.

~

Inside skeletal muscles are a group of receptors, called spindles, that feed information back to the central nervous system about how the muscle is stretching. They work in conjunction with similar receptors called Golgi tendon organs found in the tendons at the ends of a muscle. However, these groups produce opposite responses to stretch.

When muscle fibers are actively tensing, they usually shorten or contract. The spindles are part of that process.

The Golgi tendon organs also sense the tension in the muscle, but they relax to protect the whole muscle unit from overstretching.

Additionally, the Golgi tendon organ signals its own related muscle to relax, via a signal to the spine. This by-passes the signaling to and from the brain. The neurotransmitter GABA is already in the interneurons in the spine. Golgi tendon organs can activate GABA through a neuron called a Type 1b neuron. A second pathway from an interneuron will activate the opposing muscle to contract so that movement becomes normal.

A proprioceptive neuromuscular facilitation stretch, often called a PNF stretch, exploits these differing responses. This stretch is mainly a topic explored in evidence-based sports medicine. Sometimes it gets a mention in rehabilitation research.

The first time Luksy used a PNF stretch on me, I was lying on my back. She placed herself at the end of the table and asked me to lift one leg and set my ankle on her shoulder. Then I pushed my foot, gently but firmly, down against her shoulder for about the count of eight. This created a strong sense of tension in my leg muscles. After that, I relaxed. When I had taken as much tension out of my leg as I was likely to, she lifted my leg and started to stretch the hamstrings. When she determined that I had reached my limit, she moved her position to accommodate my leg at the end of its range, and we repeated the exercise. When she stretched my hamstrings again, they effortlessly went further than the old limit. We repeated this several times; then she made me raise my leg without any assistance from her. My leg felt weightless and almost flew past its usual limits.

The PNF stretch relies on creating muscle tension without changing the length of a muscle. As Luksy is pushing back against the force I create, the muscle is neither shortening nor lengthening. It is in an isometric contraction. The Golgi tendon organs in the tendons at the ends of the muscle group sense the tension and create relaxation to protect the muscle from overstretching. In truth, there is no stretch, but the stretch receptors have been fooled. This results in an improvement in the range of motion of the whole muscle group. You become more flexible, and the tension across the muscle group disperses. Done often enough, in many parts of the body, it will release the endless sense of muscles pulling you in the wrong direction. Exercising will become easier, even the next day, as the effect lasts for some time.

~

Prior to a PNF stretch, you will first need a traditional massage technique to be applied. You should not use a PNF stretch without first relaxing the muscles as much as possible. At the start of a massage, my muscles can be so tight that Luksy's grip can feel like I am being bitten by the lovechild of a crocodile and a bulldog clip. This pain is unavoidable. She is trying to make the stretch receptors in the muscle itself think the speed of muscle movement is equal to the force of the contraction. The amount of pain I feel from the pressure is due to the degree of tetanus already in the muscle. After releasing the muscle as much as possible by massage, a PNF stretch can then be applied. The whole muscle finally relaxes when the Golgi tendon organs signal relaxation to prevent overstretching.

294

The golden mantra in modern medicine is "do no harm." Most medical people confuse harm with pain. Pain can be necessary just to get to the point where the muscle relaxes under the hands of the masseur. The more often and more easily you can release the contraction in the muscle, the less it will hurt.

The professor said, "Massage works, but it doesn't last." I think he was only half right.

Massage does work. It changes the way the muscle reacts to stretch, but it only remodels your actions over a prolonged period. Too many people give up far too soon. To get relief, you need to massage tight muscles over and over and over again.

Chapter 34

Pilates

I remember sitting at my desk one morning in 2003. A colleague wandered passed and slapped a leaflet down in front of me.

"You should do this," she said as she tapped her index finger briskly on the paper.

I looked at the notice, and nothing on it registered with me. "What is it?" I asked.

"It should be good for you," she replied.

"What do you do? Do you do this?" I yelled as she moved on through the office.

"No, but you should do it," she said as her voice trailed off in the distance.

I looked again at the leaflet. "Looks like a chick thing." I thought and pushed the paper to one side.

~

It may have been the color of the paper or the fact that I knew nothing about what it was saying, but I did not throw the leaflet in the bin. For a week, it just sat there on my desk.

During one lunch hour, I searched for the word "Pilates". It did indeed look like a "chick thing".

Even back then, I was well aware that men are not always welcome in settings where women want to drop their façade and just be themselves. Worrying about this meant I spent a long time considering whether I would be an unwelcome sight in what I thought was probably a women's space.

It was only after I found a lot of information stating that Pilates was created by a man, and that men were welcome, that I decided I should at least inquire. Pushing me to this conclusion was an ever-increasing level of tightness and discomfort in the back of my legs. I didn't want to go back to a neurologist. Doing that meant more medication, and I had already had a gutful of what I had been offered. The less I saw of them, the better.

I rang the number at the bottom of the leaflet, and a man answered the phone. That was a start I didn't expect.

Now, two decades later, I can see that Pilates is a movement dominated by women. However, unless they are naïve, they generally love a man in the class. In any Pilates session, we are all equal, all facing the same challenges.

~

Joseph Hubertus Pilates (1883 – 1967) was born in Germany and had a lifelong interest in physical health. Some instructor textbooks say that in 1913, he traveled to England to work as a circus tumbler. Upon the outbreak of World War One, he was interred as an enemy alien and held in a British concentration camp on the Isle of Man. More than 24,000 internees shared the resources of the camp. Pilates, along with others, conducted daily exercise routines for the inmates.

At some point that no one can truly determine, he developed very strong views that athletic excellence and mental discipline were the critical foundations for a happy life.

In 1919, Pilates was repatriated to Germany, where he began working with medical practitioners to rehabilitate soldiers wounded during the war. His involvement in fitness and sport was now rounded by exposure to trigger-point therapy, hydrotherapy, and work on breathing techniques. In a short-lived renaissance in Germany, he became influenced by meditation techniques, modern dance, and boxing. Again, at a juncture that remains unclear, his dissatisfaction with the prevailing training equipment of the time led to his design of apparatus that could address physical dysfunction and injuries. These became the precursors of a range of equipment now associated with Pilates, most notably the "Reformer". Some sources say that his competent approach to physical training led to an offer to train the German Military Police, but disturbed by the direction of German society, Pilates emigrated to the United States in 1926. The truth is unclear.

In the US, he modified his original training apparatus, adding straps and replacing weights with coiled springs. He called the new apparatus the

"Universal Reformer" and named his program "Corrective Exercise". Later he called the methodology "Contrology". He never called it "Pilates".

In the 1930s, Pilates became well known for his ability to deal with injuries that befell dancers. A famed modern dancer, Ted Shawn, invited Pilates to dance camps in the Berkshire Mountains between 1942 and 1947. It was here that Pilate's signature mat exercises were developed. Originally, 60% of his clientele were men.[1]

Pilates wrote two books.[2] The first in 1934 called "Your Health" is very much a book of its time. Pilates comes across as very spartan, hard, and moralistic. His second book, written in 1945, "Return to Life through Contrology," better explains his views of a systematic exercise regime for the promotion of both mental and physical health.[2] He was convinced that if the whole world adopted his philosophy, there would be less need for hospitals, sanatoriums, mental facilities, and prisons.

In his second book, Pilates introduced a series of floor exercises, sometimes now called The Foundation Series. These are seriously hard exercises. Any athlete who can do all of them would need very little additional fitness work. You can see the ghost of these exercises in nearly all modern Pilates routines.

Two things stood out to me in Pilates' 1945 book that still apply today:[2]

"Contrology is not a fatiguing system of dull, boring, abhorred exercises repeated daily "ad-nauseum.""

"If your spine is inflexibly stiff at 30, you are old; if it is completely flexible at 60, you are young."

~

Pilates starts with fundamental concepts. Probably the most important foundation is understanding that how you breathe affects how you move. If you hold your breath while you exercise, then you are bracing your torso. If you inhale when you should exhale, some movements become almost impossible to do correctly. The way you move to compensate for that can create poor posture and long-term discomfort. Recognizing that simple reality will change the pattern of how you move, and it becomes applicable in daily life.

In the real world, we rarely give the pattern of breathing any thought at all. How many people never connect breathing to sore backs, stiff limbs, bad necks, and the ubiquitous "aches and pains"?

Incorporating breathing into movement is easy to do, but when you start, you'll be amazed at how often you muck it up. Joseph Pilates grasped this concept and made breathing the core element of his program.

If MS causes stiffness, you need to fix up your breathing patterns. I've never met a physical therapist who mentions this. It is the first thing all Pilates instructors focus on.

Pilates said:

> *"Breathing is the first act of life and the last. Our very life depends on it. Since we cannot live without breathing it is tragically deplorable to contemplate the millions and millions who have never learned the art of correct breathing."* [2]

This is not fluff. Sometimes when I am tight and feel I can't possibly exercise, it is how I exhale that starts me moving through a range that I had thought was impossible to achieve.

~

Joseph Pilates had a reputation for being gruff and demanding. His wife was often considered to be the driving force who made the exercises approachable. English wasn't the Pilates' first language, so sometimes they guided the student through the exercise using their hands. They literally pushed the student in the right direction. Their hands often were placed on the body of the person exercising to ensure the muscles fired in the right order.

All proficient Pilates teachers are "hands-on". Be wary of instructors who stay away. Often, instructors can see what is going on, but by lightly placing their hands on you, both you and they receive the feedback you need. People with MS don't always know where they are in space. Something touching you can provide a reference point.

Big group classes make it impossible for an instructor to be everywhere. I have only done a few group classes. In the best classes, the instructor stayed beside me, providing that feedback that kept me on track. Watching how poor the breathing techniques are in big group sessions makes me think of them as "classes for waving your arms and legs about".

~

Once, Sarah, my instructor, had me trying to do an exercise on the floor. Every time I did it, she said, "No, do it again" and made a small suggestion. Eventually, I raised my hips off the floor, lifting my vertebrae piece by piece, and exhaled as I moved.

Her face lit up, and she extended her index finger, pointing excitedly at me, "Yes!" she exclaimed, "That's Pilates."

Small classes, passionate instructors, and correct patterns of moving and breathing all count. Otherwise, it's not Pilates.

~

Pilates is still a movement in its infancy. The medical community that Pilates tried to embrace largely ignored him. Still, a handful of orthopedic surgeons referred patients to him. As he aged, his business declined, his studio building began to deteriorate, and its location became a less than savory area of New York.

Nonetheless, his ideas had caught on, particularly amongst dance studios. The first generation of his followers began to espouse the Pilates philosophy and techniques. By the 1980s, a second-generation began formalized teacher training programs, and orthopedic doctors began to regularly refer patients to Pilates classes for rehabilitation.

A court case in October 2000 determined that the term "Pilates" was a special type of exercise system that had common features that could include unique apparatus. It was too generic a term to be trademarked. Rather than crushing the system, this decision stimulated rapid global growth in interest about Joseph Pilates' philosophies and techniques.[3]

There isn't a lot of information that gives an insight into what motivated Joseph Pilates to develop a wide range of exercise equipment. Some of the paraphernalia available today doesn't look like the equipment he proposed. There's a lot of junk that I don't really like.

The equipment that looks most like his original designs is still the best. The clearest explanation of good Pilates equipment that I can find was made by one of his first-generation disciples, Romana Kryzanowska, "*a machine does something to you, whereas with a Pilates apparatus, you are yourself guided to do the work and train your body*".[2]

I have a strong preference for working on equipment that follows his original design. It is like being invited to drive two sports cars. One is a 1950's vehicle. You have to stand on the pedals, pull the steering wheel, and deal with the elements to drive it. The other is a modern, sleek looking machine. You are cocooned inside it, surrounded in luxury, and basking in its perfection. At a flick of a switch, it will practically take you home. You have to know how to drive to enjoy the older car. The modern one has the looks, but you are kidding yourself if you think looks are a substitute for actual driving.

Real Pilates engages your muscles and relies on you to do the work. A machine will take you through the motions, but the benefit comes from you doing the work. I would prefer to try and fail on the equipment that adheres to the original concept, than to think I had succeeded on a machine that did the work for me.

~

Pilates is not easy even for the fit and well, but its genesis was in rehabilitation. That is why it is beloved by dancers, elite sportspeople, and millions of ordinary people.

~

Do you remember how the playground is where you most wanted to be when you were young? A Pilates studio is a playground. The variety it offers is endless. In the playground, you wanted to go higher or further. You wanted humor in your play. That is exactly what Pilates offers.

A good instructor points you in the right direction, but that urge to achieve something is yours. It focuses your mind, and when you achieve something, big or small, your body immediately tells you. Then, just as with the best forms of play, you choose to go again, hoping it never ends.

Rehab work, led by physical therapists, doesn't do that. It doesn't come close.

Two years after I left the hospital, an MS researcher, Brett Drummond, asked me to make a video about using Pilates with MS. It is 35 minutes long and features Sarah and me talking about Pilates and using the equipment. It was made at Sarah's studio, and all the equipment was the classical style. As we were about to begin, Brett told me to introduce myself and say how long I had known I had MS.

As the filming began, I wondered when I had first been diagnosed. It was not something I had dwelt on. I knew it was a long time ago. Scrambling to think it through on the spot, I looked into the camera and said, "1993". Of course, all the evidence points to 1994. There was only one recording of the interview, so the date has stayed as 1993 on the video. It doesn't change anything, but it's important to correct an error. You can find the video by searching for "Pilates" and "multiple sclerosis" or at https://www.youtube.com/watch?v=4lBkf3GVhEE.

References

1. *Pilates Foundation. The History of Pilates*. Available from: https://www.pilatesfoundation.com/pilates/the-history-of-pilates/. Accessed February 2021.

2. Pilates, J.H., J. Robbins and L. Van Heult-Robbins, *Pilates Evolution The 21st Century*. 2012. Presentation Dynamics.

3. Lessen, D., Editor. *The PMA Pilates Certification Exam Study Guide (Third Edition)*. 2014. Pilates Method Alliance Inc. (PMA).

A Summary of the Chapters and Notes in this Book

1. Treat any underlying infections—the essential first step

Hopefully your doctor doesn't mock you. It can happen. Too often their testing reports look impressive but are lacking.

Possible underlying infections include:

Mycobacteria, *Chlamydia pneumoniae*, *Helicobacter pylori*, periodontopathic bacteria, *Bordetella pertussis*, *Clostridium perfringens*, *Borrelia burgdorferi*, bladder infections and so on.

I have had some of these, and they have been treated, but no one ever started out by looking for them. It was not until I was quite ill that they were found.

The aim of treating them is to:

1) reduce the influence of coinfections

2) reduce the influence of Th1 cytokines (Note 7)

3) lower the levels of interferon-γ, the marker of inflammation

4) Increase the levels of the non-inflammatory marker IL10

2. If MS is confirmed

Under the guidance of a medically trained expert, introduce two doses of 500 mg per day of valaciclover.

The purpose is to control Epstein-Barr replication (Chapter 14).

Based on the work of Professor M. Pender, I believe this step is essential. This should be implemented under proper medical advice. Your prescribing physician should be aware of possible contraindicating renal issues arising from coincident use of non-inflammatory medications, and dosing levels.

3. Shift the immune response to Th2 mediated outcomes

I do this by using two 30 mg doses of curcumin daily. A shift to a Th2-mediated immune response is a move to a less inflammatory immune setting (Chapter 13, Note 7) This lowers interferon-γ and increases IL10 levels.

4. Treat fatigue

This will be helped by first following Steps 1 to 3.

Dealing with fatigue relies on improving the ability to synthesize ATP on demand. (Chapters 11 and 12, Notes 14 and 15).

1) Introduce Coenzyme Q10 soft gel capsules in a tocopherol base.

Dosing (using Stephen Sinatra's guidance on fibromyalgia, chronic fatigue syndrome and mitochondrial cytopathies) should be a minimum of 300 mg daily. I take 750 mg per day, usually all in the evening.

The greatest risk with CoQ10 supplementation is that it can change the anticoagulation properties of blood thinners. You should seek a doctor's advice on combining a high dose CoQ10 with any prescribed dosage level of blood thinners.

2) Introduce two 1,000 mg daily doses of aceytl-l-carnitine. This will improve the ability of your body's cells to burn fatty acids and produce ATP.

3) Introduce two 50 mg equivalent daily doses of elemental magnesium. To ensure a measured dose, this would preferably be delivered in tablet form as magnesium glycinate in an amino acid chelate. Magnesium will bind with ATP into a complex that improves its mobility and affinity with targets. Some magnesium will bind to the ryanodine receptor in skeletal muscles cells and improve flexibility (Chapter 13).

5. Expect your muscles may tighten

1) From as early as possible take up Pilates. Attend three times per week. Focus on small groups or solo sessions. Use classical equipment, not the latest "whiz bang" interpretation of Pilates' original concepts. The equipment should guide you, not do the work for you. Especially use the Cadillac, Reformer, High Barrel and Wunda Chair. Mat Pilates may be unsuitable if you have obvious signs of spasticity (Chapter 34).

2) Utilize massage. Preferably add PNF stretches into the massage process (Chapter 33).

3) Utilize dry needling, especially for the erector spinae group and for muscles used in flexion, as required (Chapter 32).

Ideally, follow a dry needling session (approximately 45 minutes) with a full hour of Pilates that focusses on the areas that have been needled.

6. Consider anti-spasticity medications

Always consult a medical specialist about these medications. The risk of contraindications and inappropriate dosing is high.

1) Botox, or similar, may be appropriate for targeted relief, especially for bladder conditions. Only experienced physicians who are knowledgeable about MS should be consulted. A general practitioner is not a suitable source of advice, always consult a specialist (Chapter 31).

2) Except in unusual circumstances, for chronic spasticity, the choice should be between baclofen (centrally acting) and dantrolene sodium (acts on the muscles themselves). I prefer dantrolene sodium. Specialists prefer baclofen as it is an analog of the inhibitory neurotransmitter GABA. Both have significant contraindications:

a) Baclofen is attracted to fat. Around 50% of oral baclofen is lost through the liver. Only 4% of oral baclofen reaches the spinal cord. Dosing is consequently high with consequent side effects. Complications include unintended muscle weakness and drowsiness (Chapter 30).

b) Dantrolene sodium acts by blocking the release of calcium in the muscle cells to limit excitation-contraction coupling. It is specific to skeletal muscles and spares the heart and respiratory system. This is not a well understood medication. Expect most medical practitioners to be unaware of dantrolene or fail to check for contraindications. Only deal with experts. In my own experience it contraindicates with most blood pressure medications.

Two 25 mg doses daily should be enough. Occasionally an additional 25 mg can be added between doses (Chapter 29).

7. If cramps persist in the legs despite steps 1 – 6

Consider an injection of cortisone into the piriformis muscle. It must go into the muscle, not be drizzled on it. The needle should break the fascia over the muscle. Rest the muscle for several days to allow the cortisone to be absorbed then reintroduce exercise.

Chapter 35

Do I have the Qualifications to Write this Book?

There is a pecking order in medicine. Rightfully, most practitioners of medical science defer to their peers. A professor should know more about his specialized field than a local doctor or general practitioner.

A surgeon, working on a live body, needs to know how that body works so he can protect rather than harm it. An anesthetist needs to understand how the chemicals react in the body to avoid the risk of prematurely ending a life.

A well-trained doctor should know more about the generalities of medicinal treatment than anyone just walking off the street into his practice. (At least, in the areas in which the doctor is trained.)

What happens, though, when the medical expert looks at you and says, "I know nothing about MS"?

Very few neurologists have MS. A clinical professor of medicine at the University of Iowa, Terry Wahls, has MS, and her ultimate conclusion for her own treatment was to turn away from the standard approach and follow a drug-free path.[1] Professor George Jelinek, a head of neuroepidemiology at Melbourne University, has MS.[2] He also has turned away from conventional drug treatments and follows a plan that, in some respect's mirrors Dr. Wahls, and, in others, it is diametrically opposite. Their overwhelming qualification is that they each have MS.

Here is my only relevant qualification:

In June 1995, my diagnosing neurologist wrote,

"Mr. Scott was found to be suffering from multiple sclerosis with clinical features in keeping with a brain stem pontine lesion in December '94 with a supporting MR (sic) examination.

Although much improved, Mr. Scott continues to complain of a relative weakness in the left leg, along with undue fatiguability.

…there is increased and relative slowness for repetitive left foot and ankle movement—the major persisting neurological deficit."

He had waved me goodbye after that with no more than a smile and a suggestion to come back when I needed to. Everything I did from then on was based on scant medical advice and a lot of trial and error.

In 2014, after I had drifted away from the things that kept me well, I had a far more sinister attack. The medical report I was shown said:

"…Spine -multifocal T2 hypertense lesions within the cord, especially C2/3, C7, T8 vertebral levels. These findings are in keeping with primary demyelination.

Brain – Multiple periventricular, subcortical white matter T2 hypertense lesions with some of them showing central cavitation/necrosis. Some of the lesions in the periventricular region are orientated perpendicularly. The right posterior periventricular lesion shows minimal restricted diffusion. A few T2 hypertense lesions are also noted within the pons and the left middle cerebellar peduncle. No infarcts or hemorrhage. No hydrocephalus.

Conclusion – Multiple T2 hypertense lesions within the cerebral white matter and supratentorially are likely due to primary demyelination, Some of the lesions show central cystic change/tumefaction."

So, I had cavitation in parts of my brain as my blood-brain barrier gave way. "Necrosis" meant the damage to some cells could not be reversed as they were dead. "Central cystic change" meant fluid-filled lesions were developing. "Tumefaction" meant they were in the process of swelling. "T2 hypertense lesions" just meant unidentified bright objects on an MRI. I had many, and they were typical of MS.

I have written a little about what that felt like. Above any other symptom, the effect was very isolating. It was not just the physical things that had changed. I felt like I had stood too near to an explosion, and I was still processing what that meant. That experience is my qualification.

Throughout those years I was like the World War One soldier who lived in the trenches. The medical practitioners I reported to were the Generals, five miles behind the lines. They may have seen the bigger picture, but could they live in the trenches?

When a doctor says to you, "I know nothing about MS", what will you say?

Will you say, "Neither do I", or will you open this book and say, "See what it says here?"

References

1.	Wahls, T.L. and E. Adamson, *The Wahls Protocol: A radical new way to treat all chronic autoimmune conditions using paleo principles.* 2015. Avery: New York

2.	Jelinek, G., *Overcoming Multiple Sclerosis: An evidence-based guide to recovery.* 2010. Allen & Unwin: Sydney.

A Short Introduction to the Notes Section

The Notes section is designed to give you background information. There are no test questions, and you don't need to have more than a passing knowledge of these subjects. Understanding these notes won't cure you.

This section is designed to be something you can jump in and out of. It is quite dense, so you probably need to pick and choose. Alternatively, if the information is confusing to you, just let the words wash over you and come back to the topic later. Again, there are no test questions at the end! I'm only trying to point out that MS is a challenging research topic and to give you as much information as possible.

Note 1

Neurons and Glia

When I first became ill, my discomfort was attributed to "damage to your nerves". No one ever told me what a nerve was. Somehow, I was supposed to know. Presumably, I was only expected to nod and accept a very vague explanation.

Nerves are collections of individual neurons. They are bundles of fibers, called axons, that extend from neuronal cell bodies. If you could cut across a nerve and stare down the end of it, you would see bundles of axons from many neurons. It would look like a cable full of discrete signaling tubes. A nerve is not a single thread.

~

Our nervous system consists of two major types of cells.

There are neurons, which are the precise, rapid-signaling units; supporting them are glia, the cells that provide myelin sheaths and clear up cellular debris.[1] Neurons depend on glia.

"Neurons are constantly hungry. The glia feed them. The brain is supplied by the highest density of blood vessels in the body and uses 20 percent of the body's blood-supplied oxygen and energy nutrients 24 hours a day, 7 days a week, even during sleep. The energy consumption of the newborn's brain is even more telling. As much as 40 percent of the body's energy resources are devoted to the developing brain."[2]

~

Whilst it is uncertain, there are estimates that the brain alone contains 100 billion neurons (10^{11}) with two hundred trillion contact points ($2x10^{14}$) between them.[2] Predominately, by function, the neurons are either sensory, motor or interneurons. The interneurons connect to other neurons. Not all of the roles of neurons are understood.[1]

Anatomical divisions of the nervous system

In the early stages of development, a neural plate rolls up on itself, along a crease, to create a neural tube. Some cells are outside the tube. The progenitor cells within the tube go on to form neurons and glia that will be part of the central nervous system, while those outside the tube become the foundation of the peripheral nervous system.

So, we have two anatomical divisions of our nervous system:

The central nervous system (in the brain and spinal cord), and

the peripheral nervous system (everywhere else).

Neurons

Neurons often organize themselves into circuits called neuronal pools. Signals coming to these pools arrive from varying distances. The circuits allow relay points to loop or replay signals, so they become a synchronized message that can be relayed onward.[3]

Without these circuits, the signals would be chaotic, arriving and being distributed in an uncoordinated way.

As a simple example, if you stare into a bright light, then close your eyes, you can sometimes still "see" aspects of the light continuing to be processed. The signal is arriving at different points at differing stages. We can adjust for that, but sometimes looping the circuits helps.

~

Some circuits start as a single neuron that has branching axons (called collateral axons) that can reach more than one target. That variety of neuronal circuit divides the message over and over, ultimately reaching thousands of receptors. This happens with motor neurons. A single message, by branching and involving other neurons, spreads to a whole muscle. This process is called divergence.

Other circuits start as many neurons that converge on one neuron to deliver a message. The final neuron processes the summation of all the neuronal activity. This happens with sensory neurons.

Sometimes diverging neurons synapse (or talk) with converging neurons. These circuits are called "parallel after discharge" circuits. How our eyes process signals is an example of this. They use these circuits so that we can see but do not notice our constant blinking. The signals are all moving at different speeds, but we synthesize the inputs into a consistent message.

All of us have involuntary actions going on because of our neural networks. As an example, messages to the brain (via our neurons) about our blood pressure tell us to dilate or constrict the blood vessels. We don't consciously control these actions.

Axons in circuits for involuntary actions may branch, and one branch may feed back into its own cell body to restimulate a signal until it is interrupted. This becomes a reverberating circuit that responds to its own signaling. It is not a voluntary activity that we influence.

Parts of a Neuron

A typical neuron has four distinct regions.[1]

A cell body

The neuronal cell body is called the soma. This is the metabolic center of the cell. It is the part of the cell that contains the nucleus and the machinery that synthesizes the proteins of the cell.[1] The soma is the control center of the neuron. Apart from the machinery of the cell, it contains a dense mesh of tubules and fibers that are unique to neurons.

Dendrites

These reach out from the soma like branches of a tree and are the apparatus for receiving signals from other neurons.[1] A single neuron can have many dendrites.

Axons

Typically, a neuron only has one axon. Some have none. The axon originates on one side of the cell body as a mound called an axon hillock. This is where the net charge in the cell consolidates and builds to a threshold to trigger a signal.[4] Electrical signals pass along the axon to its destination. Axons can be tiny, but some are very long, extending for meters.

Some axons can have branching networks allowing signals to be sent to different targets. These branches are called collateral axons.[4] This enhances the number of points on target cells that the neurotransmitter can reach. Near the ends, the branches can contact other neurons or interact with muscles. An axon is often covered in a fatty, insulating sheath called myelin. In the central nervous system, the sheath is provided by glial cells called oligodendrocytes. This covering allows signal strength in the axon to be maintained.[1]

Presynaptic terminals

The point where one neuron interacts with a target neuron, muscle or gland is called the synapse. The word was first used in 1897 when a neurophysiologist, Charles Sherrington, used it to describe part of the structure of a spinal cord. He used the word 'synapetein' from the Greek *syn* (together) and *haptein* (to clasp). Over time, it was felt this idea of a short union best described the point of interaction of neurons.[5]

There is a small gap between one axon terminal and the dendrite of the next neuron. They are not locked together. The signaling is performed when neurotransmitters leave one neuron and excite a reaction in the target neuron (or in a muscle plate).[1]

The number of contact points between neurons varies depending on their size and shape. A spinal motor cell might have 10,000 contacts: 2,000 on the cell body and 8,000 on the dendrites. Alternatively, a cell in the cerebellum of the brain, called a Purkinje cell, might have 150,000 contact points.[1]

Types of Neurons

Neurons are classified by their function into three major groups:

Sensory neurons

These neurons are specialized cells that can detect light, heat, pressure, chemicals, and other stimuli to transmit information to the central nervous system.[4] The information they convey helps with both perception and coordination. Some of these neurons also act as receptors for pain and smell.[4]

Another name for these cells is afferent neurons.[1] The circuit structure of sensory neurons starts with many sensory neurons, ultimately converging on one neuron.

Motor neurons

These carry commands to muscles that are responses to stimuli.[1] The circuit structure of motor neurons starts with one motor neuron generating a signal that diverges through many neurons to drive a response in a muscle from many points.

They are called efferent neurons as the signal moves away from the central nervous system.

Interneurons

This is the largest class of neurons. About 90% of our neurons are interneurons.[4] They are neither sensory nor motor. As their name suggests, they are the neurons between other neurons. They receive signals and integrate the functions of the nervous system. They process, store and retrieve information to make the decisions about how the body responds to stimuli.[4] Some can be very long, and some just operate in local circuits. Relay or projection neurons are interneurons.[1]

All known cortical interneurons, which make up less than one-fifth of the cortical neuronal population, release the inhibitory neurotransmitter γ-aminobutyric acid (GABA). Cortical interneurons make up the inhibitory cell population in the cerebral cortex. Without them, all our neuronal systems would be overexcited and out of balance.[2]

Glial Cells

Glial cells derive their name from the Greek word for glue, although they do not actually hold cells together. They do, however, provide structure to the brain by guiding the migration of neurons and directing the path axons take.[1]

Often, they insulate groups of neurons from each other. Glial cells can also act as scavengers by cleaning up debris after neuronal death. They mop up the chemical transmitters released when neurons communicate with each other.

Some glia help to form a lining in the capillaries and other small blood vessels of the brain to create the blood-brain barrier.

The Scale of Parts of a Neuron Compared to Familiar Objects

In his excellent book "Anatomy and Physiology: Unity of Form and Function," Ken Saladin eloquently describes the relative scale of a neuron:

> *"If the soma of a spinal motor neuron were the size of a tennis ball, its dendrites would form a huge bushy mass that could fill a 30-seat classroom from floor to ceiling. Its axon would be up to a mile long but a little narrower than a garden hose. This is quite a point to ponder.*
>
> *The neuron must assemble molecules and organelles in its "tennis ball" soma and deliver them through its "mile-long garden hose" to the end of the axon."* [4]

References

1.   Kandel, E.R., J.H. Schwartz and T.M. Jessell, *Essentials of Neural Science and Behavior. (International Edition)*, 1995. Prentice Hall International: London.

2.   Buzsáki, G., *Rhythms of the Brain*, 2006. Oxford University Press: Oxford.

3.   Brama, H., S. Guberman, M. Abeles, E. Stern and I. Kanter. *Synchronization among neuronal pools without common inputs: in vivo study.* Brain Structure and Function, 2015. **220**(6): p. 3721–3731.

4.   Saladin, K.S., *Anatomy & Physiology : The Unity of Form and Function (Third Edition).* 2004. McGraw-Hill Higher Education: Boston.

5.   Todman, D., *Synapse.* European Neurology, 2009. **61**(3): p. 190–191.

Note 2

How Neurotransmitters Work

Neurons communicate by converting the chemical signals they receive into electrical impulses. This stimulation leads to the release of further chemical signals by another neuron in a chain. Alternately, it can result in the activation of a process in a muscle, gland, or organ.

These chemical signals are called neurotransmitters. They are the language of the neurons. Some neurotransmitters excite, and some inhibit the pulse of messages in a neuron.

Neurotransmitter manufacture

In the cell body of the neuron, chemicals, called neurotransmitters, that can influence the behavior of target neurons, organs, glands, and muscles, are manufactured. Once constructed in the cell body, they are deposited into fluid-filled sacs, called vesicles. These vesicles still need to get from where they are made to the end of the axon. It is only from there that they can influence any target.

There is one significant exception. Although most neurotransmitters are made in the neuronal cell, there is a strong relationship between a type of supporting glial cell called an astrocyte and neurons for the production of the most ubiquitous neurotransmitter in the brain, glutamate, and its derivative, GABA. In this case, the astrocyte makes the precursor, glutamine, and transfers that to the neurons. Neurons don't build those important neurotransmitters from scratch as they lack all the enzymes to do so.[1] When neurodegeneration is considered, it is important to remember this. The astrocyte is critical.

Neurotransmitter transport

Inside the tube of the axon, a complex series of microtubules forms. Each strand of microtubule becomes a path from the beginning of the axon to its end. The structure of the ends of the microfilaments creates a distinct polarity for each strand. The polarity determines the direction of movement of the sacs of neurotransmitters. In axons, the growth of the microtubules is always outwards, away from the cell body.[2] The traffic, however, is two-way.[3]

Two odd looking transport proteins attach themselves to the sacs and pull them along the microtubules. I say odd because they look like little men with oversized feet. These little 'men' are called kinesin and dynein. Some proteins inhibit them, and others help them to select a specific cargo.[4]

Kinesin controls traffic moving outward. It carries not only the sacs of neurotransmitters, but also mitochondria, cell components, calcium ions, enzymes, glucose and amino acids along the axon.[3]

Dynein returns the rubble of used vesicles and other material to the cell body for recycling.

Sometimes pathogens and viruses use dynein to invade neurons. We see this in the time elapsed between infection and symptoms. It is the time it takes the pathogen, transported by dynein, to reach the cell body.[3]

Kinesin and dynein are highly regulated by the signals they receive inside the cells. The polarity of the microtubules determines in which direction the feet of these transporters will advance.[2]

When they have reached the end of their particular pathway, a signal makes kinesin proteins disengage their sacs. The package of neurotransmitter then floats towards the very end of the axon in search of a new home. Anything that upsets any stage of this process can lead to degradation of the whole neuron.[5–8]

The release of neurotransmitters

The very end of the axon is a bulb-like shape that resembles a round door handle. On its outermost face, there are small pores to which the sacs can bind. The sac, resting in its pore, is called a vesicle. The contents of the sacs are called neurotransmitters. At rest, a vesicle is a closed sac.

The bulb at the end of the axon has other pores in it that are known as voltage-gated channels. When the electrical signal, driven by an exchange of sodium and potassium, has traveled along the axon, its strength and duration determine if these channels will open. When they open, these channels allow calcium ions to enter the bulb.

The calcium binds to proteins in the membrane at the face of the bulb, changing their shape. This exchange allows the vesicle to directly bind to the membrane at the very end of the axon. In this process, the sac is torn open, and its contents spill out of the axon, towards receptors on the face of the target cell.[9]

The electrical impulse, coming down the axon, doesn't push the neurotransmitter. It just opens gates.[10]

The synapse: the gap between neurons

Neurons do not touch each other. They release neurotransmitters into the gap between them. A quantity of a neurotransmitter crosses the gap and binds to target receptors. Most of the chemical is in the space between the terminals, called the synapse.

The bulb at the end of the axon is called the presynaptic cleft or presynaptic terminal. The location of the target receptors is called the postsynaptic terminal or postsynaptic membrane. The energy, in the chemical release, that is delivered to the target, is called the postsynaptic potential.

If the charge coming along the axon is too sustained or repeated too often, the amount of neurotransmitter released may build up in the synapse. Not all of it can be utilized.

A neuron needs complete control over the timing of this process. The message needs to be intentional.

Many toxins and venoms work by disabling the fusion between vesicles and membranes, to immobilize, or even kill. Botox uses this aspect to disable a fusion protein called SNAP-25.

If something triggers the acceleration of the signaling process (such as uncontrolled calcium release), then the messaging between neurons becomes a series of misleading signals.

Surplus neurotransmitters are cleared away quickly

There are four ways the surplus transmitter can be removed:

1) The neurotransmitter can diffuse into the space between cells. That can be a slow process.[3]

2) A catalyst, called an enzyme, breaks down the neurotransmitter chemical into its constituent components. This process removes most of the neurotransmitter surplus.[3]

3) In the axon bulb, unique pumps activate to reabsorb the excess neurotransmitter back into the axon for reuse. These pumps are called reuptake pumps.[3]

4) In the central nervous system, glial cells called astrocytes abut the synapse. They also use pumps to absorb any surplus neurotransmitters. These can then be broken down, or the astrocyte can transfer some back to the axon for reuse.[11]

Each method helps to clear the synapse for reuse.

Neurotransmitters can excite or inhibit.

There are many neurotransmitters.

If neurotransmitters cause an influx of positive ions, such as sodium, they are called excitatory transmitters. If they cause an influx of negative ions, such as chloride, they are then delivering inhibitory transmitters. This often happens at a synapse of an interneuron and a principal neuron (a cell with a long axon and a large cell body).

Interneurons are significant players in signaling. These neurons are smaller and outnumber the principal neurons. They operate faster and with more amplitude than the excitable larger neurons.

It is the sum effect of all these influences that determines whether a neuron will fire a charge, called an action potential, along its axon or not. Positive and negative charges cancel each other out. The net balance determines if a charge will be sufficient to fire along an axon. Otherwise, nothing happens.

Inhibitory synapses, which appear symmetrical in electron micrographs, are mostly located on cell bodies. In contrast, excitatory synapses, which appear asymmetrical, form on dendritic spines and dendritic shafts.[12] They don't appear on the cell body.

The excitable neuron passes a positive signal from its axon to another's dendrite. The signal weakens as it passes through the cell body and interneurons meet it there. Inhibitory neurons can further reduce the cell's charge by triggering negative ion channels to open. As a result, inhibitory neurons can modulate the activity of the nervous system.[13] Without them, the excitatory signaling is overpowering.

~

The best known of the inhibitory neurotransmitters is γ-aminobutyric acid, better known as GABA.

The inhibition of neurons is critical to how we function. If you suppress inhibition, then each neuron will just excite the next until it builds to a crescendo that causes malfunction.

As there are so many interactions going on simultaneously, parts of the nervous system will seem to oscillate between excited and inhibited, creating a balance.[13] If the neurons that are part of the inhibitory system are damaged, then the excitatory system jams the network creating muscular and cognitive overloads.

~

Synaptic disruption is a suspicious element in many diseases. Neurodegenerative disorders, such Parkinson's, Alzheimer's, age-related hearing loss and neuropsychiatric conditions such as schizophrenia have been classed as diseases called synaptopathies since 2003.[14] In more recent times; there have been several articles looking at synaptopathies to explain multiple sclerosis.[15–17]

Reprisal: How Neurotransmission Moves Through the Neuron

In summary, neurotransmission relies on several steps:

- A chemical forms in the neuron's cell body.

- An axon builds charged pathways along its interior, from the cell body to its terminal bulb.

- Small transport proteins convey sacs of neurotransmitter along these interior charged pathways to the bulb of the axon.

- The neuron uses the differing electrical charges of ions of sodium and potassium, both inside and outside the cell, to create an electrical current. That current will move along the outside of the axon.

- Myelin sheaths sustain the electrical current along the axon in sensory and motor neurons. Without them, the charge may dissipate.

- The electrical current triggers gates on the surface of the end of the axon to open.

- These gates allow calcium ions to enter the axon bulb.

- The calcium impacts on proteins in the axon membrane causing them to fuse with the sacs.

- The sacs are torn open by this process and spill their contents into the gap known as a synapse.

- Some of the target cell's receptors react to the neurotransmitter when it crosses the synapse.

- The unused neurotransmitter is rapidly either swept away or reabsorbed from the synapse.

- In the central nervous system, astrocytes absorb some neurotransmitters and help recycle them.

References

1. Watanabe, M., K. Maemura, K. Kanbara, T. Tamayama and H. Hayasaki, *GABA and GABA receptors in the central nervous system and other organs*, in *International Review of Cytology*. K.W. Jeon Editor. 2002. **213** p. 1–47.

2. Wang, L. and A. Brown, *Rapid movement of microtubules in axons.* Current Biology., 2002. **12**(17): p. 1496–1501.

3. Saladin, K.S., *Anatomy & Physiology: The Unity of Form and Function (Third Edition).* 2004. McGraw-Hill Higher Education: Boston.

4. Fu, M.-M. and E. Holzbaur, *JIP1 regulates the directionality of APP axonal transport by coordinating kinesin and dynein motors.* The Journal of Cell Biology, 2013. **202**(3): p. 495.

5. Zhou, J., H. Wang, Y. Feng and J. Chen, *Increased expression of cdk5/p25 in N2a cells leads to hyperphosphorylation and impaired axonal transport of neurofilament proteins.* Life Sciences., 2010. **86**(13–14): p. 532–537.

6. Chu, Y., G.A. Morfini, L.B. Langhamer, Y. He, S.T. Brady and J.H. Kordower, *Alterations in axonal transport motor proteins in sporadic and experimental Parkinson's disease.* Brain, 2012. **135**(7): p. 2058–2073.

7. Chung, C., J.B. Koprich, H. Siddiqi and O. Isacson, *Dynamic changes in presynaptic and axonal transport proteins combined with striatal neuroinflammation precede dopaminergic neuronal loss in a rat model of AAV alpha-synucleinopathy.* Journal of Neuroscience, 2009. **29**(11): p. 3365–3373.

8. Kuznetsov, A., A.A. Avramenko and D.G. Blinov, *Effect of protein degradation in the axon on the speed of the bell-shaped concentration wave in slow axonal transport.* International Communications in Heat and Mass Transfer, 2009. **36**(7): p. 641–645.

9. Sudhof, T.C., *Neurotransmitter Release: The last millisecond in the life of a synaptic vesicle.* Neuron. 2013. p. 675–690.

10. Hyman, S., *Neurotransmitters.* Current Biology, 2005. **15**(5): p. R154–R158.

11. Chung, W.-S., N.J. Allen and C. Eroglu, *Astrocytes control synapse formation, function, and elimination.* Cold Spring Harbor Perspectives in Biology. 7(9): p. a020370–a020370.

12. Cheyne, J.E. and C. Lohmann, *Chapter Three - The First Hour in the Life*

of a Synapse: Contact Formation, Partner Selection, and Onset of Function, in *The Synapse*, V. Pickel and M. Segal, Editors. 2014, Academic Press: Boston. p. 111–128.

13. Buzsáki, G., *Rhythms of the Brain*, 2006. Oxford University Press: Oxford.

14. Zoghbi, H.Y., *Postnatal neurodevelopmental disorders: Meeting at the synapse?* Science, 2003. **302**(5646): p. 826.

15. Mandolesi, G., A. Gentile, A. Musella, D. Fresegna, F. De Vito, S. Bulitta, H. Sepman, G.A. Marfia and D. Centonze, *Synaptopathy connects inflammation and neurodegeneration in multiple sclerosis.* Nature Reviews Neurology, 2015. **11**(12): p. 711–724.

16. Yalın, O.Ö., T.G. Edgünlü, S.K. Çelik, U. Emre, T. GüneŞ, Y. Erdal and A.E. Ünal, *Novel SNARE complex polymorphisms associated with multiple sclerosis: Signs of synaptopathy in multiple sclerosis.* Balkan Medical Journal, 2019. 36(3): p. 174.

17. Musella, A., G. Mandolesi and F. Mori, *Linking synaptopathy and gray matter damage in multiple sclerosis.* Multiple Sclerosis Journal, 2016. **22**(2): p. 146–149.

Note 3

Common Neurotransmitters

Many substances can be classified as neurotransmitters. Some don't seem to meet all the criteria for inclusion that others might. Nitric oxide and carbon monoxide are gases so aren't stored in vesicles, but they are still neurotransmitters. Some peptides are released from the presynaptic neurons but have no known enzyme that diffuses them. Sometimes, no known receptor accepts what is released.

D-Serine is formed in astrocytes, not neurons, and affects diverse receptors but is still regarded as a neurotransmitter. Glutamate, the primary excitatory neurotransmitter, acts on some receptors quickly and others through slower processes involving biochemical functions.

Chemical groupings don't help describe neurotransmitters, as a wide variety of chemicals can activate some receptors. Classifying by function is difficult, as some neurotransmitters can be both excitatory and inhibitory.[1]

Acetylcholine

In 1921, a scientist called Otto Loewi exposed the beating hearts of two frogs. Both were kept moist with saline. He stimulated a nerve called the vagus nerve in the first frog, and its heart rate slowed. Then he transferred some of the saline solution from the first frog to the second. The second frog's heart then also slowed.

By stimulating one frog's vagus nerve, he could use its secretions to slow another's heart rate. The first frog must have released a substance. Loewi named this unknown substance Vagusstoffe (vagus substance). This was the first neurotransmitter discovered, later called acetylcholine.

Over time, acetylcholine was understood to be the transmitter used by the motor neurons of the spinal cord. It also was found to be the transmitter for neurons coming from the central nervous system to their first major junction in the peripheral nervous system.

After that junction, some neurons are influenced by a different transmitter, norepinephrine. Those neurons are concentrated in the sympathetic nervous system. The repeated stimulus of norepinephrine will trigger the release of adrenaline (epinephrine) from the adrenal glands. Both norepinephrine and adrenaline can bind to specific receptors to trigger the response we call "fight or flight".

The parasympathetic nervous system remains the domain of acetylcholine. As a neurotransmitter, acetylcholine is in a class of its own.

Glutamate and GABA

Although there are many neurotransmitters, two interlinked metabolites are the dominant signaling mediators in the brain: glutamate and γ-aminobutyric acid (GABA).

Glutamate excites, and GABA inhibits the electrical impulses in neurons.[2] Astrocytes, in the central nervous system, have a pivotal role in maintaining the pools of these two neurotransmitters as they are responsible for producing the enzyme (pyruvate carboxylase)[3] that can start the synthesis of glutamate from the glucose input.

The astrocyte exports glycine through specific transporters to the glutamatergic neurons, where enzymes reassign nitrogen atoms to make ammonia and glutamate. The ammonia is recycled to make more glutamate. How the ammonium ions pass back to the astrocyte still hasn't been completely worked out.[2] It is likely that a very similar process happens in the GABA-ergic neurons to make GABA.[4]

If the astrocytes are damaged, this balance between the primary excitatory and inhibitory modulators breaks down. If the neuron itself is damaged, or cannot pass a strong enough signal because its myelin sheath is damaged, the astrocyte will occupy the space left by the damaged neuron and become scar tissue.[5] This will affect the balance between the neurotransmitters.

Amines

Amino acids contain an amine group (a nitrogen atom connected to three other atoms) and a weak acid, made up of a carbon atom with two attached oxygen atoms and a hydrogen atom flip-flopping between them, called a carboxyl group. When this carboxyl group splits from amino acids, what is left is a class of neurotransmitters called monoamines. The major products of this division are epinephrine, norepinephrine, dopamine, histamine, and serotonin. The first three belong to a subclass called catecholamines.

This group can act as hormones in the fight or flight response. They stimulate not only oxygen consumption but triglyceride breakdown, the transformation of glycogen into glucose, and the regulation of hormones. Some of this group forms in the adrenal glands.

If the carboxyl group does not cleave, amino acids can form other potent neurotransmitters, such as glycine, glutamate, aspartate, and GABA.[5]

Neuropeptides as Neurotransmitters

Neuropeptides are chains of between two and 40 amino acids. They tend to act at lower concentrations. Some act as hormones. In some cases, they are produced not only in the neuron but in the digestive tract and are known as gut-brain peptides.[5]

References

1. Hyman, S., *Neurotransmitters.* Current Biology, 2005. **15**(5): p. R154–R158.

2. Schousboe, A., L.K. Bak and H.S. Waagepetersen, *Astrocytic control of biosynthesis and turnover of the neurotransmitters glutamate and GABA.* Frontiers in Endocrinology, 2013. **4**: p. 102.

3. Hertz, L. and H. Zielke, *Astrocytic control of glutamatergic activity: Astrocytes as stars of the show.* Trends in Neurosciences, 2004. **27**(12): p. 735–743.

4. Watanabe, M., K. Maemura, K. Kanbara, T. Tamayama and H. Hayasaki, *GABA and GABA receptors in the central nervous system and other organs*, in *International Review of Cytology*. K.W. Jeon Editor. 2002. **213** p. 1–47.

5. Saladin, K.S., *Anatomy & Physiology: The Unity of Form and Function (Third Edition).* 2004. McGraw-Hill Higher Education: Boston.

Note 4

Glial Cells of the Central Nervous System

There are four main types of glial cells in the central nervous system.

Astrocytes

Astrocytes are found only in the central nervous system. These are star-shaped cells that have extensions coming from the cell body that wrap around both neurons and blood vessels. Oxygen and glucose traveling through the blood vessels can get to neurons via astrocytes.

Astrocytes are the "stars of the show".[1] As neurons cannot synthesize glucose to create the primary excitatory neurotransmitter glutamate, that role falls to the astrocytes. They also absorb the bulk of spent glutamate for reuse, returning it to the neurons as glutamine.[1] If the astrocyte is damaged, it cannot perform this function.

Glutathione is a major antioxidant and as such, plays a significant neuroprotective role. It is synthesized from glutamate, cysteine, and glycine. Not only is glutathione produced by astrocytes; they also supply neurons with cysteine to make further glutathione and thereby boost their antioxidative capacities.[2]

The depletion of glutathione in neuronal cells is a feature of early Parkinson's disease.[3] It is a hallmark of apoptosis (natural cell death)[4] and possibly both a marker and cause of oxidative stress.[5] Consequently, damage to astrocytes will have numerous knock-on effects.

If neurons fire repeatedly, they can adversely affect other neurons. To modulate this, an astrocyte will absorb any extra potassium released by the firing neuron and store it to protect neighboring neurons.

Astrocytes also secrete factors that significantly increase the number of structural synapses that neurons form. [6]

There are two kinds of astrocytes:[7]

a) Fibrillary astrocytes

This type is usually found in white matter. They have many filaments in a radial pattern.

b) Protoplasmic astrocytes

These are found in grey matter and contain few, if any, glial filaments. They are more delicate and veil-like.

Both perform the same function.

When neurons are damaged, astrocytes form hardened masses of scar tissue and fill the space formerly occupied by neurons. This process is called astrocytosis or sclerosis.[8]

Ependymal cells

These cells line the spinal cord and parts of the brain. They help generate cerebrospinal fluid.

There are several types of ependymal cells. They create a lining throughout the interconnected cavities of the brain where cerebrospinal fluid is produced. They also cover the walls of the central canal of the spinal cord. There is no extracellular space between them, so they form a barrier between the blood and the spinal fluid.[7]

Ependymal cells contain cilia that move fluid around the system.

Oligodendrocytes

These are small cells with little function except to wrap their membranous extensions (myelin) around the axons of neurons. This insulates the axon. As the electrical current generated in the neuron can move more quickly if the axon is thicker and has an enlarged surface area, the myelin will speed up the signal. One oligodendrocyte can myelinate several axons simultaneously.

Microglia

These cells make up 10–15% of all the cells found within the brain. They act as the first line of immune defense in the central nervous system. They are the scavengers who will consume faulty neurons and attack any invader. They are highly sensitive to changes in intracellular potassium levels, which is an early sign of inflammation.

If the central nervous system is damaged by infection or trauma, it becomes challenging to distinguish between microglia and cells of the immune system called macrophages. They have very similar roles.[7] There is some speculation that microglia can become macrophages, but it is unproven.

References

1.   Hertz, L. and H. Zielke, *Astrocytic control of glutamatergic activity: Astrocytes as stars of the show.* Trends in Neurosciences, 2004. **27**(12): p. 735–743.

2.   Wang, X. and M.S. Cynader, *Astrocytes provide cysteine to neurons by releasing glutathione.* Journal of Neurochemistry, 2000. **74**(4): p. 1434–1442.

3.   Mytilineou, C., B.C. Kramer and J.A. Yabut, *Glutathione depletion and oxidative stress.* Parkinsonism & Related Disorders, 2002. **8**(6): p. 385–387.

4.   Franco, R., W.I. DeHaven, M.I. Sifre, C.D. Bortner and J.A. Cidlowski, *Glutathione depletion and disruption of intracellular ionic homeostasis regulate lymphoid cell apoptosis.* The Journal of Biological Chemistry, 2008. **283**(52): p. 36071–36087.

5.   Won, S.J., J-E. Kim, G.F. Cittolin-Santos and R.A. Swanson, *Assessment at the single-cell level identifies neuronal glutathione depletion as both a cause and effect of ischemia-reperfusion oxidative stress.* The Journal of Neuroscience, 2015. **35**(18): p. 7143–7152.

6.   Chung, W.-S., N.J. Allen and C. Eroglu, *Astrocytes control synapse formation, function, and elimination.* Cold Spring Harbor Perspectives in Biology. 7(9): p. a020370–a020370.

7.   *2 - Neuron-Glial Cell Cooperation*, in *Cellular and Molecular Neurobiology (Second Edition)*, C. Hammond, Editor. 2001, Academic Press: London. p. 24–35.

8.   Saladin, K.S., *Anatomy & Physiology: The Unity of Form and Function (Third Edition).* 2004. McGraw-Hill Higher Education: Boston.

Note 5

Glial Cells of the Peripheral Nervous System

The other broad part of the nervous system, the peripheral nervous system, has two main types of supporting cells:

Satellite cells

These cells are similar in function to astrocytes (Note 4). They cover the neurons in the peripheral nervous system, supplying nutrients and cushioning the neurons from damage. Their covering provides structure and support to the neuron.

Schwann cells

Schwann cells are very similar to oligodendrocytes (Note 4). Where the oligodendrocytes send out membranous extensions to cover the axon of the neuron, the Schwann cell wraps its whole self around the axon and secretes a myelin covering. Unlike the oligodendrocytes of the central nervous system, each Schwann cell forms only one myelin segment.[1]

Schwann cells in the peripheral nervous system can regenerate nerve cells. Oligodendrocytes in the central nervous system do not regenerate neurons.[1] Damaged neurons in the central nervous system need to be replaced.

~

MS is primarily a problem with the functioning of the central nervous system, but it is helpful to be able to distinguish which types of cells belong where.

336

1.   *2 - Neuron-Glial Cell Cooperation*, in *Cellular and Molecular Neurobiology (Second Edition)*, C. Hammond, Editor. 2001, Academic Press: London. p. 24–35.

Note 6

The Relationship Between Blood Vessels and Nerves

The central nervous system has networks of both blood vessels and neurons running through it. Viewed together, they are called a neurovascular unit.

What formed first, blood vessels or nerves?

~

How do the blood vessels know where to go, and how do the neural cells organize themselves into patterns involving an emerging vertebra?

The development of these systems relies on communication between them.[1]

~

The organs of the body require oxygen and nutrients to be delivered. Blood vessels have to develop to meet this need.

Within the brain, the blood vessels form almost as fast as the neural tissue grows.

There is an order of precedence. The neuronal network precedes the blood vessels that then invade it.

Ultimately the brain receives blood from two sources:

1) the carotid arteries which branch to form cerebral arteries, and

2) the vertebral arteries which join at the pons to supply the cerebellum and the brain stem.[2]

The blood vessel development is a response to the needs of the tissue that forms in the neural networks.

~

To properly vascularize the spinal cord, the blood vessels have to follow a precise pattern. Blood vessels enter the spinal cord at specific locations and follow particular paths.[1] There is no oxygen involved in determining the path.

Nonetheless, each path is regulated.

What guides the path of blood vessels?

Before the blood vessels arrive, tissue has little access to oxygen. In this hypoxic environment, the neural cells express a factor called vascular endothelial growth factor or VEGF. Initially, this is expressed into the tissue and attracts the developing blood vessels, which then penetrate and vascularize the region. This signaling turns off when the tissue cells receive an appropriate oxygen supply.[3] In simple terms, when tissues grow beyond the limit of oxygen diffusion, they trigger the release of 'hypoxia-inducible transcription factors' from nerve cells. The best understood of these is VEGF.[4]

What guides the path of nerve cells?

Nerves grow almost as quickly as tissue cells form. Axons rely on a nerve growth factor to guide them, as the target cells are immature. When an electrical stimulation of cells finally takes place, the nerve growth factor is downregulated. Where the nerve goes is determined by the needs of its target cells.[3] By comparison, what guides the blood vessels is the VEGF expressed by neurons.[3]

~

A wide range of signals stimulates VEGF transcription. They include inflammatory cytokines and oncoproteins, including interleukins IL-1 and IL-6, insulin-like growth factor 1, transforming growth factor 1, and many others.[5]

The factor initially identified as stimulating the formation of new blood vessels was called VEGF-A. However, VEGF-A can also be elevated in disease situations. Some studies suggest that this factor is upregulated in the central nervous system in the presence of inflammatory cytokines. Other studies don't confirm this.

One research article[5] felt this was just a timing issue. It noted that the data suggested that VEGF-A in an experimental autoimmune encephalitis

338

(EAE) mouse model (an animal model of MS) increased inflammation in the central nervous system. The report assumed that it was VEGF-A-activated receptors that made the blood-brain barrier permeable.

Many models suggest that the blood/brain barrier breakdown occurs well before the onset of clinical EAE symptoms. Some assume that this same process may happen in MS. The study argued that the VEGF-A-induced barrier breakdown precedes damaging inflammation.

The study also showed VEGF-A protected lower motor neurons (outside the central nervous system) while upper motor neurons deteriorated. That is, VEGF-A was elevated when damage was observed in the central nervous system of the mouse model.

~

A study looking at post-mortem material reported that the hypoxia-inducible transcription factors and receptors for VEGF had been upregulated in MS brains.[6] They didn't know if this happened because cells were adapting to MS or were being neuroprotective. What was concluded was that the white matter of the MS brains showed evidence of hypoxia-like damage.

Another study looked at 27 MS patients where the optic nerve and spinal cord were selectively involved (they called it opticospinal MS) plus 23 conventional MS patients.[7] All 50 MS patients were compared to 33 healthy control subjects.

The serum VEGF levels in the MS patients were well above the controls, irrespective of the type of MS. In relapsing patients, it was most pronounced. There was also a strong correlation between the length of the spinal cord lesion and the level of VEGF.

In 2017, a study looking at the well-known relationship between Epstein Barr Virus and Hodgkin's Lymphoma, noted that an EBV protein called LMP1 helped promote the unfavorable growth of new blood vessels in tumors by stimulating VEGF and the inflammatory cytokines IL-1 and IL-6.[8] This observation adds weight to Professor Michael Pender's view that a link exists between the inability to control EBV and an illness like MS.[9]

References

1. Himmels, P., I. Paredes, H. Adler, A. Karakatsani, R. Luck, H.H. Marti, O. Ermakova, E. Rempel, E.T. Stoeckli and C.R. De Almodóvar, *Motor neurons control blood vessel patterning in the developing spinal cord.* Nature Communications, 2017. **8**: p. 14583.

2. Tata, M., C. Ruhrberg and A. Fantin, *Vascularisation of the central nervous system.* Mechanisms of Development, 2015. **138 Pt 1**: p. 26–36.

3. Carmeliet, P. and M. Tessier-Lavigne, *Common mechanisms of nerve and blood vessel wiring.* Nature, 2005. **436**(7048): p. 193.

4. Carmeliet, P., *Angiogenesis in health and disease.* Nature Medicine, 2003. **9**(6): p. 653.

5. Lin, W., *Neuroprotective effects of vascular endothelial growth factor A in the experimental autoimmune encephalomyelitis model of multiple sclerosis.* Neural Regeneration Research, 2017. **12**(1): p. 70.

6. Graumann, U., R. Reynolds, A.J. Steck and N. Schaeren-Wiemers, *Molecular changes in normal appearing white matter in multiple sclerosis are characteristic of neuroprotective mechanisms against hypoxic insult.* Brain Pathology, 2003. **13**(4): p. 554–573.

7. Su, J.J., M. Osoegawa, T. Matsuoka, M. Minohara, M. Tanaka, T. Ishizu, F. Mihara, T. Taniwaki and J. Kira, *Upregulation of vascular growth factors in multiple sclerosis: Correlation with MRI findings.* Journal of the Neurological Sciences, 2006. **243**(1): p. 21–30.

8. Koh, Y.W., J-H. Han, D.H. Yoon, C. Suh and J. Huh, *Epstein-Barr virus positivity is associated with angiogenesis in, and poorer survival of, patients receiving standard treatment for classical Hodgkin's lymphoma.* Hematological Oncology, 2018. **36**(1): p. 182–188.

9. Pender, M.P., *The essential role of Epstein-Barr virus in the pathogenesis of multiple sclerosis.* Neuroscientist, 2011. **17**(4): p. 351–67.

Note 7

T Cells, B Cells, and Cytokines

"..because the regulation of the immune system is not completely understood. It is assumed that cytokines hold the 'key' of the remaining unknowns in immune responses, as well as diseases related to disorders of immunity."

Zlatco Dembic

The Cytokines of the Immune System[1]

To understand any illness, you need to understand how cells communicate.

In a healthy body, there is a balance between cells that ensures the normal, proper functioning of the entire being. We are dynamic organisms, and the fulcrum of this balance keeps moving.

Our body is affected by our environment, the stresses we bear, and our state of health before a new influence arises.

All our body wants to do is maintain an equilibrium. This constant regulation to find balance is called homeostasis. Sometimes, the body gets it wrong. Not all the responses achieve the maintenance of a stable, healthy internal environment. This body's delicate stability is easily upset.

Cytokines

The primary messengers that cells produce to communicate with each other are called cytokines.

Cytokines are glycoproteins: proteins with simple sugars attached to them. They generally act locally and have a short life. Hormones, by comparison, diffuse through the whole body, to have a broad influence and are produced by a dedicated gland or tissue.[2]

There are some cytokines that seem to behave like hormones and can produce effects across the whole body. They include transforming growth factor (TGF) and tumor necrosis factor (TNF).

You may have experienced a fever. This is an indirect influence of two cytokines: interleukin-1 in combination with TNF. Those cytokines are affecting your whole body.[1]

Cytokines in Detail

Some cytokines are named after their original discovered function. Some names are quite outdated and refer to only part of the actual role of the molecule. They haven't been renamed, although their title doesn't adequately describe them.[1] Others are known by a number.

When cytokines are produced, they bind to receptors that can relay messages to the nucleus of the target cell; sometimes this changes the behavior of the cell.

The main groups of cytokines are interleukins, chemokines, and interferons.

Interleukins

The most common group of cytokines are interleukins. They are the cytokines that act on the general class of white blood cells called leukocytes.[2] Scientists numbered them as interleukin (IL)-1 to 40 and on. When more are discovered, they are added to the list.

Chemokines

Another subset of cytokines, called chemokines, also act on leukocytes (the white blood cells) by attracting them to the site of infection. Chemokines can help facilitate the entry of B cells into the central nervous system during demyelination or inflammation.[3]

Interferons

The third group of cytokines is called interferons. As their name suggests, they interfere with virus-infected cells to limit their replication.[2] Two types, interferons α and β, inhibit virus replication. The third type, interferon-γ, helps place a molecule, called an antigen, on the surface of the infected cell that can be recognized by the immune system. The B cells and plasma cells can respond each time they see this signal. If interferon-γ levels are elevated, it is a marker of inflammation.

All cells express cytokines and also have receptors that can bind to them. That allows cells to communicate with each other. Receptors that bind to cytokines are found in abundance on the surface of cells, including the T and B cells. These cells are the heavyweight prize fighters of the immune system. Many MS treatments are specifically targeting the way these cells behave.

T and B Cells are Lymphocytes

In a typical response by the immune system, lymphocytes (subtypes of the white blood-cell group) scan for, and respond to, abnormalities. Cells of this type that develop in the thymus gland are called T cells. Those that originate in the bone marrow are called B cells.[4]

Both are lymphocytes because they migrate to and then reside in lymph nodes and other organs of the lymphatic system.

They can also travel through the bloodstream and are found at the site of infections.

Antigens

An antigen is often the marker of an infection. It can be a toxin or foreign substance that induces an immune response.

T cells don't need to see a whole antigen. A fragment, called a peptide, is sufficient. The T cells use a "T cell antigen receptor". This receptor gives them the ability to see when cells are infected.

Two of the types of T cells are helper T cells and killer T cells.

Helper T cells undergo two pathways to develop specialized properties.

They are generally designated as 'Th' cells. They work in different ways:

1) Th1 cells orchestrate cell mediated immunity to clear pathogens from within the cell, and

2) Th2 cells, by evoking antibody responses, remove pathogens that arrive from outside the cell.

If you become ill, for whatever reason, the immune response will activate an inflammatory response. When I pick up a virus, my MS symptoms noticeably worsen. I have to pay more attention to recovering quickly to shift the bias in my body to a Th2 mediated response as the MS symptoms will then lessen. How I do this is discussed in Chapter 13.

When antigens cluster on the surface of cells and can then be recognized by the immune system, they are named by a reference system called the "cluster of differentiation" or CD nomenclature.[7]

The CD number refers to both the antigen and the antibody that will bind to it. The antibodies are generally known as polyclonal antibodies because they are clones of unique parent antibodies. Typically, the antibodies are made by a series of B cells that have been simultaneously exposed to the antigen. One lonely B cell doesn't have to do all the work.

During inflammation Th1 cells expand in number

When demyelination occurs, it is speculated that something has either become an antigen (a toxic substance) or is recognized as one. The Th1 cells, then copy themselves (clonally expand) and release proinflammatory cytokines such as IL-1, interferon-γ, and TNF-α.

The Th1 response triggers the monocytes, the largest of the white blood cells, to transform into macrophages that can engulf invaders. A macrophage is as subtle as an atom bomb. If it attacks a pathogen, it destroys it, but it can leave a lot of collateral damage.

Some of the microglia (the glia that make up 10–15% of the brain) also are assumed to be stimulated by the Th1. They respond by scavenging for invaders.[5]

Antibodies

As discussed earlier, the immune system reacts to antigens. An antigen can be a toxin or a foreign substance. When an antigen appears, it can lead to the generation of a specific protein designed to stop it, called an antibody. It is a B cell that makes an antibody.

When an antigen binds to a B cell, it stimulates the cell to divide and create clones of itself. This division creates a group of cells that mature to become plasma cells. The process allows vast numbers of antibodies to establish themselves in the bloodstream and lymphatic system.[6]

Both T and B cells can recognize pathogens. A T helper cell introduces the pathogen to a cytotoxic T cell and/or a B cell.

A cytotoxic T cell is a "hitman." It is a contract killer. The B cell is like an army general. It remembers the invader and will orchestrate attacks if it returns.

Both Th1 and Th2 helper cells express the molecule called CD4. The name CD4 refers to both the group of antibodies that recognize the CD4 molecule on the cell surface and the molecule itself.

The cytotoxic T cells express CD8 molecules.

The Relationship Between Pro- and Anti-inflammatory Cytokines

One reaction can trigger another. T cells can produce interferon-γ. This cytokine can activate cells called macrophages. The macrophages are stimulated to consume and destroy anything unwanted in a healthy body.

These activated macrophages can produce other cytokines. One of these may be interleukin 12 (IL-12). In turn, this cytokine causes T cells to make even more interferon-γ. So, one cytokine can induce a cascade of reactions.

A T cell can also produce IL-4, which suppresses interferon-γ, to keep a balance.

If interferon-γ levels seem elevated, then inflammation, and all its knock-on effects, is likely.[2] A high level of interferon-γ is a hallmark of inflammation.

A Russian study published in 2017 described interferon-γ as, "a pivotal participant in the pathogenesis of central nervous system manifestations of MS."[8]

~

Numerous studies, looking at a range of illnesses, have noted an inverse relationship between the cytokine IL-10 and interferon-γ. In MS, low levels of IL-10 coincide with more significant disability, a higher lesion load, and more elevated markers of inflammation such as interferon-γ.[9]

Although pro-inflammatory cytokines such as tumor necrosis factor and interferon-γ are elevated in MS patients, there is not a meaningful relationship between their levels and patient disability. However, high levels of IL-10 seem to coincide with minimal deficits for patients.

In other words, high levels of non-inflammatory cytokines such as IL-10 seem more beneficial in MS than proinflammatory cytokines seem detrimental. There is not a magic ratio between these markers. It has long been known that interferon-γ dosing of MS patients is linked with increases in attacks.[10]

References

1.   Dembic, Z., *The Cytokines of the Immune System*. 2015. Elsevier Science: Burlington.

2.   Knox, B.A., *Biology: an Australian Focus (Fifth Edition)*. P.Y. Ladiges, B.K. Evans and R. Saint, Editors. 2014. McGraw-Hill Education: North Ryde, N.S.W.

3.   Nikbin, B., M.M. Bonab, F. Khosravi and F. Talebian. *Role of B cells in pathogenesis of multiple sclerosis.* International Review of Neurobiology, 2007. **79**: p. 13–42.

4.   *T cells.* National Multiple Sclerosis Society, 2018.

5.   Agrawal, S.M. and V.W. Yong, *Immunopathogenesis of multiple sclerosis.* International Review of Neurobiology, 2007. **79**: p. 99–126.

6.   Panawala, L., *Difference Between T Cells and B Cells*. 2017.

7.   *CD Nomenclature.* 2018; Available from: https://www.immunopaedia. org.za/immunology/basics/cd-nomenclature/. Accessed February 2021.

8.   Khaibullin, T., V. Ivanova, E. Martynova, G. Cherepnev, F. Khabirov, E. Granatov, A. Rizvonov and S. Khaiboulina, *Elevated levels of proinflammatory cytokines in cerebrospinal fluid of multiple sclerosis patients.* Frontiers in Immunology, 2017. **8**: p. 531.

9.   Petereit, H.F., R. Pukrop, F. Fazekas, S.U. Bamborschke, S. Röpele, H.W. Kölmel, S. Merkelbach, G. Japp, P.J.H. Jongen, H.P. Hartung and O.R. Hommes, *Low interleukin-10 production is associated with higher disability and MRI lesion load in secondary progressive multiple sclerosis.* Journal of the Neurological Sciences, 2003. **206**(2): p. 209–214.

10.   Panitch H.S., R.L. Hirsch, A.S. Haley and K.P.,Johnson, *Exacerbations of multiple sclerosis in patients treated with gamma interferon.* Lancet, 1987. **Apr 18;1**(8538): p. 893–895. doi: 10.1016/s0140-6736(87)92863-7. PMID: 2882294.

Note 8

White Blood Cells and the Immune System

This note describes how the immune system is structured.

The Overarching Immune System

About a century ago, scientists became interested in transplanting cancerous tumors from sick mice into healthy substitutes. They aimed to extend their study of particular cancers beyond the life of the ill mouse. Initially, they were unsuccessful as the healthy mice rejected the transplants and died.

The scientists discovered that if tumors were transplanted into mice that were from the same inbred strains as the donor mouse, the recipient did not reject the graft. Researchers concluded that one or more factors controlled acceptance or rejection of the graft.

Trials with healthy tissue transplants (instead of cancers) produced similar negative reactions in unrelated mice. These outcomes helped formulate the idea that an immune response was what led to tissue being rejected.

In time, all these results led to a concentrated effort to create strains of mice that were so inbred that they were genetically identical. As the understanding of chromosomes and genetics improved, the concepts of genetic markers and coding genes developed. Some factors, called genetic loci, were seen as key to determine if tissue would or would not be rejected.

~

While 10 to 20 loci might be involved in determining tissue compatibility, there was often a dominant, defining factor, while the other elements made smaller contributions. The dominant factors were called the major histocompatibility complex (MHC), and the lesser loci became known as the minor histocompatibility complex.[1]

The MHC was further divided into two classes, according to the molecules expressed by the cells.

Class I molecules are expressed by most immune-related cells.

Class II molecules are only expressed by specialist cells.

The Human Leukocyte Antigen Complex

In humans, the red blood cells do not produce any of the ubiquitous Class I molecules. They can't because they don't have a nucleus. Their function is just to carry hemoglobin.

Class I molecules are only produced by leukocytes, the white blood cells. They do have a nucleus. The gene complex that controls the histocompatibility complex is called the human leukocyte antigen (HLA) complex.[1]

The HLA complex consists of about four million base pairs of DNA. There are over 200 genes in this complex, but they represent only a small part of the whole system. Only 10–20% of those genes have a function in defense or immunity.[1]

Types of White Blood Cells

On the surface of all cells, proteins will present themselves as antigens. They are recognized by the broad group of white blood cells as either "self" or "non-self" antigens. In response to the antigens, the leukocytes differentiate themselves into subgroups that perform specific tasks.

The recognized groups are:

Neutrophils, which are like the first responders at an accident, quick to respond but lacking in any special skills. The bulk of pus is made up of dead neutrophils.

Eosinophils, which are like hazard control cleaners that release chemicals to control pests.

The Major Histocompatibility Complex Classes

Scientists learned, through trial and error, that cells need to be compatible.

Compatibility is classified by an overarching program called the major histocompatibility complex. (MHC)

The complex divides into several classes.

MHC Class I genes take antigens that are made inside the cell and presents them on the surface of the cell. These antigens tell the immune system if there is a problem inside the cell. The antigen is made up of fragments exported from inside the cell.[3] If the immune system regards the protein as foreign, or "non-self", it triggers the cell to self-destruct. Examples of antigens made inside the cell that are "non-self" are cancers or some viruses. The MHC Class I molecule tells the immune system that the cell needs to be destroyed because it houses something corrupt. Otherwise, if the antigen is perceived as a "self" antigen then the cell is compatible and is not destroyed.

MHC Class II genes make proteins that are exclusively from outside the cell. Their molecules are responsible for presenting proteins or fragments from invaders to the immune system. The white blood cells that make these molecules engulf an antigen, chop it up and display bits of the invader on their cell surface. The piece of the molecule they present alerts the T cells to hunt down the invader. The fragment is like a scented rag to a bloodhound. The T cell will go after the scent it has been instructed to recognize.

MHC Class III and Class IV genes don't present antigens at all. They belong to a gene-rich area where inflammatory cytokines such as tumor necrosis factor and heat shock proteins arise. There is a considerable discussion that autoimmune diseases may be related to the cytokines released from this area.[4]

Basophils, the firefighters that "back burn" to contain inflammation and strengthen defenses.

Monocytes, which are either macrophages that behave as riot police to control bad behavior, or dendritic cells which operate like senior detectives to identify the culprit and direct the neutrophils and potent lymphocytes to respond.

Lymphocytes, which behave like superheroes that activate when danger is greatest. They are slow to engage but highly skilled responders that can multiply to meet the challenge.[2] They are the weapons used for major warfare.

In models of MS, researchers don't always specify what form a leukocyte has taken. In that case, they generally mean lymphocytes.

The main point is that white blood cells can differentiate into many subgroups.

T Cells

T cells (white blood cells called lymphocytes that develop in the thymus gland) are divided into groups based on the surface molecules they express—CD4+ or CD8+. All T cells begin as naïve cells that have no instruction to activate. They go on to become effector T cells, which can respond to a stimulus.

There is a large group of activated cells called T helper cells. When an immune response has achieved its goal, another T cell, called a regulatory T cell, shuts down the reaction.

T Helper Cells

When the inflammatory cytokine, interferon-γ, triggers the conversion of naïve (antigen free) T cells into T helper 1 (Th1) cells, interleukin12 (IL-12) and interleukin18 (IL-18) maintain that development.[5]

T helper 2 (Th2) cells require the cytokine IL-4 to kick-start them. Activated Th2 cells then produce more IL-4 and IL-10. Those two cytokines inhibit IL-12 and IL-18.

In other words, when non-inflammatory Th2 expands, its cytokines will inhibit proinflammatory Th1 development.

T Cells that Respond to Antigens Outside the Cell

Th1 and Th2 are both CD4+ cells. They have a delayed type of hypersensitivity. These immune cells are not first responders. They are good at recognizing something they have seen before, but if the pathogen is something new, they need instruction.

Their roles are diverse: they help B cells differentiate, and they assist other white blood cells to respond and activate cytotoxic and scavenging immune cells. Hence, they are called T helper cells.[6]

Both Th1 and Th2 molecules can bind to the MHC Class II proteins and instruct the immune system to attack those invaders from outside the cell. The cytokine messages the naïve T cell receives determines if it will be either an inflammatory (Th1) or a non-inflammatory (Th2) cell.

T Cells that Respond to Antigens from Inside the Cell

CD8+ T cells are restricted to responding to MHC Class I proteins, those that come from inside the cell. If the cell is faulty, these T cells become cytotoxic and destroy that cell.

~

In simple terms, MHC Class I molecules mainly interact with cytotoxic CD8+T cells, and MHC Class II molecules mostly interact with CD 4+ T cells.

References

1. Marsh, S.G.E., P. Parham and L.D. Barber, *The HLA Factsbook*. 2000, Academic Press: San Diego.

2. Bioninja. *Types of Leukocytes*. Available from: http://ib.bioninja.com.au/standard-level/topic-6-human-physiology/63-defence-against-infectio/types-of-leukocytes.html. Accessed February 2021.

3. *Human Leukocyte Antigens*. U.S. National Library of Medicine, Genetics Home Reference, Your Guide to Understanding Genetic Conditions: Human leukocyte antigens. Available from: https://ghr.nlm.nih.gov/primer/genefamily/hla. Accessed February 2021.

4. Gruen, J. and S.M. Weissman, *Human MHC class III and IV genes and disease associations*. Frontiers in Bioscience, 2001. **6**: p. D960–972.

5. O'Garra, A. and N. Arai, *The molecular basis of T helper 1 and T helper 2 cell differentiation*. Trends in Cell Biology, 2000. **10**(12): p. 542–550.

6. Chitnis, T., *The role of CD4 T cells in the pathogenesis of multiple sclerosis*. International Review of Neurobiology, 2007. **79**: p. 43–72.

Note 9

The Standard MS Theory: The CD4+T Cell Model and Other Issues

The main theory, which has prevailed for years, is that MS is an inflammatory disease.[1] The standard view is that the disease is mediated by the Th1 cells that express a cell surface protein classed as a CD4 molecule. In other words, the focus has been on proinflammatory T cells tuned to invaders from outside the cell.

As well as the Th1 cells, a developmentally different subset of T cells, called Th17, has been observed to increase in number alongside the CD4+ T cell expansion.

Some argue that Th17 is initially protective but requires anti-inflammatory cytokines, such as Il-23, to stay that way.[2] An alternative view is that IL-23 forms an axis with Th17 to produce the interleukin IL-17.

IL-17 is implicated in psoriasis. Dimethyl fumarate, which is used to treat both MS and psoriasis, seems to shift the cell's production away from IL-23 towards the noninflammatory IL-10 to reduce inflammation.[3] However, there is no particular link between MS and psoriasis.[4]

A high IL-17 count is associated with MS. This fact is noted, but not focused on, in the CD4+ T cell model.

The Standard MS Theory

Tethering and breaching basement membranes in blood vessels

The inside layer of the walls of your blood vessels has a one-cell-thick veneer of flat endothelial cells. When proinflammatory cytokines, such as tumor necrosis factor-α, appear in the central nervous system's associated blood vessels, they promote other cytokines that then adhere to this internal lining of the blood vessel.

The most important point to remember about MS disease-modifying drugs

All the medications discussed in this note only have one purpose—to slow the rate of demyelination. They are not intended to repair the damage that already exists. Some claim benefits if patients start to exhibit fewer symptoms. The assumption is that if you stop the cause of damage, the body has a chance to begin to repair itself. Maybe there is a chance of that.

The reality is that when myelin is destroyed in the central nervous system, it does not recover to its original state. Myelin builds in layers. If there is no first layer left, a scar will form.

The treatments vary from smashing the whole immune system (chemotherapy) to selectively targeting the mechanisms of specific cell types. Interferons, by comparison, change the profile of the signals that immune cells receive.

No drug has been proven to promote remyelination in humans. None is a cure. Some can help some people.

There is an argument that remyelination is possible, though not assured.[5] It comes down to whether precursor cells will differentiate into new oligodendrocytes. Just one of those cells can myelinate forty central axons.[5]

Two adhering cytokines are commonly found on the wall of the blood vessels: the chemokines, CCL19, and CCL21. These are known as lymphoid cytokines.

They are seen as the likely candidates to lock onto and tether the leukocytes that would otherwise just travel on through the blood vessel.

Other adhesion molecules are also known to be able to tether cells to the walls of blood vessels. The best known are called intercellular adhesion molecule (ICAM-1), vascular cell adhesion molecule (VCAM-1) and the lymphocyte function-associated antigen (LFA-1).

This tethering prompts the (now captured) infection-fighting cells (the leukocytes), to roll along the endothelial layer of the blood vessel and gradually be drawn through it.[1]

Once through the endothelial layer, the leukocytes bind to part of the basement membranes of the blood vessel wall called laminin.[7] Here they produce enzymes that are accelerated by metal complexes called metalloproteinases.[8]

These leukocytes stick to the basement membrane barriers and create access to the central nervous system.

The theory is that this leads to massive local inflammation, which degrades the local myelin and eventually destroys the axons.[1] When the neuron is irreparably damaged, the astrocytes fill the degraded space, creating a scar called a sclerosis.[9]

This theory is just a variant on the basic concept of how immune cells are recruited to the site of inflammation to fight infection.

The role of lymphoid cytokines is to organize the tissue responsible for producing lymphocytes (T and B cells). They are thought to help with antibody production. They are commonly found in the lymph nodes, thymus, tonsils, spleen, and the nasopharynx-associated lymphoid tissue. CCL19 also helps, in other ways, to traffic both B and T cells.[6]

Th1 cells are thought to see an antigen

Th1 cells only last a short time in the central nervous system unless they are stimulated to expand in number. The standard MS theory is that microscopic supporting cells in the central nervous system, called microglia, or antigen-presenting cells, prompt an expansion of Th1 cells. The Th1 cells then release more proinflammatory cytokines.

In turn, the new cytokines then activate the large wandering cleansing white blood cells called macrophages and a class of cells called the scavenging microglia. These release neurotoxic elements (free radical derivatives of oxygen, more metalloproteinases, and nitric oxide) to continue the cycle of inflammation.

356

Traditional MS Model

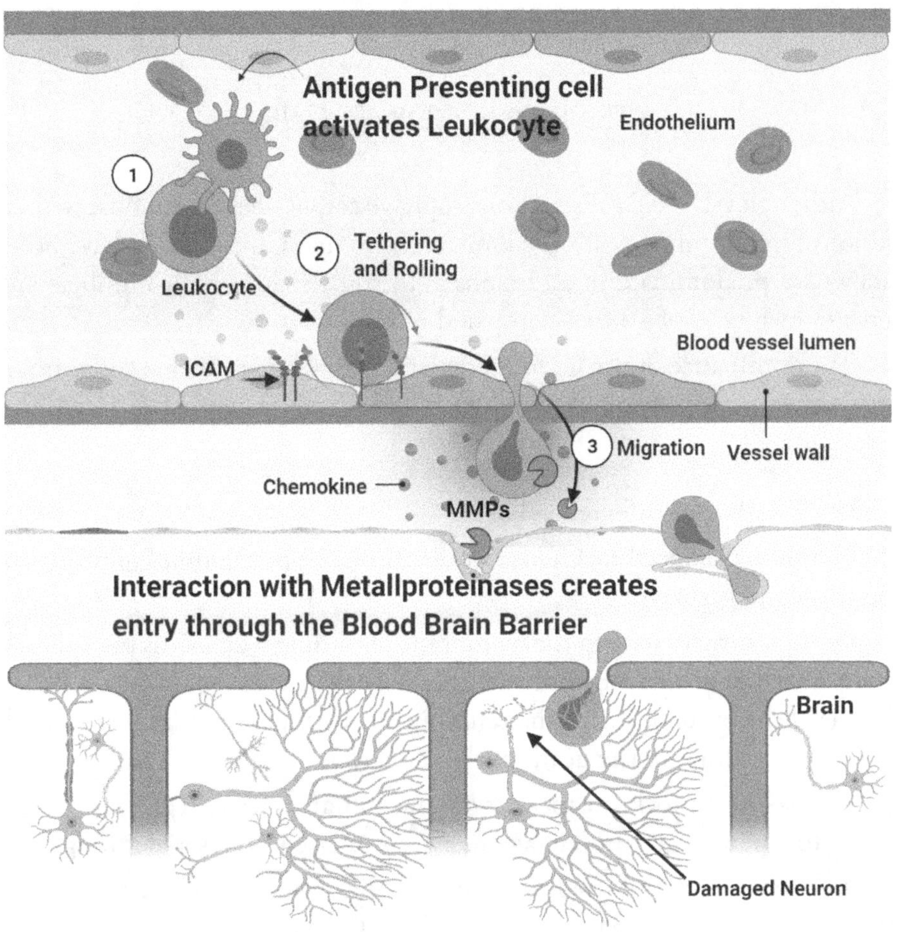

Figure IX.1

1. A white blood cell, such as a lymphocyte, is primed by interacting with an antigen presenting cell.

2. An adhesion molecule (ICAM) anchors the primed cell to the wall of the blood vessel and it is gradually drawn through.

3. The activated cell interacts with metalloproteinases which enhance its ability to pass through the blood/brain barrier.

This model is just a variation on the way immune cells are transported in other settings.

Created with BioRender.

What drives experiments with this model is the similarity between MS and the CD4+ T cell driven mouse model called experimental allergic encephalomyelitis (EAE). This is the most commonly studied model.[10]

The Role of CD8+ T Cells

Although CD4+ T cells and macrophage activity have been observed in lesions for some time, it is only more recently that CD8+ T cells have been shown to predominate in all lesions.[10] In some lesions their numbers are greater by a ratio of 10 to 1 compared to CD4+.

The dominance of the CD4 model and the lack of available tissue from MS patients has transpired to reduce research interest in CD8+ T cells for a long time.[10]

CD8+ T cells and infected cells

Granules produced by CD8+ T cells consist of two families of proteins: perforin and granzymes.

Perforin forms a pore in the membrane of the target cell. This pore allows the granzymes to enter the infected cell. They then break apart the chemical bonds of the proteins inside the cell, shutting down the production of viral proteins, resulting in the death of the target cell.

CD8+ T cells lock on to a target and kill an infected cell. Then they move to a new target and kill again. This is referred to as serial killing.[11]

A review in 2004 showed, in autopsies, that cases of acute, chronic, and inactive MS all displayed evidence of MHC Class I molecules, the markers of CD8+ T cells. These molecules appeared on astrocytes, oligodendrocytes, neuron bodies, and axons.[12]

Further studies showed a correlation between axonal damage and CD8+ T cell infiltration and noted that the infiltration was strongest at the early stages of disease development.[13, 14]

The role of CD8+ T cells is not well understood. There have been numerous studies showing that cytokines related to CD8+ T cells, such as interferon-γ, are elevated in the blood of MS patients.[10]

Some T-Cell Targeted Therapies

Glatiramer acetate, also known as Copolymer 1, Cop-1, or Copaxone, is a therapy for remitting-relapsing MS. It is a sequence of the amino acids glutamic acid, lysine, alanine, and tyrosine, designed to crudely resemble myelin basic protein. When tested in an animal model (EAE), T cells that were reactive to the medication produced Th2 (non-inflammatory) cytokines, which accumulated in the central nervous system. This led researchers to speculate that the medication may exert a bystander suppression of inflammation.[15]

Natalizumab, also known as Tysabri, is a humanized mouse monoclonal antibody. It breaks the link on the leukocyte called $\alpha4\beta1$ integrin that joins the leukocyte to the adhesion molecule ICAM-1 so that it can no longer tether to the endothelial layer of the blood vessel. Tests of natalizumab showed a reduction in disease activity and progression.[16] One study showed a prolonged decrease in T lymphocytes six months after treatment ceased. However, the patient in that study with the highest T cell counts still experienced relapses.[17]

An opportunistic infection, called John Cunningham virus, can be activated by natalizumab to result in progressive multifocal leukoencephalopathy. This is an infection of oligodendrocytes in the central nervous system. It is better known as PML and is usually fatal. Other disease-modifying therapies have now also been identified as catalysts for PML. Natalizumab was the first identified.

The interferons (interferon-β-1a (Avonex, Rebif, Plegridy) and interferon-β-1b (Betaseron)) act as cytokines to modulate some T cell functions and downregulate the Th1 cytokine production.[15] They are only modulators and are not regarded as a cure for MS.

Interferon-β-1a is produced in mammalian cells (Chinese hamster ovaries) while interferon-β-1b is produced in bacterial cells (*E. Coli*). The latter is more likely to be perceived by the immune system as a foreign protein and generate an antibody response that negates the effect of the medication.

Several studies supported the concept that interferon-β's primary mechanism in MS is to decrease the level of metalloproteinases or, alternately, to increase the inhibition of their transmigratory pathways.[1]

Daclizumab was voluntarily withdrawn from the market in March 2018 after 12 reports of severe inflammatory disorders worldwide.[18] It is a mouse-human chimeric monoclonal antibody against the IL-2 receptor. IL-2 is also known as the T-cell growth factor, which plays a significant part in the expansion of stimulated T cells. Daclizumab is also used to prevent renal graft rejection.[19]

Minocycline is a semisynthetic tetracycline derivative. Its action has been described as reducing a metalloproteinase called MMP-9 in T cell activity. Serum samples from patients in a trial showed reduced MMP-9 activity within two months. This reduction in activity persisted for 18 months until the end of the trial. Apart from the improvement at the blood-brain barrier, microglial activity and glutamate cytotoxicity were inhibited.[20] There are, however, reports that some central nervous system functions are worsened by minocycline when other drugs are co-administered. Animal models given the dopamine neurotoxin MPTP, fared worse from Parkinson's disease when minocycline was administered.[21]

Fingolimod, known as Gilenya, was the first oral disease-modifying therapy to be approved for multiple sclerosis in the United States. It is described as a receptor modulator for remitting-relapsing MS. It binds to the lymphocytic S1P1 receptors and degrades them. This has the effect of trapping central memory T cells, which are believed to be auto aggressive, in the lymph nodes.

Fingolimod can cross the blood-brain barrier, where the drug may down-modulate S1P receptors on neural cells, particularly astrocytes, to reduce astrogliosis, a phenomenon associated with neurodegeneration in MS.[22] In 2019, the European Medicines Agency issued a restriction on the use of Gilenya when pregnancy occurred or when no effective contraception was in use by women with MS who can have children. Their argument was that the risk of *in utero* congenital abnormalities for the heart, kidneys, bones, and muscles for the fetus was double that of the general population.[23]

Siponimod is similar to fingolimod. It causes a dose-dependent decrease of the peripheral blood lymphocyte count within six hours of the first dose. The lymphocytes, particularly the T cells, are trapped in lymphoid tissues. This results in a decrease in inflammation.

The siponimod manufacturer's note mentions it can cause a temporary decrease in heart rate and atrioventricular conduction at the beginning of treatment.[24]

B Cells

The stem cells that go on to become B cells first arise in the human embryo at about the seventh week of development. By the second trimester, they can be found in the bone marrow. When these cells are exposed to specific cells, generated in the lymphoid organs, they commit to becoming B cells in either the fetal liver or bone marrow. In the adult bone marrow, B cells continue to be produced throughout life.

B1 cells are produced from the fetal liver but not so readily from bone marrow. These cells have a role in self-recognition and the development of high incidence, non-exclusive, or "public" antibodies.[25]

B2 cells are the "conventional" B cells.[25] When they are still immature, they leave the bone marrow to reside in the spleen. Here, they differentiate into two varieties: B-MZ cells that can respond to antigens without the involvement of T cells in the bloodstream, and FO-B cells that act as antigen-presenting cells for the T cells.

As the FO-B cells have a high affinity for antigens, they develop into short-lived plasma cells. They can clone at an intense rate. When this replication happens, they seek the help of a specialized T helper cell to release cytokines. This triggers their survival as memory B cells. This type of cell can live for years in humans.

B cells can regulate responses

All types of B cells produce the surface molecule CD5, which seems to downregulate T cell activity. CD5 plays a similar role in B cells to help them self-regulate.

B cells can contribute to immunity through production of antibodies, presentation of antigens to T cells, and secretion of cytokines.[26]

Antibiotics can alter B cell development as well as affect microbiota. In germ-free mouse models where certain bacteria were introduced, there were significant defects in B cell types. When these mice were treated with antibiotics, healthy biota developed, and normal cell numbers were restored. The microbiota of the gut and B cells have a profound effect on each other. Cytokine pathways on this topic are still being explored.[27]

B cells that produce Interleukin 10 reduce chronic disease in MS

Mice with a deficiency in IL-10 expression in B cells develop a chronic form of an illness that mimics MS, called EAE. This illness arises after they are immunized with mouse myelin oligodendrocyte glycoprotein (MOG).[26]

In 2007, researchers reported that MS patients showed a decreased average rate of production of the B-cell derived cytokine IL-10.[28] This decrease correlated with worsening disease. The researchers found that the majority of proinflammatory cytokines came from memory B cells. The naïve B cells, those without exposure to an antigen, played little part. They concluded that IL-10 has a role in promoting tolerance to antigens.

In 2008, researchers observed that when MS patients were infected with a parasitic worm (Helminth infection), their IL-10 levels rose, and exacerbations declined, disability scores reduced, and there was less activity on MRIs.[29] They concluded that Helminth infection created a B-cell population producing high levels of IL-10, dampening harmful immune responses.

Some B-Cell Targeted Therapies

Rituximab is an FDA approved monoclonal antibody for treating B cell non-Hodgkin's lymphoma. It is a B-cell depleting agent that causes fast elimination of B cells carrying the CD20 antigen. Plasma B cells do not express the CD20 antigen, so those B cells persist in peripheral circulation and continue to produce antibodies. Adverse effects of rituximab include fever, chills, nausea, vomiting, headache, and fatal reactions.[19] There is debate about whether the treatment reaches the central nervous system as effectively as elsewhere, leading to speculation that treatment results for remitting-relapsing and primary progressive MS may differ.[30]

Ocrelizumab, known as Ocrevus, is presumed to bind to CD20 on the surface cell antigen on pre-B and mature B cells. It is a recombinant, humanized, monoclonal antibody. Dosing at various intervals resulted in a 77–81% relative reduction in enhancing lesions and a 46–47% relative reduction in the annualized primary endpoint relapse rate.

The Effect of MS Drugs on the Unborn

In 2018, a study from the Department of Neurology, Aarhus University Hospital surveyed 590 Danish patients with MS (488 female, and 102 male) about their knowledge of whether T and B cell therapies affected unborn children.[48]

Only 16% of the females and 19% of the males were not on any T or B cell treatment. Many of the others had tried up to five different medications.

Of the participants without children, 50% wanted to start a family. And 91% of the females planned to discontinue treatment during pregnancy.

While 53% felt they were well informed about treatment effects, the internet was the primary source of information for both sexes.

The study concluded that any understanding of the risk factors for the unborn from MS therapies was low. There was almost no knowledge of any risk factors arising for fetuses via males on treatment. About half the respondents said their reliance on a neurologist for guidance was roughly equal to their reliance on browsing the internet.

Pregnancy seems to have almost no discernible negative impact on MS. The rate of relapses, particularly in the third trimester, appears to be reduced by pregnancy. There is, however, an increase in the rate of relapse post-pregnancy.[49]

In terms of the familial risk of MS, the results are not conclusive. The correlation between MS and family membership is proportional to the latitudinal risk (i.e., where you live is just as significant as who you are related to). There are numerous reporting problems in assessing this.[50]

Interferon-β exposure has been associated with lower mean birth weight, shorter mean birth length, and preterm birth. It has not been associated with congenital abnormalities or spontaneous abortion.[51]

~

Most drug testing for T and B cell-based therapies exclude pregnancy, and there is not a suitable database from real-world experience to draw on. In animal studies, some of the newer disease-modifying drugs are clearly contraindicated in females during pregnancy, and some even carry a risk of being transmitted via semen from a male to the female and on to the fetus.[52]

In 2019, the European Medicines Agency issued a restriction on the use of fingolimod during pregnancy. This advice also covered its use when no effective contraception was employed by women able to have children. Their argument was the risk of congenital abnormalities for the heart, kidneys, bones, and muscles of the fetus was double that of the general population.[23]

~

In addition to a daughter, who was born before diagnosis, I have two boys. One was born post-diagnosis while I was not on any treatment, and the other while I was using interferon-β. They are both now in their 20s. I am, at least, five inches shorter than my sons. Both are fit, well adjusted, quick-witted, and a joy to be around. My wife was in good health when they were born. No one ever discussed whether a medication was a risk factor at any stage with me.

Treatments that Aim to Target the Immune System to Reset it Nonspecifically

Plasma exchange or plasmapheresis, is a three-step technique.

1) Whole blood is withdrawn from the patient.

2) A machine separates the red and white blood cells from the liquid portion (plasma) of the blood.

3) The immune cells are transfused back into the patient using a replacement plasma.

It is thought that circulating antibodies that exacerbate attacks and cytokines that signal inflammation are removed. The intention is to modify the progression of the disease. There is no suggestion that this treatment is a cure.

Usually, the disorders that are treated with plasma exchange are associated with presumed aberrant humoral (antibodies from B cells) immune responses, including myasthenia gravis, Guillain-Barré syndrome, and chronic inflammatory demyelinating polyneuropathy.[31]

A study, published in 2006, called *Plasma Exchange in Neuroimmunological Disorders* looked at a large number of clinical studies of the use of plasmapheresis. They rated the quality of the evidence using the rating system of the Therapeutics and Technology Assessment Subcommittee of the American Academy of Neurology and the MS Council for Clinical Practice Guidelines. They could not determine a clear role for the procedure in the management of MS. It may have some usefulness in acute attacks where corticosteroids have failed, but they found no evidence it assisted the progressive forms of MS.[31]

The guidelines, published in *Neurology* in 2002 by the same subcommittee, state,

"On the basis of consistent Class I, II, and III studies, plasma exchange is of little or no value in the treatment of progressive MS"[32]

However, at that time (2006), there was evidence that most plasma exchange studies lacked follow-up with MRIs, there was a lack of control groups in the analysis, and the usefulness of the treatment in early demyelinating attacks was yet to be determined. It is still a treatment in use today.

Intravenous gammaglobulin (IVIg) is a blood product made from many, potentially thousands, of donors. Most preparations contain some Immunoglobulin A and that can cause severe reactions.[33]

The goal of immunoglobulin replacement in patients with primary immunodeficiency is to provide adequate antibodies to prevent infections and long-term complications.[34] It is unknown how this may impact on MS. Some suggest it may modulate T cell or cytokine activation.[33]

There was a report in *Neurology* in 2008 of a study that tested two different formulations of IVIg.[35] Two cohorts made up of 44 and 42 patients who took differing doses of immunoglobulin treatment were compared with a placebo control of 41 patients. There was no statistical difference between the different group's relapses or lesion developments after 48 weeks. MRI reviews were performed on a six-weekly basis throughout the study, and there were no significant differences between the patterns of adverse events.

To quote from the study, "*This result seriously questions the utility of IVIg for the treatment of relapsing-remitting multiple sclerosis.*"[35]

Methotrexate is an immunosuppressant drug used in the treatment of cancer, arthritis and psoriasis. It is a toxic drug derived from folate.[36] It should never be used if pregnancy occurs or if it is possible. Do not use when breastfeeding.

This drug has numerous side effects.[37] It converts folic acid to tetrahydrofolic acid. This impacts on both purine and pyrimidine synthesis, making it highly toxic and impacting cellular synthesis.

Methotrexate is thought to slow the rate of MS progression and has been trialed in France as a co-treatment with Prednisolone. Usually, it is not a first line treatment.[38]

Azathioprine or Imuran is a drug that comes with the risk of skin malignancies and lymphoma. It should not be used during pregnancy or if there is an underlying risk of malignancy. Cases of PML have been reported to the FDA following its use.[39] It is toxic on many levels. Its mechanisms are obscure, but it does suppress T cells.

Mycophenolate mofetil (CellCept) inhibits the guanosine nucleotides in T and B cells, reducing the proliferation of the cells. It also limits the formation of nitric oxide by depleting the substrate tetrahydrobiopterin. It reduces the number of T and B cells and the markers of inflammation.[40] As it suppresses primary antibody responses it is often used in preventing the rejection of grafts.[41]

Cyclophosphamide or Cytoxan is a chemotherapy treatment in many cancers. It is cytotoxic due to its ability to cross-link RNA and DNA strands leading to the inhibition of protein synthesis. This capability extends beyond the normal cell cycle. It predominately targets rapidly dividing cells. In multiple sclerosis, cyclophosphamide has been shown to decrease the secretion of the pro-inflammatory cytokines interferon-γ and interleukin (IL)-12 and to increase the secretion of the anti-inflammatory Th2 cytokines IL-4 and IL-10 in cerebrospinal fluid (CSF) and peripheral blood.[42] The major safety issues include bladder cancer and gonadal toxicity.

A 2003 study of 112 MS patients who received cyclophosphamide for 12 months with monthly dosing and then a further 12 months with bimonthly dosing reported that 21.4% of patients discontinued treatment due to serious side effects. They reported that 33% of the fertile women ceased menstruation (a condition called amenorrhoea). This early menopause did not seem reversible, whereas the remainder recovered from their side effects. The researchers concluded that "the therapy turned out to be relatively safe".[43]

Mitoxantrone (Novantrone) is a chemotherapy drug that indiscriminately attacks both T and B cells as a cytotoxic agent.[15] Researchers found mitoxantrone used in conjunction with methylprednisolone decreased B cell proinflammatory cytokines and increased anti-inflammatory IL-10 levels.[28]

Treatments that Specifically Target Both T and B Cells

Alemtuzumab, also known as Lemtrada or Campath, is a humanized monoclonal antibody which attacks the surface molecule CD52. While this molecule is expressed on T and B cells, it is not expressed on stem cells or plasma cells. Its first use was for the treatment of B cell chronic lymphocytic leukemia. The concept supporting its use for MS is that the severe lymphocyte depletion leaves a pool of reconstructed T cells that don't have any CD4 expression. Pilot clinical trials showed a reduction in both CD4 expression (for 61 months) and CD8+ T cell expression. B cell expression increased to 124% of pre-treatment levels at 27 months. Post-treatment, exacerbations declined, and MRIs showed that lesions reduced sharply. After an average follow up of 7.5 years, the majority of patients had deteriorated clinically. Alemtuzumab is a potent immunosuppressive but comes with similar problems to other drugs like it, such as immune-mediated thyroiditis.[19]

Teriflunomide or Aubagio is believed to interfere with the cycle of cell reproduction. When lymphocytes divide, there are two phases 1) The DNA is copied, and 2) the dividing cell splits into daughter cells.

The building blocks of DNA are either purines or pyrimidines. Both are necessary. Teriflunomide blocks a mitochondrial enzyme needed to make the pyrimidines (called dihydro-orotate dehydrogenase). This interrupts the inflammatory expansion of lymphocytes.

The resting T and B cells that were not activated in an MS attack use a different mechanism (called homeostatic proliferation) to self-renew.

As the treatment only affects rapid, antigen-induced proliferating cells, other less aggressively expanding cells are presumed to be less affected. This makes the medication specific to inflammatory T and B cells.[44]

Cladribine or Mavenclad belongs to a class of cancer drugs called anti-metabolites.[45] They can stop cells from making and repairing DNA. The drug is an analog of a critical element of DNA called deoxyadenosine. As an analogue of this molecule, it is functionally useless and resists being broken down by the enzyme adenosine deaminase. It becomes cytotoxic against DNA formation in T and B cells. Ultimately use of cladribine will affect ATP synthesis resulting in cell death.[46]

According to the National Multiple Sclerosis Society, there is a warning for increased risk of cancers and congenital disabilities/fetal harm from cladribine. Women and men should use birth control before, and at least six months after the last dose of cladribine. The most common adverse reactions reported during clinical trials included upper respiratory tract infections, headaches, and low white blood counts.[47]

T Cell Autoproliferation

T cells develop in the thymus. This is where HLA Class II molecules (from the antigen-presenting cells) are involved in shaping the selection of T cells.[53, 54] Tiny proteins, called peptides, play a role in this. While the pathway is unknown, some CD4+ T cells and the HLA Class II molecules continue to interact outside the thymus, rather than being deleted.

People with MS have higher levels of T cells that are reactive against "self" antigens

Whereas T cells that may be autoreactive (react against "self" antigens) are supposed to have been deleted in the thymus, there is evidence that some are not. In particular, the human heat-shock protein and myelin oligodendrocyte glycoprotein seem to trigger these T cells.[55, 61] This spontaneous T cell proliferation is termed "autoproliferation".[56]

A study in *Cell* in September 2018 described evidence of higher levels of autoproliferation in MS groups than healthy donors.[56] There was a higher proportion of CD4+ T cells following this route than CD8+ T cells.

Brain Homing CD4+ T Cells

There are four interconnected cavities in the brain that together make up a network of ependymal cells where the cerebrospinal fluid is produced. This region of the brain is called the choroid plexus. A study in 2009, again using the EAE mouse model, determined that the route of entry of the Th17 cells into the central nervous system was via the choroid plexus.[61] Several studies had shown that the maintenance of Th17 in the central nervous system was necessary to sustain EAE in mice.

The study noted that lymphocytes could also enter the central nervous system through the choroid plexus. It suggested that T cells may use these structures to enter the cerebrospinal fluid and disseminate.

The researchers thought the Th17 cells that expressed the chemokine CCR6 entered, in a small first wave. The Th17 cells that had crossed then expressed a different cytokine, CCL20, and a much larger second wave began. This second wave was characterized by increased expression of the inflammatory marker, interferon-γ. While the exact determinants that let the lymphocytes home into the choroid plexus are uncertain, these cells are now known as brain homing CD4+T cells.

Genes and the Activation of Specific T Cells

The basic units of our physical and functional makeup as humans are our genes. A gene is a short section of DNA that codes how amino acids should join together to make proteins.

About 1% of our DNA is made up of coding genes. Some genes are made up of a few hundred DNA pairs, and others run to millions of pairs. The Human Genome Project estimates we each have between 20,000 and 25,000 genes.[57]

In the nucleus of each cell, there are long strands of DNA that make up our chromosomes. Each chromosome may contain hundreds or thousands of genes. The location of each gene on the chromosome is called its locus. Each chromosome coils around proteins called histones that preserve its structure. Every chromosome has a constriction point, called a centromere, that divides the chromosome into two arms. The location of this point creates the shape of the chromosome and helps describe the location of specific genes. The arms are generally of unequal length. The short arm is called the "p arm," and the longer section is called the "q arm."

~

Healthy humans have 23 pairs of chromosomes, one of each pair from each parent. Twenty-two of these pairs are called autosomes and look the same in males and females. If one chromosome is slightly different because the gene make up differs, it may present as the dominant or recessive gene. The 23rd pair constitute the sex chromosomes. Females have two "x" chromosomes, and males have one "x" and one "y."

If a group of genes on a chromosome regularly appear together, they are classified as a haplotype and can determine inherited features. When MS is considered, the most common haplotype is designated "DR." In Caucasians with MS, the haplotype "DR2" regularly appears.[58]

~

Chromosome 6 is the home of the human leukocyte antigen (HLA) genes. Living somewhere on the short arm of Chromosome 6, a haplotype, DR15, appears to increase the risk of MS in many studies.[59]

> *"The association between human leukocyte antigen HLA-DR15 and multiple sclerosis was first noticed in 1973. Since then, this has been among the most reproduced findings in major histocompatibility complex (MHC) genetics".[53]*

A research paper in 2011 showed that when infectious triggers that were ubiquitous in the population (e.g., EBV, smoking, low vitamin D), were matched with the antigen HLA-DR15, the combination predisposed individuals towards MS development.[60]

B Cells and Autoproliferation

In 2018, a study from the journal *Cell,* noted that B cells could upregulate the genes involved in the expression of the multiple sclerosis-associated genetic haplotype HLA-DR.[56] These B cells appeared in substantial numbers in the presence of autoprolific CD4+ T cells. A review of cell lines in another study also supported the evidence that B cells could express significant amounts of the DR haplotype.[53] This second article noted that predominately, it was memory B cells, the activated B cells, that expressed HLA-DR.

This research gave support to an anti-CD20 therapy as a means of depleting the activated B cell population and resetting the immune system with naïve B cells. Consequentially, this would lower the output of pro-inflammatory cytokines. The study concluded that the autoproliferation of CD4+ T cells depended on memory B cells. They noted CD8+ T cells might become involved as bystanders.

Significantly, this study, *"Memory B cells activate brain-homing, autoreactive CD4+ T cells in multiple sclerosis"*, linked the activity of T and B cells with a genetic disposition.[56]

B Cell Involvement in Secondary and Primary Progressive MS

In our brain and wrapped around our spinal cord are three layers of membrane called meninges. The innermost layer is called the pia mater. It adheres to the brain and fuses with the tissue that forms the choroid plexus, where the cerebrospinal fluid is made.

The tough and inflexible outermost layer of the meninges is called the dura mater. This holds the brain in place and creates sinuses for blood and fluid.

The middle layer projects into the sinuses. This segment aids the transfer of cerebrospinal fluid back to the bloodstream.

In a postmortem study of brain tissue, B cell follicles were found in the meninges, adjacent to lesions in the cortex.[62] These unusually placed cells were found in the brains of secondary progressive MS (SPMS) cases but not primary progressive samples. The study was only performed on a small sample. The history of the patients was unclear, and the SPMS cases were predominantly female. However, the study confirmed that B cells can migrate into the central nervous system.

References

1. Agrawal, S.M. and V.W. Yong, *Immunopathogenesis of multiple sclerosis.* International Review of Neurobiology, 2007. **79**: p. 99–126.

2. Zambrano-Zaragoza, J.F., E.J. Romo-Martinez, M. d-J Durán-Avelar, N. Garcia-Magallanes and N. Vibanco-Pérez, *Th17 cells in autoimmune and infectious diseases.* International Journal of Inflammation, 2014. **2014**: p. 651503–651503.

3. Schön, M.P. and L. Erpenbeck, *The interleukin-23/interleukin-17 axis links adaptive and innate immunity in psoriasis.* Frontiers in Immunology, 2018. **9**(1323).

4. Kwok, T., W. Jing Loo and L. Guenther, *Psoriasis and multiple sclerosis: is there a link?* Journal of Cutaneous Medicine and Surgery, 2010. **14**(4): p. 151–155.

5. Mason, P., *Medical Neurobiology (Second Edition).* 2017, Oxford University Press: New York.

6. Yoshida, R., T. Imai, K. Hieshima, J. Kusuda, M. Baba, M. Kitaura, M. Nishimura, M. Kakizaki, H. Nomiyama and O. Yoshie, *Molecular cloning of a novel human CC chemokine EBI1-ligand chemokine that is a specific functional ligand for EBI1, CCR7.* Journal of Biological Chemistry 1997. **272**(21): p. 13803–13809.

7. Domogatskaya, A., S. Rodin and K. Tryggvason, *Functional diversity of laminins.* Annual Review of Cell and Developmental Biology, 2012. **28**: p. 523–553.

8. Nagase, H., R. Visse and G. Murphy, *Structure and function of matrix metalloproteinases and TIMPs.* Cardiovascular Research, 2006. **69**(3): p. 562–573.

9. Saladin, K.S., *Anatomy & Physiology: The Unity of Form and Function (Third Edition).* 2004. McGraw-Hill Higher Education: Boston.

10. Johnson, A., G.L. Suidan, J. McDole and I. Pirko, *The CD8 T cell in multiple sclerosis: Suppressor cell or mediator of neuropathology?* International Review of Neurobiology, 2007. **79**: p. 73–97.

11. Wissinger E., CD8+ T cells; Available from: https://www.immunology. org/public-information/bitesized-immunology/cells/cd8-t-cells. Accessed February 2021.

12. Hoftberger, R., F. Aboul-Enein, W. Brueck, C. Lucchinetti, M., Rodriguez, M. Schmidbauer, K. Jellinger and H. Lassmann, *Expression of Major Histocompatibility Complex Class I molecules on the different cell types in multiple sclerosis lesions.* Brain Pathology, 2004. **14**(1): p. 43–50.

13. Bitsch, A., J. Schuchardt, S. Bunkowski, T. Kuhlmann and W. Brück, *Acute axonal injury in multiple sclerosis. Correlation with demyelination and inflammation.* Brain, 2000. **123**(6): p. 1174–1183.

14. Kuhlmann, T., G. Lingfeld, A. Bitsch, J. Schuchardt and W. Brück, *Acute axonal damage in multiple sclerosis is most extensive in early disease stages and decreases over time.* Brain, 2002. **125**(10): p. 2202–2212.

15. Chitnis, T., *The role of CD4 T cells in the pathogenesis of multiple sclerosis.* International Review of Neurobiology, 2007. **79**: p. 43–72.

16. Hoepner, R., S. Faissner, A. Salmen, R. Gold and A. Chan, *Efficacy and side effects of natalizumab therapy in patients with multiple sclerosis.* Journal of Central Nervous System Disease, 2014. **6**: p. 41–49.

17. Stüve, O., C.M. Marra, K.R. Jerome, L. Cook, P.D. Cravens, S. Cepok, E.M. Frohman, J.T. Philips, G. Arendt, B. Hemmer, N.L. Monson and M.K. Racke, *Immune surveillance in multiple sclerosis patients treated with natalizumab.* Annals of Neurology, 2006. **59**(5): p. 743–747.

18. *"Drug Safety and Availability - FDA working with manufacturers to withdraw Zinbryta from the market in the United States".* Available from: https://www.fda.gov/Drugs/DrugSafety/ucm600999.htm. Accessed February 2021.

19. Korniychuk, E., J.M. Dempster, E. O'Connor, J.S. Alexander, R.E. Kelley, M. Kenner, U. Menon, V. Misra, R. Hoque, E. Gonzalez-Toledo, R.N. Schwendimann, S. Smith and A. Minagar, *Evolving therapies for multiple sclerosis.* International Review of Neurobiology, 2007. **79**: p. 571–88.

20. Zabad, R., J.M. Dempster, E. O'Connor, J.S. Alexander, R.E. Kelley, M. Kenner, U. Menon, V. Misra, R. Hoque, E. Gonzalez-Toledo, R.N. Schwendimann, S. Smith and A. Minagar, *The clinical response to minocycline in multiple sclerosis is accompanied by beneficial immune changes: a pilot study.* Multiple Sclerosis, 2007. **13**(4): p. 517–26.

21. Yong, V.W., J. Wells, F. Giuliani, S. Cahsa, C. Power and L.M. Metz, *The promise of minocycline in neurology.* The Lancet Neurology, 2004. **3**(12): p. 744–751.

22. Brinkmann, V., A. Billich, T. Baumruker, P. Heining, R. Schmouder,

G. Francis, S. Aradhye and P. Burtin, *Fingolimod (FTY720): Discovery and development of an oral drug to treat multiple sclerosis.* Nature Reviews Drug Discovery, 2010. **9**: p. 883.

23.   European Medicines Agency, *Updated restrictions for Gilenya: Multiple sclerosis medicine not to be used in pregnancy.* Available from: https://www.ema.europa.eu/en/news/updated-restrictions-gilenya-multiple-sclerosis-medicine-not-be-used-pregnancy. Accessed February 2021.

24.   European Medicines Agency, *Assessment Report Mayzent.* Available from: https://www.ema.europa.eu/en/documents/assessment-report/mayzent-epar-public-assessment-report_en.pdf. Accessed March 2021.

25.   Hardy, R.R., *B-1 B Cell Development.* The Journal of Immunology, 2006. **177**(5): p. 2749.

26.   Shen, P., E. Eilgenberg, A.C. Lino, V.D. Dang, S. Ries, I. Sakwa and S. Fillatreau, *Chapter 13 - B Cells as Regulators*, in *Molecular Biology of B Cells (Second Edition)*, F.W. Alt, T. Honjo, A. Radbruch and M. Reth, Editors. 2015, Academic Press: London. p. 215–225.

27.   Vale, A.M., J.F. Kearney, A. Nobrega and H.W. Schroeder, *Chapter 7 - Development and Function of B Cell Subsets*, in *Molecular Biology of B Cells (Second Edition)*, F.W. Alt, T. Honjo, A. Radbruch and M. Reth, Editors. 2015 Academic Press: London. pp. 99–119.

28.   Duddy, M., M. Niino, F. Adatia, S. Herbert, M. Freedman, H. Atkins, H.J. Kim and A. Bar-Or, *Distinct effector cytokine profiles of memory and naive human B cell subsets and implication in multiple sclerosis.* The Journal of Immunology, 2007. **178**(10): p. 6092–6099.

29.   Correale, J., M. Farez and G. Razzitte, *Helminth infections associated with multiple sclerosis induce regulatory B cells.* Annals of Neurology, 2008. **64**(2): p. 187–199.

30.   Monson, N.L., *Effective suppression of cerebrospinal fluid B cells by rituximab and cyclophosphamide in progressive multiple sclerosis—reply.* Archives of Neurology, 2005. **62**(10): p. 1642–1642.

31.   Lehmann, H.C., H-P., Hartung, G.R. Hetzel, O. Stüve and B.C. Kieseier, *Plasma exchange in neuroimmunological disorders: Part 1: Rationale and treatment of inflammatory central nervous system disorders.* Archives of Neurology, 2006. **63**(7): p. 930–935.

32.   Goodin, S.D., E.M. Frohman, G.P. Garmany Jr, J. Halper, W.H. LIkosky, F.D. Lublin, D.H. Silberberg, W.H. Stuart and S. van den Noort, *Disease modifying therapies in multiple sclerosis: Report of the*

Theapeutics and Technology Assessment Subcommittee of the American Academy of Neurology and the MS Council for Clinical Practice Guidelines. Neurology, 2002. **58**(2): p. 169–178.

33. Fernández Liguori, N., J.I. Rojas, D.S. Kajin and A. Ciapponi, *Intravenous immunoglobulin to prevent relapses during pregnancy and postpartum in multiple sclerosis.* Cochrane Database of Systematic Reviews, 2013(7).

34. Ballow, M., *Safety of IGIV therapy and infusion-related adverse events.* Immunologic Research, 2007. **38**(1–3): p. 122–132.

35. Fazekas, F., F.D. Lublin, D. Li, M.S. Freedman, H.P. Hartung, P. Rieckmann, P. Soelberg Sørensen, M. Maas-Enriquez, B. Sommerauer, K. Hanna, PRIVIG Study Group and UBC MS/MRI Research Group, *Intravenous immunoglobulin in relapsing-remitting multiple sclerosis.* Neurology, 2008. **71**(4): p. 265–271.

36. Inoue, K. and H. Yuasa, *Molecular basis for pharmacokinetics and pharmacodynamics of methotrexate in rheumatoid arthritis therapy.* Drug Metabolism and Pharmacokinetics, 2014. **29**(1): p. 12–19.

37. *drugs.com monograph on methotrexate.* Available from: https://www.drugs.com/monograph/methotrexate.html. Accessed February 2021.

38. Multiple Sclerosis Trust, *Methotrexate (Maxtrex).* Available from: https://mstrust.org.uk/a-z/methotrexate-maxtrex. Accessed March 2021.

39. *FDA Approved Drug Products: Imuran Azathioprine Oral Tablets.* Available from: https://www.accessdata.fda.gov/drugsatfda_docs/label/2011/016324s034s035lbl.pdf. Accessed February 2021.

40. Allison, A.C., *Mechanisms of action of mycophenolate mofetil.* Lupus, 2005. **14** Suppl 1: p. s2–8.

41. Allison, A.C. and E.M. Eugui, *Mycophenolate mofetil and its mechanisms of action.* Immunopharmacology, 2000. **47**(2–3): p. 85–118.

42. Awad, A. and O. Stüve, *Review: Cyclophosphamide in multiple sclerosis: scientific rationale, history and novel treatment paradigms.* Therapeutic Advances in Neurological Disorders, 2009. **2**(6): p. 357–368.

43. Portaccio, E., V. Zipoli, G. Siracusa, S. Piacentini, S. Sorbi and M.P. Amato, *Safety and tolerability of cyclophosphamide 'pulses' in multiple sclerosis: a prospective study in a clinical cohort.* Multiple Sclerosis, 2003. **9**(5): p. 446–450.

44. Bar-Or, A., A. Pachner, F. Menguy-Vacheron, J. Kaplan and H. Wiendl, *Teriflunomide and its mechanism of action in multiple sclerosis.* Drugs,

2014. **74**(6): p. 659–674.

45.   *Drug Bank- Cladribine.* 2020; Available from: https://www.drugbank.
ca/drugs/DB00242. Accessed February 2021.

46.   Leist, T.P. and R. Weissert, *Cladribine: Mode of action and implications
for treatment of multiple sclerosis.* Clinical Neuropharmacology, 2011.
34(1): p. 28–35.

47.   *National MS society.org FDA approves cladribine – brand named
Mavenclad.* 2020; Available from: https://www.nationalmssociety.org/
About-the-Society/News/FDA-Approves-Cladribine-Brand-named-
Mavenclad%C2%AE-for. Accessed February 2021.

48.   Rasmussen, P.V., M. Magyari, J.Y. Moberg, M. Bøgelund, U.F.A.
Jensen, K.G. Madsen, *Patient awareness about family planning represents
a major knowledge gap in multiple sclerosis.* Multiple Sclerosis and
Related Disorders, 2018. **24**: p. 129–134.

49.   Confavreux, C., M. Hutchinson, M.M. Hours, P. Cortinovis-Tourniare,
T. Moreau,and the Pregnancy in Multiple Sclerosis Group, *Rate of
pregnancy-related relapse in multiple sclerosis.* The New England Journal
of Medicine, 1998. **339**(5): p. 285–291.

50.   O'Gorman, C., R. Lin, J. Stankovich, S.A. Broadley, *Modelling genetic
susceptibility to multiple sclerosis with family data.* Neuroepidemiology,
2013. **40**(1): p. 1–12.

51.   Lu, E., et al., *Disease-modifying drugs for multiple sclerosis in pregnancy.*
Neurology, 2012. **79**(11): p. 1130.

52.   Amato, M.P. and E. Portaccio, *Fertility, pregnancy and childbirth in
patients with multiple sclerosis: Impact of disease-modifying drugs.* CNS
Drugs, 2015. **29**(3): p. 207–220.

53.   Mohme, M., C. Hotz, S. Stevanovic, T. Binder, J-H. Lee, M.
Okoniewski, T. Eiermann, M. Sospedra, H-G. Rammensee and R.
Martin, *HLA-DR15-derived self-peptides are involved in increased
autologous T cell proliferation in multiple sclerosis.* Brain, 2013. **136**(6): p.
1783–1798.

54.   Ashton-Rickardt, P.G., A. Bandeira, J.R. Delaney, L. Van Kaer, H.P.
Pircher, R.M. Zinkernagel and S. Tonegawa, *Evidence for a differential
avidity model of T cell selection in the thymus.* Cell, 1994. **76**(4): p.
651–663.

55.   Danke, N.A., D.M. Koelle, C. Yee, S. Beheray and W. W. Kwok,
Autoreactive T cells in healthy individuals. The Journal of Immunology,

2004. **172**(10): p. 5967–5972.

56. Jelcic, I., F.A. Nimer, J. Wang, V. Lentsch, R. Planas, I. Jelcic, A. Madjovski, S. Ruhrmann, W. Faigle, K. Frauenknecht, C. Pinilla, R. Santos, C. Hammer, Y. Ortiz, L. Opitz, H. Grönlund, G. Rogler, O. Boyman, R. Reynolds, A. Lutterotti, M. Khademi, T. Olsson, F. Piehl, M. Sospedra and R. Martin, *Memory B cells activate brain-homing, autoreactive CD4(+) T cells in multiple sclerosis.* Cell, 2018. **175**(1): p. 85–100.e23.

57. National Human Genome Research Institute. *The Human Genome Project 2019*; Available from: https://www.genome.gov/10001772/. Accessed February 2021.

58. Sospedra, M., P.A. Muraro, I. Stefanová, Y. Zhao, K. Chung, Y. Li, M. Giulianotti, R. Simon, R. Mariuzza, C. Pinilla and R. Martin, *Redundancy in antigen-presenting function of the HLA-DR and -DQ molecules in the multiple sclerosis-associated HLA-DR2 haplotype.* The Journal of Immunology, 2006. **176**(3): p. 1951–1961.

59. Zivadinov, R., L. Uxa, A. Bratina, A. Bosco, B. Srinivasaraghavan, A. Minagar, M. Ukmar, S. yen Benedetto and M. Zorzon, *HLADRB1*1501, DQB1*0301, DQB1*0302, DQB1*0602 and DQB1*0603 alleles are associated with more severe disease outcome on MRI in patients with multiple sclerosis.* International Review of Neurobiology. 2007. **79**: p. 521–535.

60. Kakalacheva, K., C. Münz and J.D. Lünemann, *Viral triggers of multiple sclerosis.* Biochimica et Biophysica Acta, 2011. **1812**(2): p. 132–140.

61. Reboldi, A., C. Coisne, D. Baumjohann, F. Benvenuto, D. Bottinelli, S. Lira, A. Uccelli, A. Lanazavecchia, B. Engelhardt and F. Sallusto, *C-C chemokine receptor 6-regulated entry of T-H-17 cells into the CNS through the choroid plexus is required for the initiation of EAE.* Nature Immunology, 2009. **10**(5): p. 514–523.

62. Magliozzi, R., O. Howell, A. Vora, B. Serafini, R. Nicholas, M. Puopolo, R. Reynolds and F. Aloisi, *Meningeal B-cell follicles in secondary progressive multiple sclerosis associate with early onset of disease and severe cortical pathology.* Brain, 2007. **130**(4): p. 1089–1104.

Note 10

The Experimental-Animal-Model Basis of the Standard Theory

There are two major animal models of MS.

1) Experimental Allergic Encephalomyelitis (EAE)

Fragments of spinal cord cells or a protein called myelin oligodendrocyte glycoprotein (MOG), along with an agent that speeds up antigen presentation known as an adjuvant, are injected into a mouse or other experimental animal.[1] The T cells, stimulated by this, induce neuropathological disease and paralysis. Sometimes, activated T cells from such an animal are transferred to another mouse to induce disease.

There is no single model of EAE. Since 1933 there has been a range of models reported in more than 5,000 publications. Advocates of this model argue that it is justified as it led to advanced clinical trials from which the FDA approved glatiramer acetate, mitoxantrone and natalizumab after they showed promise in EAE models.[2]

Critics argue that current EAE models are mainly based on inflammation and are biased toward auto-reactive CD4+ T cells. By comparison, pathological data and results from clinical trials in MS indicate that CD8+ T cells and B lymphocytes may play an important role in propagating inflammation and tissue damage in established MS.[3]

Another criticism of the EAE model is that while MS is an immune-mediated disease, the model lacks many features of classic autoimmunity.[4]

EAE remains the dominant animal model of MS in studies.

2) Theiler's Murine Encephalomyelitis Virus

In 1951, Max Theiler of the Rockefeller Foundation received the Nobel Prize in Physiology or Medicine for his discovery of an effective vaccine against yellow fever.[5] This was something he had developed in 1937. Also, in the 1930s, he had discovered an encephalomyelitis virus while working on a polio-like virus in mice. When this virus was introduced, it caused chronic inflammation in the brain of the mouse, similar to MS in humans.

Its demyelinating lesions are evident as early as three weeks after infection. These lesions progress and reach a plateau at around one hundred days post-infection. At that time, infected mice begin to present with neurological symptoms, including hind limb weakness, spasticity, and gait abnormalities. After this time, spinal cord atrophy continues to progress. Hind limb paralysis and bladder incontinence occurs six to nine months after infection.[4]

A study using TMEV in 1998 was the first to implicate CD8+ T cells in neurological disease.[6]

References

1.   Shen, P., E. Eilgenberg, A.C. Lino, V.D. Dang, S. Ries, I. Sakwa and S. Fillatreau, *Chapter 13 - B Cells as Regulators*, in *Molecular Biology of B Cells (Second Edition)*, F.W. Alt, T. Honjo, A. Radbruch and M. Reth, Editors. 2015, Academic Press: London. p. 215-225.

2.   Steinman, L. and S.S. Zamvil, *How to successfully apply animal studies in experimental allergic encephalomyelitis to research on multiple sclerosis.* Annals of Neurology, 2006. **60**(1): p. 12–21.

3.   Lassmann, H. and M. Bradl, *Multiple sclerosis: Experimental models and reality.* Acta Neuropathologica, 2017. **133**(2): p. 223–244.

4.   Denic, A., A.J. Johnson, A.J. Bieber, A.E. Warrington, M. Rodriguez and I. Pirko, *The relevance of animal models in multiple sclerosis research.* Pathophysiology, 2011. **18**(1): p. 21–29.

5.   Norrby, E., *Yellow fever and Max Theiler: the only Nobel Prize for a virus vaccine.* The Journal of Experimental Medicine, 2007. **204**(12): p. 2779-2784.

6.   Rivera-Quiñones, C., D. McGavern, J.D. Schmelzer, S.F. Hunter, P.A. Low and M. Rodriguez, *Absence of neurological deficits following extensive demyelination in a Class I-deficient murine model of multiple sclerosis.* Nature Medicine, 1998. **4**(2): p. 187–193.

Note 11

Dendritic Cells

The problem with therapies targeting T cell and B cell activity in MS is they often fail.

Call it early stage, mild, remitting-relapsing, or whatever you choose, the non-progressive form of MS often seems to respond positively to these treatments. When the disease moves to a progressive form, the treatments don't consistently work.

The approach to T and B cells in MS research is a focus on the adaptive immune system. This is our second line of defense. It is preceded by the innate immune system's responses to signals.

It follows that, as many drugs fail, a focus just on the responses of the adaptive immune system can only have limited application. In MS research, our primitive immune response, the innate system, hasn't received nearly as much commercial attention.

~

To activate the first T cell in the chain of adaptive immune reactions requires a prompt from the innate system. The adaptive immune system is introduced to antigens when cytokines produced by a class of specialist cells present them to T cells. While any cell with a nucleus can make an MHC (major histocompatibility complex) Class I molecule, only the real professionals can make Class II antigens and present them to a T cell.

Some cells, such as macrophages, engulf pathogens and present fragments of them on their cell surface attached to an MHC Class II molecule. This stimulates T cells and triggers an adaptive immune response. Activated B cells can also act as antigen-presenting cells.

However, the most critical cell in antigen presentation is the dendritic cell. It has pattern recognition receptors that, when triggered, express not only MHC Class II molecules but the stimulatory molecules that activate T cells.

Dendritic cells are the gold medalists among antigen presenting cells. They can take the smallest amount of an antigen and use it to stimulate Tcell responses. They are the cells that can home into the lymphatic system to activate the T cells.

If a naïve T cell has not been stimulated by a dendritic cell, it will not respond to a pathogen. The naïve T cell will be blind to the pattern of the pathogen if the dendritic cell does not interact first.

The dendritic cell is also the gatekeeper that controls compatibility. It decides which antigens are foreign.

Rather than release toxins against pathogens, dendritic cells create peptides (chains of amino acids) that T cells can understand and react to. By responding to patterns from pathogens, dendritic cells can translate the early responses of the innate immune system into the language of the Tcells of the adaptive immune system.

Dendritic cells exist in a variety of forms. Initially, they are immature cells living in our tissues. In this form, they capture the signature of pathogens.

While they are immature, dendritic cells are incapable of stimulating Tcells. In this state, all the MHC class II molecules are inside the dendritic cells rather than being expressed on the cell surface. When the dendritic cells have migrated to the lymphatic system, they rapidly mature.

As mature cells, they relocate their MHC class II molecules to their cell surface. The shape of the cells changes, and they extend long arms called dendrites. When this happens, they express co-stimulatory molecules that activate the T cells. Dendritic cells can mature within hours. A receptor on the immature dendritic cell called a Toll-like receptor drives this maturation.

Toll-Like Receptors

In 1989, an article in the *Journal of Immunology*[2] by Charles A. Janeway Jnr presented a new theory on how the immune system operated. He proposed that T cell activation was a two-step process. A first step would "see" an antigen but could not distinguish if it was "self" or 'non-self.' It could not trigger a response from a T cell. Only the second signal could trigger an immune response. Janeway believed his conceptual, unknown receptor would control immune response by pattern recognition.

In 1994, the same year I was diagnosed with MS, a young Russian scientist, Ruslan Medzhitov, joined Janeway's laboratory and began looking for proof that this receptor existed.

Both scientists felt that the unknown receptor must influence a protein called a transcription factor. This protein controls how DNA is passed to messenger RNA by binding to a specific sequence. A known common transcription factor was called NFκB (pronounced NF kappa B). Their goal was to find what stimulated NFκB.

Medzhitov eventually found a receptor that looked remarkably like one called "Toll" from the fly species "Drosophila."

In 1997, which is not long ago, Janeway and Medzhitov reported in *Nature*[3] that a human version of the Toll receptor activated NFκB. They showed that this receptor controlled the release of the inflammatory cytokines IL-1, IL-6, and IL-8. It also determined the release of the stimulatory molecules that activated T cells.

So far, 11 human Toll-like receptors have been discovered, and 10 have specific functions that are somewhat well understood. Some are believed to be associated with MS.

Dendritic Cell Subsets in MS

Scientists can discriminate between two subsets of dendritic cells in our blood: plasmacytoid and myeloid cells.

Plasmacytoid dendritic cells

Cytology is a branch of biology dealing with the structure, function, multiplication, pathology, and life cycle of cells. The plasmacytoid dendritic cells circulate in the blood and are found in the lymphatic organs. They share many cytological similarities with antibody-producing plasma cells.[4] Hence their name.

Studies have found these cells in increased numbers, compared to controls, in the inflamed cerebrospinal fluid of MS patients.[5] This is significant, as the brain was once considered privileged and the blood-brain barrier should block an antigen-presenting cell.

It has been noted that for patients experiencing relapses, the number of plasmacytoid dendritic cells increases compared to patients in remission.[6] These cells express Toll-like receptor 9 (TLR9), which is activated by viral DNA. Driven by TLR9, these cells express large amounts of Type 1 interferon, which should dampen the immune response in active MS. We see Type 1 interferons used as treatments for MS patients.[6]

CD123 is a marker of interferon expression

A study in 2008 concluded that interferon-β treatment (a Type 1 interferon) modulated the maturity of plasmacytoid dendritic cells, resulting in a lower secretion of proinflammatory cytokines and a reduced ability to stimulate T cells. They also noted that the higher expression of CD123 might be a confirming signal that interferon expression has become elevated.[16]

Non-inflammatory and inflammatory plasmacytoid dendritic cells

A study in 2010 noted there are two types of plasmacytoid dendritic cells with very different cytokine expressions.[12] Type 1 expressed high levels of CD123 and low levels of CD86, as well as displaying low levels of TLR2. These cells also directed T cells to produce the non-inflammatory IL-10, which has been noted to reduce MS symptoms.

By contrast, Type 2 plasmacytoid dendritic cells had the inverse response. They were characterized by low levels of CD123, and high CD86. Also, TLR2 expression levels in these cells were elevated. Additionally, these cells secreted inflammatory IL-6 and tumor necrosis factor-α. T cells associated with these dendritic cells are Th17 class and are often observed in MS lesions.[12]

Dendritic cells taken from the blood of people with MS have been found to secrete more proinflammatory cytokines than those found in healthy people.[8]

The 2011 Nobel Prize was awarded to Ralph Steinman, who first identified dendritic cells in 1973.[1] In a sad twist, he died three days before the award was announced. As a mark of respect, the committee, which only awards the prize to living nominees, made the unprecedented decision to let the award stand.

Myeloid dendritic cells

Myeloid dendritic cells, sometimes called conventional dendritic cells, strongly express Toll-like receptor 2 (TLR2), which seems to set up protective pathways against viruses. Possibly, TLR2 forms a complex with the protein MyD88 and triggers the release of the transcription factor NFκB, leading to Type 1 interferons being expressed.[7]

Toll-like receptor 4 is also activated in MS patients by myeloid dendritic cells. This receptor is associated with endotoxins in the outer membrane of gram-negative bacteria. It's activation also precedes the activation of the transcription factor NFκB.[9]

Both types of dendritic cells (plasmacytoid and myeloid) have been noted to accumulate in and between the inner two layers of meninges through which the spinal fluid circulates. The occurrence of myeloid dendritic cells is highest in early disease or in clinically isolated syndrome. It seems to decrease with time. Plasmacytoid dendritic cells follow a different pattern. During relapses, their levels in lesions and spinal fluid rise compared to the levels in patients in remission.[5]

A little bit of DNA makes a big difference

In our DNA, when a molecule called a cytosine triphosphate deoxynucleotide is joined to a guanine triphosphate deoxynucleotide, the tiny strands of DNA that surround these molecules are called CpG DNA.

The actual structure of these CpG motifs has been divided into three subgroups with differing profiles.

1) B-class CpG has vigorous anti-tumor activity. When transcribed, it stimulates a strong B cell response, activates natural killer cells, and promotes the expression of many cytokines. It boosts the inflammatory

Th1 type responses and produces a weak Type 1 interferon response.

2) Transcription of A-class CpG activates dendritic cells to produce high levels of Type 1 interferon (interferon-α).[13] This creates a non-inflammatory response.

3) C-class CpG stimulates robust B cell proliferation where A-class doesn't.[14]

CpG motifs are an area of intense interest in the field of epigenetics. Epigenetics explores which genes are turned "on" and which are turned "off". The understanding of how gene expression interacts with the dendritic cells needs a lot of work.

~

A report in 2012 noted that the CpG DNA strands should stimulate TLR9 to direct T cells and B cells to produce non-inflammatory IL-10 as well as anti-inflammatory Type 1 interferons.[15] The review noted that with Type 2 plasmacytoid dendritic cells, this stimulus does not occur, and proinflammatory cytokines predominate. The study also noted that treatment with MS interferon medication might help offset this.

Type 1 plasmacytoid dendritic cells don't seem to fully mature. They have low levels of the surface marker CD86. This might be low due to the expression of large amounts of Type 1 interferon that may occur because of the transcription of A-class CpG DNA.

The difference is significant; Type 1 plasmacytoid cells are producing a healthy regulatory response from interferon expression, Type 2 are producing an inflammatory cytokine response. As a complication, the type of CpG DNA can modulate the outcome.

All this suggests that when Toll-like receptors in dendritic cells encounter viruses, they trigger those cells to mature so they can activate T cells. The path they take depends on whether or not the nature of a DNA strand, called CpG, prompts TLR9 to release the dampening, non-inflammatory Type 1 interferons.

It may be that if interferon is released early, the plasmacytoid dendritic cell does not fully mature, so its surface marker CD86, which stimulates T cells, stays low while the marker of interferon release, CD123, appears elevated.[4]

Plasmacytoid dendritic cell model for MS

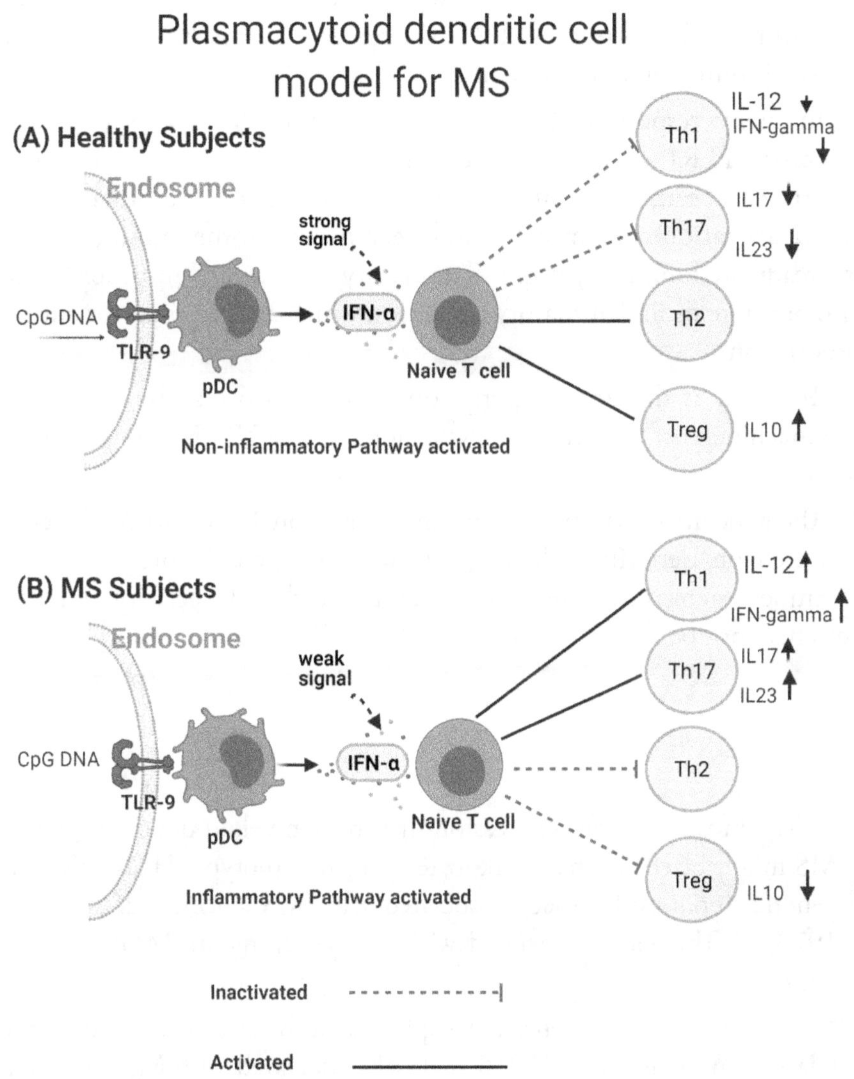

Figure XI.1 TLR9 preferentially binds to unmethylated gene sequences called CpG. These unmethylated motifs are mostly viral or bacterial, as CpG in humans is mostly methylated. The plasmacytoid dendritic cell (pDC) interacts with TLR9 and then releases Type 1 interferon which dampens inflammatory pathways. In MS subjects, this signal is weaker leading to the activation of inflammatory pathways.

Created with BioRender.

If virus-activated TLR9 is not stimulated, the dendritic cell continues to mature, and if instead, TLR2 is the receptor that is stimulated, there is a more proinflammatory outcome.

In many responses, TLR2 forms a complex with another toll-like receptor (TLR1 or TLR6). The exact role of TLR2 is challenging to determine because the outcome is co-dependent on the other receptor. TLR2 activation may improve viral clearance when the immune response is already predominately non-inflammatory (i.e., in early infection). It may also promote proinflammatory responses, which are necessary for antibody production.[17]

The issue is that the transcription factor NFκB may be released into the machinery of the cell by these actions. What NFκB does is discussed in Note 12.

The majority of MS treatments are focused on T cell and B cell activity. Research on dendritic cells suggests what happens before the adaptive immune system is triggered is important, and that the activity of T and B cells may not be the main driver of MS.

The most pertinent expression driven by myeloid dendritic cells in MS might be the human leukocyte antigen haplotype, HLA-DR. This genetic signature has been associated with MS since its discovery in 1973.[5, 10] The genes associated with this grouping are MHC Class II antigens.

It takes dendritic cells, macrophages or B cells to express MHC Class II antigens. HLA-DR15 is closely associated with MS, and there seems to be a link between that phenotype and other MHC Class II molecules associated with MS.[11]

References

1. Prize, T.N. *The Nobel Prize in Physiology or Medicine 2011*. Available from: https://www.nobelprize.org/prizes/medicine/2011/steinman/biographical/. Accessed February 2021.

2. Janeway, C.A., *Approaching the asymptote? Evolution and revolution in immunology.* Cold Spring Harbor Symposia on Quantitative Biology, 1989. **54**: p. 1–13. Also, The Journal of Immunology, 2013. **191**(9): p. 4475.

3. Medzhitov, R., P. Preston-Hurlburt and C.A. Janeway, *A human homologue of the Drosophila Toll protein signals activation of adaptive immunity.* Nature, 1997. **388**(6640): p. 394–397.

4. Manuel, C., X. Montalban, C. Münz and J.D. Lünemann, *Targeting dendritic cells to treat multiple sclerosis.* Nature Reviews Neurology, 2010. **6**(9): p. 499–507.

5. Nuyts, A., W.P. Lee, R. Bashir-Dar, Z.N. Berneman and N. Cools, *Dendritic cells in multiple sclerosis: key players in the immunopathogenesis, key players for new cellular immunotherapies?* Multiple Sclerosis Journal, 2013. **19**(8): p. 995–1002.

6. Longhini, A.L.F., F. von Glehn, C.O. Brandão, R.F.O. de Paula, F. Pradella, A.S. Moraes, A.S. Farias, E.C. Oliveira, J.G. Quispe-Cabanillas, C.H. Abreu, A. Damasceno, B.P. Damasceno, K.E. Balashov and L.M.B. Santos, *Plasmacytoid dendritic cells are increased in cerebrospinal fluid of untreated patients during multiple sclerosis relapse.* Journal of Neuroinflammation, 2011. **8**: p. 2.

7. de Oliviera Nascimento, L., P. Massari and L. Wetzler, *The role of TLR2 in infection and immunity.* Frontiers in Immunology, 2012. **3**: p. 79.

8. Huang, Y.M., B.G. Xiao, V. Ozenci, M. Kouwenhoven, N. Teleshova, S. Fredrikson and H. Link, *Multiple sclerosis is associated with high levels of circulating dendritic cells secreting pro-inflammatory cytokines.* Journal of Neuroimmunology, 1999. **99**(1): p. 82–90.

9. *Invivogen TLR4 ligands*. Available from: https://www.invivogen.com/tlr4-ligands. Accessed February 2021.

10. Thorsby, E., *A short history of HLA.* Tissue Antigens, 2009. **74**(2): p. 101–116.

11.   Harbo, H.F., B.A. Lie, E.G. Celius, K-Z Dai, A. Oturai, J. Hillert, A.R. Lorentzen, M. Laaksonen, K-M. Myhr, L.P. Ryder, S. Fredrikson, H. Nyland, P.S. Sørenson, M. Sandberg-Wollheim, O. Anderson, A. Svejgaard, A. Edland, S.I. Mellgren, A. Compston, F. Vartdal and A. Spurkland, *Genes in the HLA Class I region may contribute to the HLA Class II associated genetic susceptibility to multiple sclerosis.* Tissue Antigens, 2004. **63**(3): p. 237–247.

12.   Schwab, N., A.L. Zozulya, B.C. Kieseier, K.V. Toyka and H. Wiendl, *An imbalance of two functionally and phenotypically different subsets of plasmacytoid dendritic cells characterizes the dysfunctional immune regulation in multiple sclerosis.* Journal of Immunology, 2010. **184**(9): p. 5368–5374.

13.   Menon, M., P.A. Blair, D.A. Isenberg and C. Mauri, *A regulatory feedback between plasmacytoid dendritic cells and regulatory B cells is aberrant in systemic lupus erythematosus.* Immunity, 2016. **44**(3): p. 683–697.

14.   Vollmer, J., R. Weeratna, P. Payette, M. Jurk, C. Schetter, M. Laucht, T. Water, S. Tluk, M. Liu, H.L. Davis and A.M. Krieg, *Characterization of three CpG oligodeoxynucleotide classes with distinct immunostimulatory activities.* European Journal of Immunology, 2004. **34**(1): p. 251–262.

15.   Hirotani, M., M. Niino, T. Fukazawa, H. Yaguchi, M. Nakamura, S. Kikuchi and H. Sasaki, *Decreased interferon-α production in response to CpG DNA dysregulates cytokine responses in patients with multiple sclerosis.* Clinical Immunology, 2012. **143**(2): p. 145–151.

16.   Lande, R., V. Gafa, B. Serafini, E. Giacomini, A. Visconti, M.E. Remoli, M. Severa, M. Parmentier, G. Ristori, M. Salvetti, F. Aloisi and E.M. Coccia, *Plasmacytoid dendritic cells in multiple sclerosis: Intracerebral recruitment and impaired maturation in response to interferon-β.* Journal of Neuropathology & Experimental Neurology, 2008. **67**(5): p. 388–401.

17.   Oliveira-Nascimento, L., P. Massari and L.M. Wetzler, *The role of TLR2 in infection and immunity.* Frontiers in Immunology, 2012. **3**: p. 79.

Note 12

NFκB in Cell Signaling and Gene Expression

Another name for an antibody is "immunoglobulin".

Chains of polypeptides make up immunoglobulins. Characteristically, they consist of two heavy chains and two light chains. Each chain consists of constant regions and variable regions.

The constant region of the heavy chains determines the five classes of immunoglobulins: IgG, IgM, IgA, IgD, and IgE. However, there are thousands of different amino acid sequences in immunoglobulins because of the inherent hypervariability in the bonds formed between the regions.

The light chains bind to the heavy chains to complete the antibody. They are called either kappa (κ) or lambda (λ) light chains. In humans, serum antibody light chains are about 60% κ and 40% λ.[1] The receptors on B and T cells rearrange as the cells develop and mature, and the type of antigen receptor rearrangement depends a lot on the light chains of the antigens. The receptor rearrangement is dictated by a protein called an enhancer.

When first discovered in B cells, the factor that triggered the enhancer of the immunoglobulin kappa light chain (IκE) was called "the nuclear factor kappa-light-chain-enhancer of activated B cells" or NFκB.[2] The name stuck.

Now it is recognized that NFκB is in all cells. When it is activated, it enters the nucleus of the cell, inducing the transcription of of genes by binding to promotors and, ultimately causing the activation of genes. The messenger RNA created from this transcription is taken to ribosomes in the cytoplasm for new protein production. If NFκB is activated in response to stress, then the proteins made are designed to help the cell survive. If misleading signals cause the activation, then the proteins produced may be unhelpful.

NFκB is one of the master switches that regulate inflammation in T cells, macrophages, and microglia. Depending on which pathway is activated, it will influence the development of lymphoid organs as well as B and T cell development.

Numerous studies have shown that NFκB is noticeably activated in the brain tissue of patients with MS.[7]

A study in 2010 of MS patients found that naïve CD4+T cells (those that had not been exposed to an antigen) already had hyperactivated levels of NFκB. This raised the question of whether there was a genetic variation of NFκB involved in MS.[8]

The study found that when tumor necrosis factor-α (TNF-α) stimulated two MS-associated genes (rs228614 and rs7665090) located very near the NFκB gene, there was a 20-fold increase in a component of the transcription factor, called p50 NFκB, and a reduced expression of the regulators that keep NFκB out of the cell nucleus. So inflammatory cells can express TNF-α, resulting in loops and cascades that increase the amounts of NFκB released in the cell.

Nuclear factor kappa B (NFκB) has a diverse set of functions in the nervous system. In neurons, it may enhance memory. By comparison, the supporting cells of the nervous system, called glia, may be induced to activate NFκB in brain inflammation.[3] This activation may be a defensive response to regulate the infiltration of immune cells into lesions.[3]

A study in 2007 concluded that persistent pain might rely on the activation of NFκB by an inflammatory stimulus, while acute pain depends on regular NFκB activity.[4]

Constitutive NFκB does not appear to play a negative role in healthy animal test subjects. However, when NFκB was induced in the glial cells of the brain, the spinal cord and the peripheral nerves of animals, the inflammatory marker IL-6 was significantly upregulated and motor function became impaired. By contrast, inhibiting NFκB reduced glial scarring.[5]

Proinflammatory cytokines, bacteria, viruses, physiological stress, oxidative stress, modified proteins and a range of other agents can all trigger NFκB.[6]

One of NFκB's most significant roles is its ability to rapidly upregulate the gene that leads to the expression of Inducible Nitric Oxide Synthase (iNOS).[9] This is a form of the oxidoreductase that leads to the formation of large quantities of nitric oxide. This outcome can be positive if it is a response to acute septic damage but the presence of iNOS can also be detrimental. Although nitric oxide is the central regulator of the vascular response (acting as a vasodilator), overexpression can be involved in neurodegenerative, autoimmune, cardiovascular and inflammatory disorders.[10] Its expression in response to shock can also result in hypotension.

Activation of NFκB is an essential step for iNOS induction in most cell types.[11] When activated, NFκB will increase the amount of nitric oxide in the cell, sometimes to abnormal levels.

References

1.   Passos Jr., G.A.S., *Physical map and one-megabase sequencing of the human immunoglobulin lambda locus.* Genetics and Molecular Biology, 1998. **21**: p. 281–286.

2.   Sen, R., *NF-kappaB and the immunoglobulin kappa gene enhancer.* The Journal of Experimental Medicine, 2004. **200**(9): p. 1099–1102.

3.   Kaltschmidt, B. and C. Kaltschmidt, *NF-kappaB in the nervous system.* Cold Spring Harbor Perspectives in Biology, 2009. **1**(3): p. a001271–a001271.

4.   Niederberger, E., A. Schmidtko, W. Gao, H. Kühlein, C. Ehnert and G. Geisslinger, *Impaired acute and inflammatory nociception in mice lacking the p50 subunit of NF-kappaB.* European Journal of Pharmacology, 2007. **559**(1): p. 55–60.

5.   Brambilla, R., V. Bracchi-Ricard, W-H. Hu, B. Frydel, A. Bramwell, S. Karmally, E.J. Green and J.R. Bethea, *Inhibition of astroglial nuclear factor kappaB reduces inflammation and improves functional recovery after spinal cord injury.* The Journal of Experimental Medicine, 2005. **202**(1): p. 145–156.

6.   Yue, Y., S. Stone and W. Lin, *Role of nuclear factor κB in multiple sclerosis and experimental autoimmune encephalomyelitis.* Neural Regeneration Research, 2018. **13**(9): p. 1507-1515.

7.   Leibowitz, S.M. and J. Yan, *NF-κB pathways in the pathogenesis of multiple sclerosis and the therapeutic implications.* Frontiers in Molecular Neuroscience, 2016. **9**: p. 84.

8.   Housley, W.J., S.D. Fernandez, K. Vera, S.R. Murikainati, J. Grutzendler, N. Cuerdon, L. Glick, P.L. De Jager, M. Mitrovic, C. Cotsapas and D.A. Hafler, *Genetic variants associated with autoimmunity drive NFκB signaling and responses to inflammatory stimuli.* Science Translational Medicine, 2015. 7(291): p. 291ra93–291ra93.

9.   Jia, J., Y. Liu, X. Zhang, X. Liu and J. Qi, *Regulation of iNOS expression by NF-κB in human lens epithelial cells treated with high levels of glucose.* Investigative Ophthalmology and Visual Science, 2013. **54**(7): p. 5070–5077.

10.   Taylor, S.B. and A.D. Geller, *Molecular regulation of the human inducible nitric oxide sythase (iNOS) gene.* Shock, 2000. **13**(6): p. 413–424.

11.   Mendes, A.F., A.P. carvalho, M.M. Caramona and M.C. Lopes, *Role of nitric oxide in the activation of NF-κB, AP-1 and NOS II expression in articular chondrocytes.* Inflammation Research, 2002. **51**(7): p. 369-375.

Note 13

NO! OO, NO!

The role of Nitric Oxide, Superoxide, and Peroxynitrite in Inflammation

The Immune System

The human immune response divides into two classes: our natural, unlearned immune response called the innate immune system, and our acquired, learned response called our adaptive immune system.

Even before these two systems are engaged, our immunity against pathogens involves our basic physiology, the barriers of our skin, the self-clearing mucous pathways, the acidity of our digestive system, and the antibacterial chemistry of our secretions.

The next barrier is the innate system, which responds immediately to pathogens. Speed is its defining characteristic. The innate system recruits the adaptive immune system.

The adaptive immune system is slow. It both depends on and interacts with the innate system. The adaptive immune system encompasses the T and B cells. The T and B cell populations can expand and sustain an immune response by developing and harnessing antibodies. It can take days for the T and B cells of the adaptive immune system to clone themselves sufficiently to mount a serious challenge to a pathogen.[1]

The Innate System

Our innate immune system relies on receptors. In particular, a type of lymphoid killer cell (that is not antigen-specific) recognizes when a cell has lost certain receptors and can no longer inhibit an invader. This lymphoid cell is a natural killer cell. It is the ancient form of immunity. It should be

398

our first defense against viral infection, and many cancer therapies try to recruit this cell.

The innate immune system relies on receptors that recognize differences in patterns. These patterns determine what is "self" or "non-self". Innate immunity looks for damage in molecular patterns. To the innate immune system, damage represents danger. Damage-associated molecular patterns (DAMPs) indicate infection and inflammation.

Examples of markers of danger include heat-shock proteins, uric acid levels, and molecules associated with cell stress or necrosis (unplanned cell death).[2] These molecules are similar to cytokines but are called endokines or alarmins. Sometimes they are simply called "danger signals."

Innate immune receptors also detect the "missing self"; they look for the absence of molecules expressed by healthy cells. When cells are damaged or perhaps when microbes roam unchecked, molecules may be missing. If the right proteins are not expressed from inside a cell, the innate immune system uses natural killer cells to destroy what it will regard as a damaged cell.

Ten receptors are critical to the function of recognition and response by the innate immune system.[1] Collectively, they are called Toll-like receptors. As a family, through sentinel cells such as dendritic cells, they drive proinflammatory responses by activating the protein complexes (called transcription factors) that can switch genes on or off.

When inactive, the transcription factor NFκB sits in the cytosol of the cell, held in place by a series of inhibitors. Toll-like receptors can block factors that inhibit NFκB. This unlocks NFκB and allows it to modify gene expression by entering the nucleus of the cell and binding to DNA. Targeting NFκB is seen as a possible therapy in many diseases. Over 800 compounds can affect NFκB. Some appear in non-medical therapies (e.g., curcumin, green tea), and others are being investigated in clinical trials.[3]

So, not everything that happens in our immune system depends on T and B cell activity. The Toll-like receptors, the natural killer cells, the transcription factors and how DNA is expressed can all determine proinflammatory activity.

Inflammation

Inflammation is a response to injury. It may be related to toxins brought by invading organisms, noxious chemical stimulus, physical trauma, other environmental stressors, or a breakdown in autoregulation.

The primary immune response can be either specific to the irritant or nonspecific. If there is an irritant, the immune system wants to remove it. If it is an invading pathogen, the immune system wants to destroy it.

~

The bloodstream distribution of arteries, veins, and capillaries varies throughout the body. This causes variation in how much oxygen becomes available to each type of tissue. The inflammatory response is tied to the level of oxygenation.

In the upper airways, the oxygen level is closest to the content in the atmosphere at around 19%; in the bone marrow, it is about 6.4%; in the intestinal tissue, it might be 7%; and in the hollow tube of our gut it can be as low as 0%.[4] The brain has the highest oxygen requirement of any organ of the body. It needs about 25% of all the body's oxygen requirement, yet it makes up less than 3% of our mass.[5] If oxygen is deprived, the brain can be damaged in less than five minutes, but the heart can go on to function for roughly 30 minutes.

Just as the supply of oxygen can vary, the oxygen demand also varies. The brain has a consistent need. Large organs are definitely oxygen hungry. The oxygen demands of the tissues of the liver or the bowel vary according to the changing demands on them. In simple terms, each organ and part of the body has a different oxygen requirement.[6]

Nitric oxide and inflammation

Nitric oxide is a compound made up of one atom of nitrogen and one atom of oxygen. As it has an unpaired electron in its structure, it is a free radical. Unlike many free radicals, nitric oxide has a comparatively long half-life (around one second). Its roles in the body are diverse; it is involved in the immune system, the circulatory system, and the nervous system.[9]

When nitric oxide concentrations are low, it reacts with the metal complexes in cells and other free radicals. However, when its concentration level rises, it reacts more vigorously with molecules, such as superoxide and oxygen to create more potent free radicals, such as nitrogen dioxide and other nitrogenous oxides.

Among these oxides, the DNA-damaging radical peroxynitrite is particularly disruptive. It is formed when nitric oxide (NO) combines with superoxide (O_2^-). The chemical formula for peroxynitrite is $ONOO^-$.

Enzymes Critical to Making Nitric Oxide

Enzymes that catalyze nitric oxide formation are collectively called nitric oxide synthases. The name "synthase" is outdated. A real synthase catalyzes two molecules to join together. This is not what these enzymes do. However, they are still called synthases for historical reasons.

Each of these enzymes consists of two proteins joined together to form an oxidoreductase. The two domains are an oxygenase domain that accepts an electron from oxygen, and a second domain called a reductase domain that donates an electron.

There are three different enzymes involved in making nitric oxide:[9]

nNOS (neuronal nitric oxide synthase) predominates in both the central and peripheral nervous systems but is also found in other cells.

eNOS (endothelial nitric oxide synthase) predominates in the endothelial cells that line the blood vessels but is also found in other cells.

iNOS (inducible nitric oxide synthase) is only found in meager amounts except when inflammatory cytokines or similar signals spark a rapid increase in production. Macrophages are prolific producers of iNOS when they are activated.

Constitutive nitric oxide synthases

The forms nNOS and eNOS are usually found in roughly constant volumes in particular cell types. They are classified as constitutive forms. They are part of our regular physical makeup. Their activity is tightly regulated and depends on the presence of calcium ions. Calcium access into the cytoplasm of a cell is limited, irrespective of diet. Usually, a cell will pump out excess calcium or shift it into a store that cannot be accessed by the nitric oxide synthases.[9]

Inducible nitric oxide synthase

iNOS is typically induced to proliferate under inflammatory conditions.[9] As its structure differs from the constitutive forms, it doesn't require calcium ions to activate it. Expression of the cytokines IL-1, IL-6, IL-8, TNF-α, and interferon-γ are all a "call to arms" for iNOS. Its gene is activated by the transcription factor NFκB.

iNOS is the critical enzyme expressed by macrophages. These are the white blood cells that have the role of cleaning up the unhealthy debris at a cellular level. NFκB triggers genes inside macrophages to rapidly expand iNOS production. The expression of nitric oxide by this path is about one thousand times faster than expression of the constitutive forms. It dominates during inflammation.

A loop can develop: The iNOS stimulates nitric oxide formation. That combines with superoxide to make peroxynitrite. The peroxynitrite encourages NFκB to enter the nucleus of the cell and alter the DNA. If this leads to the expression of inflammatory cytokines, then a new cycle of iNOS is induced, stimulating more nitric oxide.

iNOS induction is particularly high in the immune cells and the glial cells of the brain.[9]

Nitric oxide levels are challenging to measure, but they can be indirectly measured by measuring its breakdown products—nitrite, and nitrate.[9]

When challenged, the immune system will draw on the normal processes of the body to create a burst of inflammatory cytokines. The response will act locally and will also go further. In a hormone-like manner, these molecules will recruit smooth muscles, glands, nerves, platelets, and other tissues.

Collectively the agents involved are called autacoids. They are associated with regulatory messengers called eicosanoids, neurotransmitters such as epinephrine, neurotransmission, neuroendocrine regulation, neurophysiology, vasoconstriction and vasodilation, peptides, and a whole network of chemical responses.[7]

Nitric oxide plays a role in most stages of inflammation development.[8]

Oxygen and Blood

There is an interplay between oxygen (O_2) and nitric oxide (NO). Nitric oxide inhibits the uptake of oxygen (O_2) in mitochondria. This forces oxygen to be diffused and distributed into the tissues of the body. So, in a healthy system, nitric oxide will help extend the zone of adequate cellular oxygenation away from a blood vessel.[10]

~

If oxygen is to reach all parts of the body, it needs hemoglobin to carry it via the bloodstream.

Hemoglobin, a protein molecule in red blood cells, is made up of chains called globulins. In fetuses and children, the chains are known as alpha (α) and gamma (γ) chains. By adulthood, the γ chain is replaced by a beta (β) chain. Each chain contains an iron atom embedded inside a substance that attracts protons to make a compound called porphyrin. The entire compound, the porphyrin and the iron, is called heme. The heme and the globin, together called hemoglobin, is responsible for transporting oxygen from the lungs to the tissues of the body and carrying carbon dioxide back through the system. As well as the lack of a nucleus, the hemoglobin also helps maintain the characteristic, almost donut shape of red blood cells.

Blood flow and tissue oxygenation

The classical view of oxygen delivery to tissues focused on the oxygen content transported by the hemoglobin in red blood cells. Changes in local blood flow (known as tissue perfusion) regulate the respiratory cycle. These changes are coupled with metabolic demand. A runner, for example, demands more oxygen than a sedentary person. The physiological response is called "blood flow autoregulation." How that worked was unknown.[11]

Research in 2015 showed that three amino acids are conserved in hemoglobin by both mammals and birds.[11] Only two are required to carry oxygen. The third, called βCys93, has the role of carrying nitric oxide.

In a challenge to the orthodox view, the research[11] showed that the entire respiratory cycle of blood flow and tissue oxygenation requires the third amino acid to carry nitric oxide. The researchers showed that respiration is a "three in one" system encompassing nitric oxide, oxygen, and carbon dioxide rather than a simple two-step process. βCys93 becomes critical as the transporter of nitric oxide.

Without βCys93, mortality increases as the cells of the heart struggle for oxygen, impacting its muscle contraction, blood vessels fail to dilate, and the normal flow of blood is impaired. When blood does not flow properly, the tissues of the body are starved of oxygen, creating the conditions of ischemia and hypoxia.

A broad base of research has shown that astrocytes wrap their extensions around both neurons and blood vessels to allow the transport of oxygen and glucose to the neurons.[12] If blood flow is impeded by the lack of βCys93, it is not inconceivable that the nourishment of neurons is compromised.

Neurons and astrocytes are both involved in neurotransmitter production.[13] The primary excitatory neurotransmitter, glutamate, starts its synthesis in astrocytes. They pass it, as glycine, to the neurons which complete the conversion. The glycine is made from glucose and is supplied through the blood flow.

As well as driving excitatory neurotransmission, the glutamate also is the feedstock for the primary inhibitory neurotransmitter, GABA. If the blood flow is compromised, the astrocytes will struggle, not only to supply oxygen and glucose to neurons, but also to modulate the availability and activity of the dominant neurotransmitters.

Superoxide

Superoxide, like nitric oxide, fulfills some functions in cells.[9] It forms when an oxygen molecule (O_2) loses an electron to become a negatively charged free radical. Due to its negative charge, it does not move easily through membranes and remains in the locality of its formation. As a free radical, it is not particularly potent but it does react with metals such as iron and copper to produce very reactive oxidants. The destructive hydroxyl radicals which damage macromolecules, lipids, carbohydrates, amino acids, and nucleic acids are formed when this reaction with metals occurs.[14]

Oxygen is a critical molecule in the electron transport chain. It is essential as the final acceptor of electrons in the process that allows us to make the energy molecule ATP. The negatively charged oxygen then combines with two hydrogen ions to make water.

If oxygen is not perfused into the tissue, it may struggle to do its job. It may either be absent or replaced with the superoxide radical. The hydrogen ions will build up in the cell, decreasing the pH level, and creating an acidic environment. This impacts on ATP formation.

As superoxide is potentially so damaging, cells create enzymes called superoxide dismutases (SODs) to control its formation. A specific gene encodes each form. One form is found in the cytoplasm of the cell, and another is secreted outside the cell. The third, perhaps most significant form, exists in the mitochondria of the cell where ATP is created. It helps modulate the superoxide by-product in the electron transport chain. The series of steps in electron transport is fundamental to energy metabolism.[9]

An overabundance of superoxide in the mitochondria will cause lethal damage.[9] Uncontrolled superoxide production in the mitochondria breaks down the entire chain of energy formation. It interrupts the production of ATP. The consequence is enduring fatigue, or worse.

Peroxynitrite

Peroxynitrite is produced when nitric oxide reacts with superoxide. The ability of nitric oxide to diffuse through membranes is inherited by peroxynitrite, giving it the ability to influence surrounding cells. The pH of those cells affects peroxynitrite reactivity as well as its breakdown products in reactions with metals, carbon dioxide, and nitrogen radicals.[15]

The ratio of superoxide to nitric oxide determines the reactivity of peroxynitrite. A predominance of nitric oxide reduces oxidation caused by peroxynitrite.[16]

Peroxynitrite is most clearly an oxidant. When it reacts with major antioxidant stores such as cysteine and glutathione, it converts them to a disulfide form, increasing the measure of oxidative stress. The sulfur amino acid methionine, which is found in fish, meat and dairy products, can be converted by peroxynitrite into a disulfide, which can then be oxidized to formaldehyde. Alternately, the methionine disulfide can be fragmented into ethylene and dimethyl disulfide. Purine nucleotides, which are critical to DNA and RNA synthesis, can be oxidized by peroxynitrite. The amino acids, tyrosine and tryptophan, are each degraded by the loss of an electron to peroxynitrite.

The enzyme glyceraldehyde-3-phosphate dehydrogenase is critical to the pathway that breaks glucose into smaller components, and is necessary for the formation of ATP. The enzyme is easily degraded and inactivated by even low levels of peroxynitrite. When it fails, energy production is disrupted.[17]

In short, peroxynitrite is highly reactive and damaging.[16]

The oxidation products of peroxynitrite also stimulate the transcription factor NFκB. This allows it to enter the nucleus of the cell and bind to DNA. Peroxynitrite's influence also stimulates another transcription factor, called AP-1.[9] While not specific to MS, there is evidence that the AP-1 complex plays a vital role in how cells proliferate and differentiate, with implications for disease management.

When people talk about inflammation in MS, molecules called reactive oxygen species or reactive nitrogen species, which include the overproduction of nitric oxide, superoxide, and peroxynitrite, are really at the heart of what they mean. They are all normal elements of a healthy system but their production should not be disorderly.

References

1.   Turvey, S.E. and D.H. Broide, *Innate immunity.* The Journal of Allergy and Clinical Immunology, 2010. **125**(2 Suppl 2): p. S24–S32.

2.   Foell, D., H. Wittkowski and J. Roth, *Mechanisms of disease: a 'DAMP' view of inflammatory arthritis.* Nature Clinical Practice Rheumatology, 2007. **3**: p. 382.

3.   Gilmore, T.D. *NF-kB Transcription Factors.* Available from: http://www.bu.edu/nf-kb/. Accessed March 2021.

4.   Zenewicz, L.A., *Oxygen levels and immunological studies.* Frontiers in Immunology, 2017. **8**: p. 324–324.

5.   Mason, P., *Medical Neurobiology (Second Edition).* 2017, Oxford University Press: New York.

6.   Carreau, A., B.E. Hafny-Rahbi, A. Matejuk, C. Grillon and C. Kieda, *Why is the partial oxygen pressure of human tissues a crucial parameter? Small molecules and hypoxia.* Journal of Cellular and Molecular Medicine, 2011. **15**(6): p. 1239–1253.

7.   *Journal of Autacoids and Hormones.* Available from: https://www.omicsonline.org/autacoids-and-hormones.php. Accessed March 2021.

8.   Guzik, T.J., R. Korbut and T. Adamek-Guzik, *Nitric oxide and superoxide in inflammation and immune regulation.* Journal of Physiology and Pharmacology, 2003. **54**(4): p. 469–87.

9.   Pall, M.L., *Explaining '"Unexplained Illnesses" : Disease Paradigm for Chronic Fatigue Syndrome, Multiple Chemical Sensitivity, Fibromyalgia, Post-traumatic Stress Disorder, Gulf War Syndrome, and Others.* 2007, Harrington Park Press: Binghamton, NY.

10.   Boveris, A., M. Carreras and J. Jose Poderoso, *The Regulation of Cell Energetics and Mitochondrial Signaling by Nitric Oxide*, in *Nitric Oxide Biology and Pathobiology (Second Edition).* L.J. Ignarro Editor. 2010. Academic Press: San Diego. pp. 441-482.

11.   Zhang, R., D.T. Hess, Z. Qian, A. Hausladen, F. Fonseca, R. Chaube, J.D. Reynolds and J.S. Stamler, *Hemoglobin βCys93 is essential for cardiovascular function and integrated response to hypoxia.* Proceedings of the National Academy of Sciences U.S.A, 2015. **112**(20): p. 6425–6430.

12.   Hertz, L. and H. Zielke, *Astrocytic control of glutamatergic activity:*

Astrocytes as stars of the show. Trends in Neurosciences, 2004. **27**(12): p. 735–743.

13.   A. Scousboe, L.K. Bak and H.S. Waagepetersen, *Astrocytic control of biosynthesi and turnover of the neurotransmitters glutamate and GABA* Frontiers in Endocrinology, 2013. **4**: p. 102.

14.   Hines, I.N. and M.B. Grisham, *Reactive Metabolites of Oxygen and Nitrogen in Liver Ischemia and Reperfusion Injury*, in *Nitric Oxide Biology and Pathobiology (Second Edition)*, L.J. Ignarro, Editor. 2010, Academic Press: San Diego. pp. 773-794.

15.   Szabó, C., H. Ischiropoulos and R. Radi, *Peroxynitrite: Biochemistry, pathophysiology and development of therapeutics.* Nature Reviews Drug Discovery, 2007. **6**: p. 662.

16.   Szabó, C., *Multiple pathways of peroxynitrite cytotoxicity.* Toxicology Letters, 2003. **140–141**: p. 105–112.

17.   Buchczyk, D.P., T. Grune, H. Sies and L-O. Klotz, *Modifications of glyceraldehyde-3-phosphate dehydrogenase induced by increasing concentrations of peroxynitrite: Early recognition by 20S proteasome.* Biological Chemistry, 2003. **384**(2): p. 237–241.

18.   Angel, P. and M. Karin, *The role of Jun, Fos and the AP-1 complex in cell-proliferation and transformation.* Biochimica et Biophysica Acta, 1991. **1072**(2): p. 129–157.

Note 14

ATP and Cellular Respiration

ATP—the Source of Energy

Baron Justus Freiherr von Liebig was a German scientist in the 1840s. He wanted to know what substances were combined in animal muscle. It was generally accepted that flesh was made up of solid fiber, cells, and membranes in an organized structure. Fat was regarded as separate from this. The large amount of liquid in fresh meat was known as "the juice of the flesh".

Liebig minced 10 pounds of freshly killed flesh, added water, and squeezed as much liquid from the mixture through a linen bag as he could. He deduced that the liquid had an acid character, but that didn't tell him if it was one or more acid substances. His next step was to use a technique called distillation, which separated the components of the liquid into layers.

His first finding was that the liquid was rich in phosphates and he concluded that phosphoric acid was an essential component of the juice of muscle. He used a technique called precipitation to separate the phosphates from the rest of the liquid. Then he evaporated what was left. The residue that remained appeared as colorless needles on the bottom of the flask. This substance had already been discovered and was known as "Kreatine".

Liebig looked again at the liquid. This time he added alcohol to it and by filtration found another substance which he called inosinic acid.

A note on this discovery in Chambers Journal of Edinburgh of 1847 described the acid.

"This is a very remarkable element. The flavor of meat seems to reside in it: when it is acted on by a high heat, it gives off the very smell of roasting meat."[1]

Liebig was a prodigious contributor to agriculture and biological chemistry. He is considered to be the "father of the fertilizer industry", but you are probably more familiar with the result of his inosinic acid discovery. A company was established to exploit his process. Originally called the *Liebig Extract of Meat Company*, it introduced the Oxo brand of beef bouillon cubes to household kitchens.

~

In 1929, the German scientist, Karl Lohmann,[2] isolated a substance from muscle and liver cells, which he also called inosinic acid.[3] This compound is very close in structure to adenosine triphosphate and is a breakdown product that was formed as ATP went through Lohmann's isolation process.

~

When the nucleobase adenine reacts with the sugar called ribose, it becomes adenosine. The ribose acts like glue, holding the adenosine together with phosphate molecules. When three phosphates form a tail on this molecule, it is known as adenosine triphosphate or ATP.

Magnesium is almost always in a complex with the phosphate groups of ATP.[4] The magnesium ion partially diminishes the negative electrochemical charge of ATP. It helps ATP move around the cell and attracts it to structures that need energy to function.[5]

~

In 1941, a German-born scientist, Fritz Albert Lipmann,[6] wrote a seminal paper, "*The metabolic generation and utilization of phosphate bond energy*".[7]

In it, he introduced a new term that started with a squiggle (~P). He referred to energy-rich phosphate as the driving force behind many biological processes. These include the contraction of muscles and the transport of ions and other molecules across membranes. Other processes that involve phosphate include the chemical reactions for the biosynthesis of proteins, nucleic acids, and other large molecules.

~

Lipmann had already moved to the United States in the early 1930s. His paper stamped his ability, and he found a senior position in the laboratory of the Department of Surgery at the Massachusetts General Hospital in

Boston. There Lipmann discovered a vital molecule that linked several steps in protein synthesis. He called this "co-enzyme A" (CoA). The "A" stood for the activation of acetate.

This work on CoA led to a Nobel prize in 1953.[8] Lipmann shared the award with another giant of research, Hans Kreb,[9] who had established the existence of a cycle in metabolic respiration called the citric acid cycle.

Soon after, Lipmann turned his attention back to phosphate. By 1955 he was writing papers that described how cleaving a phosphate molecule from adenosine triphosphate drove reactions that occurred all through the metabolism.

Inosinic acid discovered by Lohmann had led the way to the discovery of ATP. The phosphate tail on this molecule contained the trigger for energy in metabolism.[10] If ATP donates a phosphate molecule to another molecule, the process is called phosphorylation. Sometimes, the receiving molecule is augmented and changed by this transfer. In other reactions the phosphate is used and then discarded.

ATPase—Breaking Down ATP

In 1953, an Austrian born biochemist, Efraim Racker,[11] working with others in the Public Health Research Institute in New York, demonstrated that the process of breaking down glucose (glycolysis) depended on a type of enzyme called an ATPase to break down ATP.

An ATPase[12] is a molecule that is sufficiently positively charged to remove a negatively charged oxygen ion from a phosphate attached to ATP. This action allows a new oxygen atom from water (or another donor) to bind to the now exposed phosphate molecule. The displaced oxygen from the phosphate molecule, now faces another negatively charged oxygen bound to the next phosphate. The two negatives repel each other, and the phosphate molecule disassociates from the phosphate tail. ATP becomes ADP plus a phosphate.

Racker noted that the phosphate molecule lost by ATP to make adenosine diphosphate could be restored to create a three-phosphate bond again. This step allows a sustainable cycle to be established.

The ATPase enzymes that catalyze the removal of a phosphate from ATP are found in the membranes of cells. They harness the ATP/ADP transformation to modify their structure. The process allows them to act as mediums of exchange for charged ions moving from one side of a membrane to another. Sometimes, these proteins act as a pump, and sometimes they just allow a movement of ions.

If ATP is totally depleted and the phosphate tail is lost entirely, if it degrades to a purine ring, it is washed from the cell, forever lost. When this happens in a concentrated burst, that degradation creates a metabolic disaster. When oxygen is missing, ischemic or hypoxic conditions develop, and this disaster is precisely what happens.[4]

In MS, there are signs that oxygen metabolism is awry.

~

Racker became fascinated by how ATP was synthesized. Although he did not discover the mechanism, he was able to prove the theory that ATP formation requires the transfer of protons across a membrane. The metabolic unit that permits the synthase of ATP uses the protons like they are water on a waterwheel to rotate a molecular machine to bind ADP to a phosphate.

Phosphate

If phosphate breaking apart from ATP releases metabolic energy, what is the source of the phosphate? Apart from some coming directly from our diet, our most sustainable source is from our bones. We cannot, however, just rip phosphate from bone whenever we instantly need it.

In 1832 a brilliant French scientist, Michel Eugene Chevreul[13] isolated creatine[12] in skeletal muscle. He had named the crystallized substance after the Greek word for meat, "Kreas".

It took until the 1920s before scientists realized that the creatine from ingested meat was stored in human muscle rather than being excreted. Researchers from both sides of the Atlantic, late in that decade, simultaneously reported that creatine had a phosphate attached to it and could better be described as phosphocreatine.[14]

In 1927, two scientists published an article, *The nature of the inorganic phosphate in voluntary muscle*.[14] They showed that phosphate decreases during muscle contraction and is restored during recovery. Therefore, it was known that phosphate played a role in muscle activity, but how it was replenished was unknown.

In time, it was understood that phosphocreatine donates a phosphate molecule to adenosine diphosphate (ADP) to restore the three-phosphate structure of ATP. When the phosphate disassociates from ATP, the phosphocreatine holds the phosphate in its structure.

This ability of creatine to act as a sink to store phosphate is probably the end of the trail in terms of impacting on the development of multiple sclerosis. Supplementing with creatine won't change the path of the disease. However, the phosphate is where the metabolic impact lies. It is the cleaving of phosphate from ATP that drives energetic action.

Phosphocreatine is like a bank account of phosphate. ATP and ADP shuttle through metabolic actions, either releasing energy when phosphate is released or replenishing energy when ATP is restored.

What triggers that exchange?

Creatine kinase—the enzyme behind phosphate storage

In 1934, Lohmann discovered a new enzyme, now known as creatine kinase.[12] In 1936, another scientist, Lehmann,[16] noted that each phosphate transfer involved this enzyme. In time, it became clear that different forms of this enzyme exist in various tissues. In muscle, it was denoted as MM-CK and in the brain as BB-CK. Later, creatine kinase was discovered inside the mitochondria of the cell (denoted as MtCK). The forms found in the mitochondria are different from the types in the cytosol of the cell. The variety found in muscles has residues of the amino acid lysine, but the form found in the brain does not.

The mitochondrial forms react three or four times more slowly than those found in the cytosol.

Phosphate is stored as a phosphoryl group

A phosphoryl group is transferred from ATP during its conversion to ADP. This group is sometimes called a "high energy phosphate". This phosphoryl group is stored attached to creatine.

The process is easily reversed.[17] The intermediate step involves an oxygen molecule.[18] Oxygen is important, as its radical forms, such as peroxynitrite, treat creatine kinase as a priority target.[19]

Peroxynitrite will inactivate creatine kinase. The result is that the phosphate stored as a phosphoryl group cannot be utilized.[20] If it is not available, you can't spend energy.

An analogy for the transfer of the phosphoryl group to ADP

Imagine there are two cats in a room, a black cat sleeping on a cushion, and a white cat sitting nearby.

In the morning, the black cat wakes. He stretches and moves off the cushion. As he does that, the white cat leaps onto the cushion and takes the comfy space.

In the afternoon, the black cat, fed up with just sitting, jumps on the white cat and pushes him off the cushion. The white cat goes somewhere else in the room and sits, waiting for the black cat to vacate the cushion.

This is what happens when phosphate is moved to and from creatine, converting ATP to ADP and back again. Peroxynitrite, a potent free radical, is a third, more unfriendly cat that interferes and displaces the other cats. It upsets the exchange. They cannot continue their routine.

What about non-meat eaters?

Creatine is mainly delivered to the body by eating muscle meat. Organ meat has very little creatine. The three amino acids that make up creatine are glycine, arginine, and methionine.[15] Without creatine, phosphate cannot be stored in our muscles.

Vegetarians will struggle to make energy if they do not have a raw plant diet rich in these amino acids. A non-meat eater must use the amino acids from plants to manufacture creatine through their kidney and liver.

The Krebs Cycle

Sir Hans Kreb, a refugee from pre-war Germany who settled in the UK, was already a noted scientist by 1933. He had, with others, previously identified the urea cycle, which allows highly toxic ammonia to be excreted from the body.

At the University of Sheffield, he ran a series of experiments aimed at establishing how oxygen consumption helped produce energy from the breakdown of glucose. To do this, he needed to discover several crucial enzymes. As new challenges to his theory developed, he worked out how to integrate them into the cycle, making his ideas more robust.

For his work, he was awarded the 1953 Nobel prize.

What happens in the Krebs cycle?

The Krebs cycle is integral to the method by which the body breaks down glucose. Glucose consists of six carbon, twelve hydrogen, and six oxygen atoms. Through glycolysis, it is split into two three-carbon molecules called pyruvate. As it prepares to enter the citric acid cycle, the pyruvate loses a carbon to become acetyl-CoA. The lost carbons bind with oxygen to become carbon dioxide, which is exhaled. The remaining carbons, at different stages, are also lost as carbon dioxide.

The Krebs cycle does not directly have oxygen added to it. Some oxygen can be utilized from water but that is not part of the respiration cycle that uses oxygen and produces ATP. Instead, the oxygen and carbon from glucose are consumed to become CO_2, and the twelve hydrogen atoms transfer to two specialized types of electron carriers.

One carrier is called NAD (nicotinamide adenine dinucleotide), an active form of niacin (vitamin B3). It becomes NADH when a hydrogen atom is attached. In this way, five hydrogen atoms per Krebs cycle leave as NADH.

The other carrier is FAD (flavin adenine dinucleotide), an active form of riboflavin (vitamin B2). It becomes FADH2 when hydrogen atoms are attached. It transports one hydrogen atom per Krebs cycle.

There are two turns of the Krebs cycle for each glucose molecule.

All the oxygen and carbon atoms from a glucose molecule are reconfigured and washed from cellular respiration as carbon dioxide or are bound up by water. All of the twelve hydrogen atoms progress to the final step.

The Electron Transport Chain, and Rebuilding ATP

The final phase of cellular respiration is called the electron transport chain. Each hydrogen atom enters the chain, bound up in FADH2 or NADH, as units made up of one proton and one electron. In a series of steps, enzymes known as complexes, split the hydrogen electron from its atom and direct the resulting proton into the space between the inner and outer membrane of the mitochondria. Inside the mitochondria, the electron is passed between the electron transport complexes by a series of molecules that can both accept and donate electrons. The most significant transporter is known as Co-enzyme Q. It can take two electrons at a time yet still move them on one at a time. Its role is to regulate the flow of electrons. Consequently, it is essential.

As this process continues, a large quantity of protons builds up in the space between the mitochondrial membranes. Each complex is a one-way street that does not allow the proton and electron to reunite. The electrons continue to be passed along the chain of complexes. As they pass from the fourth complex, they are reunited with oxygen. The fifth complex is a unique structure known as ATP synthase. It is only by passing through this that the hydrogen ions can rejoin their electrons. The oxygen and the hydrogen that passes through the ATP synthase combine to make water. If oxygen is not present, not only will the electron transport chain fail but NADH and FADH2 will be unable to be converted back into NAD and FAD and the Krebs cycle will shut down.

ATP synthase

The structure of ATP synthase is comparable to a machine. It is a complex that spans the inner membrane of the mitochondria providing an access point for the hydrogen protons to re-enter its central part, called the matrix. The complex that allows the protons to re-enter is bound to an axle or spindle so it can rotate. The action of the protons pouring back into the matrix creates something very like the movement of a water wheel in a river. The paddle spins.

The lower portion of ATP synthase is fixed. Its charge attracts ADP and phosphate molecules to bind to it. As the upper portion spins, driven by protons pouring through it, it distorts the lower portion, making it flex.

This action pushes the ADP and phosphate toward each other until they bind as ATP and dislodge from the complex.

As the protons pour back into the matrix of the mitochondria, they pick up the electrons to become complete hydrogen atoms. The oxygen and hydrogen then combine to become water, completing the steps of cellular respiration.

If oxygen is insufficient at this point, water will not be formed. The electron delivery will fail, and hydrogen ions will build up inside the mitochondria, creating a more acidic environment. The chain of delivery of electrons will back up in the earlier complexes. ATP synthase will fail.

How does ATP get out of the mitochondria and ADP get in?

Until 2019, the assumption was that on the membrane of the mitochondria, a complex consisting of two proteins, allowed an almost constant supply of ADP from the cytoplasm of the cell. It was known as ATP/ADP translocase.

In the journal, *Cell*, researchers led by the Mitochondrial Biology Unit at Cambridge University, showed this transport was, in fact, a structure that rotated around a fulcrum. It opened, either to the cytoplasm or the matrix of the mitochondria.[21] A salt bridge network at its center acted like an electrostatic gate where ATP and ADP molecules would dock. The gate would alternately swing to allow passage in or out of the mitochondria.

The researchers highlighted that this transporter would allow the recycling of each ATP molecule at least 1,000 times per day. The weight of the ADP and ATP molecules passing through all the transporters each day would roughly equal our own body weight.

~

The final products of cellular respiration are carbon dioxide, water, and ATP that has been reconstituted by the action of the final step in the electron transport chain, ATP synthase. NAD and FAD gather hydrogen atoms from the Krebs cycle for delivery to the electron transport chain. Splitting those atoms into ions and electrons and then recombining them is the function of the electron transport chain complexes.

The process will yield 38 ATP from one molecule of glucose. Some are consumed to start the process of glycolysis, so the net gain is 34–36 ATP molecules.

Fatty acids go through a different process called β-oxidation, which is much more high yielding for an equivalent number of carbon atoms. You get three Acetyl-CoA molecules from six carbons provided by fatty acids, compared to two Acetyl-CoA molecules from six carbons supplied by glucose. Additionally, fatty acids have many more carbon atoms in their structure.[22]

Despite all this activity, there is very little ATP stored. In a 250 g human heart, for example, there would be about 0.7 g of ATP at any one time. There is an absolute need to keep replenishing the ATP pool. A human heart beats 10,000 times a day. The amount of stored ATP in a heart is about enough for ten beats. The weight of ATP our heart would use is about 6,000 g a day.[4]

We need to be able to synthesize ATP on-demand rapidly. The supply always needs to meet the demand. The level of ATP should stay constant. Its concentration can't ebb and flow. The use and manufacture of ATP happen in parallel. There is not a sequence of rises and falls.[4]

All the steps of cellular respiration need to work perfectly. If they don't, you have no energy to draw on. You are fatigued, endlessly exhausted. Many systems in your body will fail.

References

1. Chambers, W. and R. Chambers, *Chambers' Edinburgh Journal, Vol V11 Jan-June 1847*. W.S. Orr: London. p. 294.

2. NNDB. *Biograpical notes on Karl Lohmann*. 2019; Available from: https://www.nndb.com/people/075/000249325/.

3. PubChem Database. Inosinic acid. Available from https://pubchem.ncbi.nlm.nih.gov/compound/Inosinic-acid. Accessed March 2021.

4. Ingwall, J.S., *ATP and the Heart*, 2002. Springer US: Boston, MA.

5. Sinatra, S., *The Sinatra Solution: Metabolic Cardiology*, 2011. Basic Health Publications: Laguna Beach, C.A.

6. *Fritz Lipmann – Biographical. NobelPrize.org.*; Available from https://www.nobelprize.org/prizes/medicine/1953/lipmann/biographical/. Accessed March 2021.

7. Lipmann, F., *Metabolic Generation and Utilization of Phosphate Bond Energy*, in *Advances in Enzymology and Related Areas of Molecular Biology*. F.F. Nord and C.H. Werkman Editors. 1969. John Wiley & Sons: New York.

8. *The Nobel Prize in Physiology or Medicine 1953*. Available from: https://www.nobelprize.org/prizes/medicine/1953/summary/. Accessed March 2021.

9. *Hans Krebs – Nobel Lecture.*; Available from: https://www.nobelprize.org/prizes/medicine/1953/krebs/lecture/. Accessed March 2021.

10. Jenks, W.P. and R. V. Wolfenden, *Fritz Albert Lipmann*. Biographical Memoirs: Volume 88. Available from: https://www.nap.edu/read/11807/chapter/14#248. Accessed March 2021.

11. *Efraim Racker, Scientist and Artist | June 28, 1913 - September 9, 1991*. Available from: https://efraimracker.library.cornell.edu/about/timeline. Accessed March 2021.

12. Hine, R. and E. Martin, *Dictionary of Biology*. 2015. Oxford University Press: Oxford, UK.

13. Lemay, P., *Michel Eugene Chevreul (1786-1889)*. Journal of Chemical Education, 1948. **25**(2): p. 62.

14. Fiske, C.H. and Y. Subbarow, *The Nature of the "Inorganic Phosphate" in Voluntary Muscle*. Science, 1927. **65**(1686): p. 401–403.

15.   Brosnan, J., R. da Silva and M. Brosnan, *The metabolic burden of creatine synthesis.* The Forum for Amino Acid, Peptide and Protein Research, 2011. **40**(5): p. 1325–1331.

16.   Lehmann, H. and L. Pollak, *The effect of amino-acids on phosphate transfer in muscle extract.* The Biochemical Journal, 1942. **36**(7–9): p. 672–685.

17.   McLeish, M.J. and G.L. Kenyon, *Relating structure to mechanism in creatine kinase.* Critical Reviews in Biochemistry and Molecular Biology, 2005, **40**(1): p. 1–20.

18.   Carusi, E.A., *It's time we replaced 'high-energy phosphate group' with 'phosphoryl group'.* Biochemical Education, 1992. **20**(3): p. 145–147.

19.   Mekhfi, H., V. Veksler, P. Mateo, V. Maupoil, L. Rochette and R. Ventura-Clapier, *Creatine kinase is the main target of reactive oxygen species in cardiac myofibrils.* Circulation Research, 1996. **78**(6): p. 1016–1027.

20.   Konorev, E.A., N. Hogg and B. Kalyanaraman, *Rapid and irreversible inhibition of creatine kinase by peroxynitrite.* FEBS Letters, 1998. **427**(2): p. 171–174.

21.   Ruprecht, J.J., M.S. King, T. Zögg, A.A. Aleksandrova, E. Pardon, P.G. Crichton, J. Steyaert and E.R.S. Kunji, *The molecular mechanism of transport by the mitochondrial ADP/ATP carrier.* Cell, 2019. **176**(3): p. 435–447.e15.

22.   Darvey, I.G., *What factors are responsible for the greater yield of ATP per carbon atom when fatty acids are completely oxidised to CO_2 and water compared with glucose?* Biochemical Education, 1999. **27**(4): p. 209–210.

Note 15

Cellular Respiration in Trouble

Hypoxia

In a conventional hypoxic (low oxygen) event, some stages are well understood.

Initially, the person becomes restless and agitated, the heart rate accelerates and breathing becomes labored. As hypoxia persists, the heart rate slows, and the person becomes far more restless. Breathing becomes very labored and eventually, the shortage of oxygen in the blood induces a bluish tinge to the skin of a troubled individual.

There are four well-understood types of hypoxia.[1] They don't, however, always follow the simple pattern described above.

1) **Stagnant hypoxia** (sometimes called ischemia) occurs when blood flow is low.

If blood flow is lowered due to an obstruction such as a plaque build-up, this is regarded as a local ischemic event.

An ischemic event can be either short term or long term. If it is short term (5–20 minutes), the body can train muscles and organs (such as the heart muscle) to withstand oxygen deprivation without significant inflammatory responses. The contractile function of the heart is impaired, but the cells adapt. In the heart, this process of adaption is sometimes called cardiac stunning.[2]

The body's response to longer-term ischemia is to release a burst of oxygen products called reactive oxygen species. These are free radicals.

In longer-term ischemia the production of hydrogen ions falls, so an exchanger called the sodium/hydrogen exchanger opens to push up the hydrogen levels. This increase makes the cells more acidic. Additionally, a protein called the mitochondrial transition pore opens to allow calcium to overload the cell. This prompts muscle contraction.

Heart muscles are conditioned to not overreact to oxygen deprivation, but not all organs are affected the same way. Often organs that are distant from the site of ischemia can be affected depending on what inflammatory markers are released into the blood.[2]

As stagnant hypoxia lowers ATP production by depriving the cells of oxygen, the muscles, particularly the heart, can switch to using carbohydrates as an energy source. This salvage mechanism usually is only seen in newborn children. Switching to this pathway is like putting the muscle into hibernation.

Stagnant hypoxia impacts ATP formation and boosts the production of reactive oxygen species. The result can be membrane and muscle damage. It causes calcium overloads, and sodium balances are affected. Pores open, trying to rescue the cell, but this can end up having the opposite effect.

The brain is particularly sensitive to oxygen deprivation. It uses 20–25% of the total body oxygen consumption. The brain doesn't have as much storage of antioxidants (such as superoxide dismutase, catalase, glutathione peroxidase, and heme oxygenase-1) as the organs of the body. It also has higher levels of polyunsaturated fats that are sensitive to being oxidized. Some neurotransmitters can be overexpressed by ischemia resulting in incorrect signaling and toxicity.[2]

2) **Hypoxic hypoxia** arises when the oxygen pressure in the blood is low. It is typically associated with breathing issues such as ventilation problems or pulmonary edema. The body's response is to open the capillaries to increase their surface area and allow greater oxygen perfusion into the tissue. As the oxygen level in the arteries is low, it will trigger the chemoreceptors in the carotid arteries to alter breathing regulation.

3) **Anemic hypoxia** occurs when blood has a reduced number of binding sites for oxygen. In response, the capillaries widen to improve oxygen delivery. This dilation will speed up blood flow to ensure the amount of oxygen reaching cells is maintained. The chemoreceptors in the carotid arteries will not be triggered to change the rate of breathing.

4) **Histotoxic hypoxia** happens when there is a change in the production of ATP caused by a defect in the cellular use of oxygen. Usually, this occurs in a profound poisoning situation.

As an example, if cyanide is introduced, it blocks an enzyme called cytochrome C oxidase. This enzyme takes the electrons in the last step of the electron transport chain and transfers them to oxygen (O_2). This step is fundamental to the reorganizing of the protons, electrons, and oxygen back into water. If this enzyme is absent, the ATP synthase step does not work. As the oxygen is no longer utilized, it stays at a higher concentration in the blood on the return journey to the heart.

~

Histotoxic hypoxia seems to have at least one parallel in the metabolism of MS patients (see below).

Stagnant hypoxia also presents useful examples of what happens to ATP itself when the oxygen supply falls.

Used blood from MS patients has higher than normal oxygen levels

A study in 2012 looked at thirty remitting-relapsing MS patients and compared them to the same number of controls. The study measured the level of blood oxygenation in the superior sagittal sinus, which funnels used blood back from cerebral sinuses to the circulatory system. The study found that the used blood of MS patients had significantly higher levels of oxygenation than the controls.[3]

By comparing the oxygen levels of arterial blood and venous blood, the study noted that lower rates of oxygen utilization strongly correlated with both EDSS measures of disability, and lesion loads. The study postulated that higher levels of nitric oxide might be outcompeting cytochrome C oxidase for oxygen and disrupting ATP synthase. However, they did not consider peroxynitrite and did not look at whether there was sufficient βCys93 to carry nitric oxide in the hemoglobin for tissue perfusion.

However, the study showed clear evidence that oxygen utilization is impaired in MS patients compared to controls.

In 2002, a professor of medicine from the Harvard Medical School, Joanne S. Ingwall, wrote an in-depth study on the biochemistry of ATP. Her focus was on heart cells, as they contain the highest concentration of mitochondria and have the greatest appetite for ATP in the human body.

While her book, *ATP and the Heart*,[4] is primarily focused on heart cells, it provides an insight into how ischemia (stagnant hypoxia) degrades ATP to simpler purines. These break down products can be lost to the cell. As the heart is just a muscle, any other muscle should have a similar profile when oxygen does not reach the mitochondria of its cells.

Ingwall saw healthy metabolic activity as a series of coupled reactions:

For ATP to be utilized, it must first react with water and then become ADP plus a phosphate and a hydrogen ion.

For ATP to be resupplied, oxygen from water must take phosphate from a phosphoryl group in a muscle's creatine store and combine it with ADP and a hydrogen ion.

In straightforward terms:

1) The body's ability to make and/or use ATP on demand depends on the availability of ADP and the availability of phosphate.

2) Even if you have adequate levels of ATP, the ADP still needs to be immediately available, and phosphate needs to be stored but available to immediately restore any ATP you use.

~

Ingwall was focusing on the viability of heart cells, called myocytes. She looked at what happened to these reactions in an ischemic environment, such as if a plaque or other event created stagnant hypoxia.

As Ingwall lowered the oxygenated arterial blood flow, the result was a rapid degrading of ATP into a spiral of purine breakdown. This degradation happened despite ischemia triggering the capillaries to widen and arteries pushing more oxygen into surrounding tissues.

~

The mitochondria are the engine rooms where most ATP is assembled. However, the degradation of ATP mainly happens outside these powerhouses, in the cytosol of the cell.[5]

If ATP is spent in the cytosol, but the lack of oxygen in the mitochondria means new ATP is not formed, a salvage mechanism kicks in.

424

Two ADP molecules will combine in the cytosol, to make one ATP and one AMP (adenosine monophosphate). This process repeats until it reaches a point of functional depletion. The enzyme adenylate kinase drives the reaction, but it is slow.

While this particular enzyme helps speed up the process during oxygen depletion, the creatine kinase that can release phosphate from phosphoryl groups in muscles becomes less active. It needs oxygen to complete its operation.

Over time, as less oxygen for the final step in the electron chain is available, the ATP concentration declines, and ADP and AMP levels increase. ATP resynthesis can keep going but at a significantly reduced rate.

If the cell has not become too acidic, the enzyme 5'-AMP-specific nucleotidase will be stimulated by AMP and start to help rebuild ATP. If that enzyme is blocked because the cell has become too acidic, then AMP continues to breakdown. Firstly, to adenosine and a phosphate. The adenosine then is washed from the cell, degrading to form inosine, then hypoxanthine, and xanthine.[6] The adenosine levels in the cell become depleted.

To rebuild ATP from scratch means a molecule-by-molecule reconstruction of the ribose ring and the binding of that to nitrogenous molecules from amino acids. Ingwall estimated that it would take more than 100 days to rebuild the ATP pool in a human heart. It would take even longer if the calculation allowed for ATP being utilized.[4]

The lack of oxygen, particularly at the final step of cell respiration, is a metabolic disaster.

What should we make of that study in 2012 that showed high levels of unused oxygen in the veins of people with MS?

Deimination Revisited

In the chapter on myelin (Chapter 6), the concept of deimination was mentioned. This is the process by which the NOS family acts on the arginine and releases nitric oxide from it to form citrulline. In a typical setting, as both nitric oxide and citrulline derive from arginine, the formation of both should be correlated.

As discussed earlier, higher demyelination levels have a positive correlation with higher deimination.

Citrulline levels can be measured in serum samples. In healthy individuals, they should be reasonably stable.[7] A study in 2018 called "*Plasma citrulline levels are increased in patients with multiple sclerosis*" looked at the hypothesis that MS was associated with a release of citrulline.[8]

The trial found no concrete proof that whatever is happening in the brain could be correlated with the plasma citrulline levels. They did, however, consider that the elevation of plasma citrulline may be a marker of multiple sclerosis. The MS group in their sample was screened to be clinically stable (i.e., no recent attacks) rather than being subjects of an active attack. However, the researchers noted that elevation of citrulline and depletion levels of arginine were statistically significant.[8]

Martin Pall, in his book *Explaining Unexplained Illnesses*, notes that people with multisystem illnesses typically have low arginine levels and concludes that the excessive production of nitric oxide may cause much of the arginine depletion. His view was that high nitric oxide levels led to a cycle of high rates of deimination.[7]

The authors of the citrulline study noted that there is a large body of evidence that high levels of iNOS are found in MS patients. They could not explain the origin of the higher citrulline level in blood plasma and speculated that it came from elevated iNOS outside the central nervous system.[9]

Nitric oxide, itself, dissipates very rapidly[10] so it cannot be measured directly.

The researchers did not explore what was happening inside the leukocytes (white blood cells), but they implied that it was the next obvious area to explore.[8]

ADMA

Citrulline forms when a nitrogen atom, known as the guanidino nitrogen, is split from arginine and replaced by an oxygen atom. The whole reaction also creates nitric oxide, and what is left over is a water molecule.

An analog of arginine is a molecule called asymmetric dimethyl arginine (ADMA). It looks similar to arginine but has two methyl structures attached to one of its two nitrogen atoms. As this happens to only one nitrogen, the structure is asymmetrical.

An enzyme expressed by endothelial cells, called dimethylarginine dimethylamino hydrolase (DDAH), combines with a water molecule to turn ADMA into L-citrulline.

In a negative feedback loop, nitric oxide inhibits DDAH. That causes a rise in ADMA when the enzyme is blocked. In turn, ADMA can inhibit all forms of NOS. As a result, nitric oxide levels decline.[11]

So, L-citrulline forms from either arginine or ADMA. However, the latter inhibits nitric oxide. This topic is an area of intense interest in cardiovascular research as a lack of nitric oxide means that blood vessels cannot dilate, resulting in a limitation on the amounts of nitric oxide available to disperse oxygen into the tissue.

The L-arginine Paradox

When isolated arterial rings have L-arginine added to them in a laboratory setting, it does not cause vasodilation. However, when L-arginine is supplemented in a living model, even when plasma levels suggest there is already adequate L-arginine, there is an improvement in vasodilation. This observation was called the L-arginine paradox.

One research group suggested in 2004 that the addition of L-arginine displaced a competitive inhibitor of NOS, improving nitric oxide production. ADMA was the inhibiting factor.[11]

There are very few studies looking at ADMA as a marker in multiple sclerosis. A study in 2015 concluded that it might be associated with both multiple sclerosis and neuromyelitis optica.[12] There's a long way to go before any conclusions can be drawn.

Protein S-Nitrosylation

When sulfur binds to hydrogen, this is called a thiol group. You can smell thiols in garlic and onions, in rotten eggs, and in the additive to natural gas that gives it an odor.

The amino acid cysteine has a side chain that is a thiol. Cysteine is found in high protein foods. It is derived from the essential amino acid methionine, found in meats, fish, eggs, dairy products, and some plants.

When nitric oxide attaches to a thiol, a process called S-nitrosylation, an S-nitrosothiol group (SNO) forms. In the body, an SNO group is often the sign of a signaling molecule. As an example, the widening of blood vessels (i.e., vasodilation) depends on an SNO group.

Many illnesses correlate with either 'hyper' (overactive) or 'hypo' (underactive) S-nitrosylation.[13]

The amino acid βCys93 carries nitric oxide in hemoglobin using an SNO group. It signals the body to dilate the blood vessel and bring oxygen into hypoxic tissue, feeding the surrounding mass.

A common problem with blood stored by the blood banking industry is that its SNO becomes depleted; therefore, transfused blood is poor at increasing blood oxygenation.[13]

Local tissue will remain hypoxic if the blood flow into the area is insufficient and/or if βCys93 is depleted.

~

When nitric oxide reacts with the antioxidant glutathione, it makes an S-nitrosothiol called S-nitrosoglutathione (GSNO). In rat models of cerebral ischemia, researchers showed that GSNO treatment led to an improvement in anti-inflammatory effects.[14]

Researchers have also concluded that the adhesion molecules found in EAE models are modulated by the S-nitrosylation of a transcription factor called P-65. In turn, this leads to the inactivation of the transcription factor NFκB.[14] If this occurs, the production of iNOS is lowered as NFκB cannot enter the nucleus of the cell to stimulate the iNOS gene.

~

Nitric oxide's role in human health is a recent discovery.[15] The 1998 Nobel prize for Medicine or Physiology was awarded to the scientists who identified its role in blood circulation. Tens of thousands of papers have now been written to include some reference to it. The focus of these has mainly been the circulatory system, while MS remains a side issue.

There are plenty of questions in this research area, but at the moment, there are not many answers!

References

1.   Pittman, R., *Oxygen Transport in Normal and Pathological Situations: Defects and Compensations.* In *Regulation of Tissue Oxygenation.* 2011. Morgan & Claypool Life Sciences: San Rafael (CA).

2.   Kalogeris, T., C.P. Baines, M. Krenz and R.J. Korthuis, *Cell biology of ischemia/reperfusion injury.* International Review of Cell and Molecular Biology, 2012. **298**: p. 229–317.

3.   Ge, Y., Z. Zhang, H. Lu, L. Tang, H. Jaggi, J. Herbert, J.S. Babb, H. Rusinek and R.I. Grossman, *Characterizing brain oxygen metabolism in patients with multiple sclerosis with T2-relaxation-under-spin-tagging MRI.* Journal of Cerebral Blood Flow and Metabolism, 2012. **32**(3): p. 403–412.

4.   Ingwall, J.S., *ATP and the Heart,* 2002. Springer US: Boston, MA.

5.   Sandhu, G.S. and G.K. Asimakis, *Mechanism of loss of adenine nucleotides from mitochondria during myocardial ischemia.* Journal of Molecular and Cell Cardiology, 1991. 23(12): p. 1423-35.

6.   Bak, M.I. and J.S. Ingwall, *Regulation of cardiac AMP-specific 5′-nucleotidase during ischemia mediates ATP resynthesis on reflow.* American Journal of Physiology-Cell Physiology, 1998. **274**(4): p. C992–C1001.

7.   Pall, M.L., *Explaining '"Unexplained Illnesses" : Disease Paradigm for Chronic Fatigue Syndrome, Multiple Chemical Sensitivity, Fibromyalgia, Post-traumatic Stress Disorder, Gulf War Syndrome and Others.* 2007, Harrington Park Press: Binghamton, NY.

8.   Vande Vyver, M., R. Beelen, J. De Keyser and G. Nagels, *Plasma citrulline levels are increased in patients with multiple sclerosis.* Journal of the Neurological Sciences, 2018. **387**: p. 174–178.

9.   Smith, K.J. and H. Lassmann, *The role of nitric oxide in multiple sclerosis.* The Lancet Neurology, 2002. **1**(4): p. 232–241.

10.   Thomas, D.D., X. Liu, S.P. Kantrow and J.R. Lancaster Jr., *The biological lifetime of nitric oxide: implications for the perivascular dynamics of NO and O_2.* Proceedings of the National Academy of Sciences, 2001. **98**(1): p. 355–360.

11.   Böger, R.H., *Asymmetric dimethylarginine, an endogenous inhibitor of nitric oxide synthase, explains the "L-arginine paradox" and acts as a novel cardiovascular risk factor.* The Journal of Nutrition, 2004. **134**(10): p. 2842S–2847S.

12.   Haghikia, A., A.A. Kayacelebi, B. Beckmann, E. Hanff, R. Gold, A. Haghikia and D. Tsikas, *Serum and cerebrospinal fluid concentrations of homoarginine, arginine, asymmetric and symmetric dimethylarginine, nitrite and nitrate in patients with multiple sclerosis and neuromyelitis optica.* The Forum for Amino Acid, Peptide and Protein Research, 2015. **47**(9): p. 1837–1845.

13.   Foster, M.W., D.T. Hess and J.S. Stamler, *Protein S-nitrosylation in health and disease: a current perspective.* Trends in Molecular Medicine, 2009. **15**(9): p. 391–404.

14.   Prasad, R., S. Giri, N. Nath, I. Singh and A.K. Singh, *GSNO attenuates EAE disease by S-nitrosylation-mediated modulation of endothelial-monocyte interactions.* Glia, 2007. **55**(1): p. 65–77.

15.   Moncada, S. and E.A. Higgs, *The discovery of nitric oxide and its role in vascular biology.* British Journal of Pharmacology, 2006. **147**(Suppl 1): p. S193–S201.

Note 16

Active and Passive Stretch

At either end of a strand of myosin, there is a protein filament anchoring it to the discs on the boundaries of the muscle unit (or the sarcomere). This filament, a giant protein called titin, acts like a spring so that the myosin can recoil, but it also has an absolute length to which it can stretch. Several mechanisms, including calcium binding the titin to the actin fiber, can change its length.

The titin filament consists of two components. One that behaves like a spring, and another part that has no stretch at all.

Look at any spring. If its length is reduced, it becomes harder to compress. It also becomes harder to stretch. In a sarcomere the effect is the same. If you shorten the titin spring, you limit how much a sarcomere can stretch to relax. The reduced length of the titin spring will also limit how how far a sarcomere can contract to exert force.

Reduction in the spring flexibility of a sarcomere creates stiffness in a muscle.[1, 2] A very flexible person will have more range in the titin protein than someone who is stiff.

The degree of stiffness determines the degree of "passive stretch" in the muscle.

Stiffness depends on what calcium is doing. Calcium doesn't just bind to troponin; it also binds to titin. The calcium links the titin to actin, reducing the spring length available to myosin.

The driver of passive muscle tension

In MS, though upper motor neurons are not functioning correctly, the lower motor neurons remain active. As they respond to a reflex, they release the neurotransmitter acetylcholine. This stimulates a constant cycle of excitation-contraction coupling.

The calcium released by this process floods the whole muscle complex.

The consequence is that calcium is always available to bind actin and titin together. Even without trying to use a muscle, the tension from a passive stretch increases because the calcium binds more titin to the actin filament. As the length of the spring in the muscle fiber unit reduces, the tension rises and rises.

Some studies show that titin can bind to actin at various points in the sarcomere, not just at the springy ends.[1] The implication is that even greater stiffness is possible.

Collagen and connective tissue add to passive tension

Several studies show it is not just titin that determines stiffness in a muscle fiber.[1, 2, 3] Collagen, a protein in the extracellular space, is just as significant. A study in 2000 showed that the degree of muscle stiffness varied from species to species in animal models, and also from region to region within a particular study subject, according to the types of titin expressed.[3] We won't all be the same.

The study noted that there was a strong relationship between the increase in collagen-based stiffness and the increase in a titin type called N2B. As this type of titin increased, so did the amount of collagen. They concluded that there was something that coordinated the simultaneous rise. It remains an unresolved observation. Nonetheless, it does support the notion that fascia grows to support the distribution of tension.

Improving the amount of passive stretch becomes critical in dealing with stiffness. I do this using a coordinated approach of massage, Pilates, and dry needling.

Passive Stretch

The only people who are taking a detailed look at muscle stiffness are bioengineers. They are interested in skeletal muscle performance at the cellular level. Everyone else is several steps removed.

These people don't meet very often. In 1996 they held the first Biomechanics and Neural Control of Movement (BANCOM) seminar. In June 2016, 148 biologists, engineers, clinicians, kinesiologists, neuroscientists, and physiologists attended the second meeting. A review of that meeting included a hope that a third meeting could be arranged 20 years from then.[4]

Nonetheless, they are still plugging away. A paper presented at a symposium in 2018 looked at what happened to the level of force generated in the excitation-contraction process as titin stiffness increased.[5] It concluded that as the stiffness increased, the efficiency of the muscle contraction significantly decreased. When a sarcomere, under laboratory conditions, was stretched considerably and the titin was already denoted as "stiff", the measured amount of ATP consumed was high, but the amount of force generated barely changed. Consequently, the contraction of a muscle became an inefficient process due to existing stiffness.[5]

These researchers noted that the active component of force, where actin and myosin overlapped, was hindered by the stiffness of the titin. Their model showed that if titin is stiff, it anchors the myosin, inhibiting its ability to crawl along the actin. The flailing arms of myosin could not move the Z-discs any closer together. The ATP expended trying to do this was wasted.

Examples of active force at its limit

When healthy people repeat an exercise, they reach a point of exhaustion. You might do as many push-ups as you can, but the next one, beyond your limit, results in you flopping to the ground.

Sometimes you can see a weightlifter effortlessly throw a weight above his head. You know he will reach a point where he starts the lift but can barely get the weight off the ground. This happens because the myosin head can no longer move along actin to complete the process of excitation-contraction coupling. Whatever energy is there does not change the action. That is when active stretch has reached its limit.

Given time to recover, the titin spring will pull the myosin back to the starting position.

~

If you have upper motor neuron damage, then your muscle units don't do what a healthy person's muscles do. Over time, you have lost the flexibility in the spring as the flood of calcium has locked the sarcomere. The length available in your titin spring has become less and less. You burn energy unnecessarily in excitation-contraction coupling and have limited flexibility to show for it.

434

Typically, researchers use graphs of fiber length or stretch plotted against force. Too often, they are trying to plot just the action of myosin pulling against actin. That is too simplistic. The relaxation phase depends on titin acting as a spring to restore a sarcomere to its relaxed length.

There is no one standard length for a sarcomere. The function of the muscle makes a big difference. A muscle fiber in your wrist has different design constraints than fiber in your lumbar region. The principal, however, is the same. What the few researchers in this area have concluded is that passive force (determined by the length of your titin and the binding of connective tissue) is the primary reason muscles are stiff.

Over time, stiffness becomes a problem. Sometimes sarcomeres are added to the chain of the muscle fibers to compensate for the reduced flexibility (this is called longitudinal hypertrophy).[2]

At the extreme, this addition of sarcomeres is a precursor for the development of bony formations around joints called heterotopic ossification. There is a history of this happening in multiple sclerosis and acquired brain injury.[6] It is often associated with brain hemorrhages but is reported more frequently with spinal cord injuries than with any other disorders. Depending on the study, heterotopic ossification is reported to occur in 16–86% of spinal cord injuries and 0.5–16% of brain injuries.[6]

Medications that target your T and B cells do not influence stretch. Controlling intracellular calcium is entirely independent of the adaptive immune processes. If you have MS and tightness is an issue, you need to disrupt the endless flooding of calcium on your muscle cells. The best way is to keep moving and use a drug like dantrolene sodium, treatments like massage and dry needling, plus an exercise program like Pilates. One thing alone is insufficient. You will need more than one intervention. If you are like me, you need them all.

References

1. Granzier, H.L. and S. Labeit, *The giant protein titin: A major player in myocardial mechanics, signaling, and disease.* Circulation Research, 2004. **94**(3): p. 284–295.

2. Brynnel, A., Y. Hernandez, B. Kiss, J. Lindqvist, M. Adler, J. Kolb, R. van der Pijl, J. Gohlke, J. Strom, J. Smith, C. Ottenheijm and H.L. Granzier, *Downsizing the molecular spring of the giant protein titin reveals that skeletal muscle titin determines passive stiffness and drives longitudinal hypertrophy.* eLife, 2018. **7**: p. e40532

3. Wu, Y., O. Cazorla, D. Labeit, S. Labeit and H. Granzier, *Changes in titin and collagen underlie diastolic stiffness diversity of cardiac muscle.* Journal of Molecular and Cellular Cardiology, 2000. **32**(12): p. 2151–2161.

4. Lieber, R.L., T.J. Roberts, S.S. Blemker, S.S.M. Lee and W. Herzog, *Skeletal muscle mechanics, energetics and plasticity.* Journal of NeuroEngineering and Rehabilitation, 2017. **14**(1): 108.

5. Powers, J.D., C.D. Williams, M. Regnier and T.L. Daniel, *A spatially explicit model shows how titin stiffness modulates muscle mechanics and energetics.* Integrative and Comparative Biology, 2018. **58**(2): p. 186.

6. Yoshimura, O., T. Murakami, R. Kobayashi, A. Minematsu, H. Sasaki, H, Maejima, S. Tanaka, N. Kanemura, K. Shirahama, T. Ueda, C. Kamoda, H. Miyamoto, K. Yata, M. Watanabe and K, Takayanagi, *Heterotopic issification associated with subarachinoidal hemorrhage.* Journal of Physical Therapy Science, 2000. **12**(2): p. 81–85.

Index

flexibility 251, 432, 434–35

flexors 192, 267, 283

frozen shoulder 157

functional independence 32

functional lines 228–35

functional systems scores 32, 34, 36–38

Funk, Casimir 130

GABA 51–53, 196, 238, 257–59, 274, 319, 328, 404

gait 84, 134, 145, 158, 161, 186, 193, 196, 232–34, 279

gastrointestinal disorders 211–12

genes *see* DNA (genes)

glandular fever 112 *see also* Epstein Barr virus

glatiramer acetate 359

glia 221, 312, 315, 316, 331–33

glucose 78, 79, 98, 121, 138, 404, 411, 415, 418

glutamate 327, 328

glutathione 331

glycine 105, 404

glycolysis 78, 98, 102–3, 138, 411, 415, 418

Golgi tendon organs 293, 294

gout 122

GPs 9–10

halothane 266

heart (cardiac) muscle 97, 222, 242, 269, 421–22

heart problems 14, 98, 106, 269–70

heat stress 84

hemoglobin 349, 403, 428

herpes family viruses 93, 96, 114–16, 125

heterotopic ossification 435

histones 66, 68, 370

uric acid 99, 122, 399

urinary tract infections 201

urodynamic studies 201

Uthoff's sign 84

UV exposure 132, 136

valaciclovir 10, 92–94, 95, 114, 120, 121, 125–26

Valium 257, 259

Valtrex 125

vascular endothelial growth factor (VEGF) 338–39

vestibulocerebellum 196

viruses 114–16

visual function 38, 41, 43

vitamin A 131

vitamin D 58, 120, 130–39

voluntary movement 104, 178, 183, 217, 256

walking 10, 11, 15, 29–35, 41, 43, 145–46, 151–52, 193, 233, 235 *see also* gait

wheelchairs 35, 145, 146, 220

white blood cells 349–52, 357

'white matter' 184

World Health Organization standard 18–19

Z-discs 244–46, 250, 434

452